Barrett Library
Allen College Campus
Waterloo, Iowa 50703

Handbook of Culturally Responsive School Mental Health

Caroline S. Clauss-Ehlers
Zewelanji N. Serpell • Mark D. Weist
Editors

Handbook of Culturally Responsive School Mental Health

Advancing Research, Training, Practice, and Policy

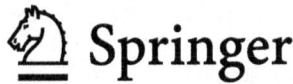

Editors
Caroline S. Clauss-Ehlers
Graduate School of Education
Department of Educational Psychology
Rutgers University
New Brunswick, NJ, USA

Zewelanji N. Serpell
Department of Psychology
Virginia State University
Petersburg, VA, USA

Mark D. Weist
Department of Psychology
University of South Carolina
Columbia, SC, USA

ISBN 978-1-4614-4947-8   ISBN 978-1-4614-4948-5 (eBook)
DOI 10.1007/978-1-4614-4948-5
Springer New York Heidelberg Dordrecht London

Library of Congress Control Number: 2012947997

© Springer Science+Business Media New York 2013
This work is subject to copyright. All rights are reserved by the Publisher, whether the whole or part of the material is concerned, specifically the rights of translation, reprinting, reuse of illustrations, recitation, broadcasting, reproduction on microfilms or in any other physical way, and transmission or information storage and retrieval, electronic adaptation, computer software, or by similar or dissimilar methodology now known or hereafter developed. Exempted from this legal reservation are brief excerpts in connection with reviews or scholarly analysis or material supplied specifically for the purpose of being entered and executed on a computer system, for exclusive use by the purchaser of the work. Duplication of this publication or parts thereof is permitted only under the provisions of the Copyright Law of the Publisher's location, in its current version, and permission for use must always be obtained from Springer. Permissions for use may be obtained through RightsLink at the Copyright Clearance Center. Violations are liable to prosecution under the respective Copyright Law.
The use of general descriptive names, registered names, trademarks, service marks, etc. in this publication does not imply, even in the absence of a specific statement, that such names are exempt from the relevant protective laws and regulations and therefore free for general use.
While the advice and information in this book are believed to be true and accurate at the date of publication, neither the authors nor the editors nor the publisher can accept any legal responsibility for any errors or omissions that may be made. The publisher makes no warranty, express or implied, with respect to the material contained herein.

Printed on acid-free paper

Springer is part of Springer Science+Business Media (www.springer.com)

To my loving husband Julian, and our wonderful daughters, Izzy and Beanie

-CC

To my father, my husband, and my sons

-ZNS

For Dana

-MDW

Foreword

Schools play a critical role in shaping the lives of children. Second only to the family, schools are where children spend most of their time; schools provide the context, direction, and support for academic, social, and emotional learning and exert significant influence on the developmental trajectory of their students. Historically, schools have been the "great" equalizer in the country, enabling students from diverse backgrounds, neighborhoods, and income levels and young immigrants to the United States to have the opportunity for success.

However, schools are changing and the pressures and expectations on schools are increasing. Driven by population changes in the last few decades, schools are facing a demographic imperative to meet the spectrum of needs for an increasingly culturally, racially, and ethnically diverse student body. In 2009, the racial and ethnic makeup of public schools in the nation was: 53.7% White, 16.6% Black, 22% Latino, 4.9% Asian/Pacific Islander, and 1.3% American Indian/Alaska Native. In some large metropolitan areas, students of color are now a majority of the student population. They bring to the classroom ever-widening academic and social/emotional experiences to which teachers and school personnel are called to respond. In contrast to the changing demographics of the student population, the ethnic/racial composition of teachers and school personnel has remained primarily White, middle class. In 2010, only 9% of elementary and middle school teachers and 8% of high school teachers were African American. For Latino teachers, these percentages were 7.3% and 6.7%, respectively. Researchers have suggested that the cultural dissonance between home and schools contributes to poor educational engagement and outcomes. Increasing student success relies on teachers to help bridge this discontinuity. Yet as the demographics of the student population change disproportionately to that of the teachers, this task becomes increasingly difficult.

Students enter public schools with a broad diversity of cultures, languages, customs, expectations, and histories. They bring individual academic, social, and emotional strengths and weaknesses; they bring histories of safe and supportive families as well as experiences of maltreatment and neglect. Students have a wide range of social and peer experiences ranging from healthy peer relationships and engagement to antisocial behaviors, interpersonal violence, bullying, and isolation. Similarly, some students have a school tenure marked by a sense of connectedness, support, and success; others are alienated and disengaged with academic histories of chronic failure and disappointment. While relevant to all students, these issues are particularly notable for students from diverse racial, ethnic, and sexual minority backgrounds. For example, we see the results of these pressures among students in California schools, one of the most diverse states in the country, in the poor high school graduation rates of 68% for Latinos, 59% for African Americans, and 56% for students who are learning English. In the USA, the percentage of individuals who do not graduate from high school is 15.5% overall: 10% for White, non-Latino; 19.7% for African Americans; 39.4% for Latinos; 14.1% for Asians; and 21.5% for American Indian or Alaska Native. Given that high school completion is a known predictor for social and economic success in adulthood, it is clear that these students, and their communities, will encounter more difficult challenges and more limited opportunities for success. These students also come from schools that are often more poorly resourced and in neighborhoods that are lower in income, some with concentrated areas of poverty and the associated, crime, exposure to violence and limited social capital.

So what does this mean for schools? Schools carry the heavy burden of dealing with all the challenges students bring into the classroom, whether health and mental health problems, and/or family and community stressors. And, given the changing demographics of the students, schools must be competent to handle these issues across diversities of culture, race, language, and ethnicity. Understanding and competently addressing the mental health needs of these diverse students will be essential to meeting the schools' goals of academic success and graduation.

Schools also face new exigencies from emerging federal and national policies. Multiple federal departments beyond the US Department of Education are targeting schools for major initiatives. The Departments of Justice and Education are partnering in a collaborative effort to address the "school-to-prison pipeline" and the disciplinary policies and practices that can push students out of school and into the justice system. The initiative aims to support good discipline practices to foster safe and productive learning environments in every classroom. Given the overrepresentation of youth of color in disciplinary actions and in the justice system and the often challenging behaviors of students with mental health problems, this has important implications for how schools handle these students. One of the most significant pieces of Congressional legislation in the current decade, the Patient Protection and Affordable Care Act, brings schools into the health reform movement. The US Department of Health and Human Services is expanding school health facilities to better meet the health and behavioral health needs of students. Continuing efforts are focused on how mental health and substance use problems are addressed in schools and emerging efforts are highlighting the association between mental health factors and school dropouts. Some of the dropout crisis may be explained by experiences of trauma and chronic exposure to high-stress environments, a particular vulnerability for ethnically and racially diverse and sexual minority youth. School-based health and mental health centers, with the appropriate resources and leadership, are well-positioned to address these issues. Additionally, the current Administration, in response to heightened bullying awareness and the recognition that bullying contributes to psychological distress and may leave physical and emotional scars as well as long-lasting academic effects, has promoted strong anti-bullying efforts and strategies to develop a sense of safety in school settings. These efforts have included a focus on lesbian, gay, bisexual, and transgender youth, as well as diverse ethnic racial youth and those with disabilities, often the targets of bullying.

Schools are at the nexus of a "perfect storm": increasing enrollment of diverse students entering with a myriad of health, behavioral health, and social concerns; pressures from national and federal policies to handle a plethora of issues, some only indirectly related to the educational mandates for schools, and a brutal economic climate that has slashed budgets of states and school districts across the country. Yet we also look to schools to produce young people ready to enter adulthood, become leaders, and ensure the competitiveness of our country on the global stage. Now, more than ever, the preparation of the whole student—academically, socially, and emotionally, is imperative. It is with this backdrop that the current volume is an important step in preparing schools, school personnel, families, researchers, and practitioners who touch upon the lives of students. Schools function in a variety of contexts—urban, rural, suburban, and military—with a variety of ethnic, racial, socioeconomic, and sexual orientations—and a wide scope of mental health competencies and needs. This comprehensive volume, expertly linking research, practice, and policy, guides us in thinking about strategies to most competently meet the mental health needs and ensure a positive trajectory of development for the students who are most often misunderstood and mistreated, yet have much to contribute to their school communities and their school success.

Larke Nahme Huang, Ph.D.
Senior Advisor, Administrator's Office of Policy Planning and Innovation,
Director, Office of Behavioral Health Equity
Substance Abuse and Mental Health Services Administration,
U.S. Department of Health and Human Services,
Rockville, MD, USA

Preface

Overview

Our idea for this project developed out of conversations about what it means to be a child in today's world. We were curious and committed to having a better understanding of the complexities, joys, and challenges that children embrace on a daily basis. Having children of our own, we have seen the many growing pains that accompany the purview of modern day school life. We have also seen the great joy and amazement children bring to the discovery of the world around them. We recognize the many resources that schools provide within classrooms as well as for individual learners. At the foundation of these supports are unbelievably committed educators, parents, family members, and neighbors. The aim of the *Handbook* was to organize scientific knowledge to address areas of growth, advocate for needed change, and make available resources known for those interested in this work.

Throughout the *Handbook of Culturally Responsive School Mental Health* our focus, and that of our contributors, is on being culturally responsive to the diverse needs and experiences of youth in schools. We found that a better understanding of what is meant by *culturally responsive training*, *practice*, *research,* and *policy in school mental health* is warranted given our changing demographic landscape, with increasingly diverse student populations.

Often children are characterized as developing along similar trajectories, when in fact the influences of culture are profound. Children enter schools with a variety of languages, customs, cultures, and historic backgrounds, and researchers have documented the disproportionality in mental health problems, as well as reduced access to referral and treatment among culturally diverse youth. Hence, the need for and considerable benefit of, a book that represents a call to teachers, school administrators, school counselors, school mental health professionals, and advocates to consider the ways in which they can be more culturally responsive. Research addressing concepts like stigma and the lack of culturally competent trained professionals and those who can speak languages other than English also highlight the fact that comprehensive approaches to culturally responsive practice are not well-defined. Associated work is in its infancy.

Rationale and Organization

The purpose of the *Handbook* is to meet gaps in the literature by organizing chapters that reflect critical themes in advancing culturally responsive school mental health promotion and intervention across key realms of training, practice, research, and policy, while exploring interconnections across these realms. Through a range of contributors, this volume addresses three main areas: (1) the status of the research on culturally responsive school mental health work with children and adolescents; (2) innovative approaches in work with diverse children and adolescents in schools; and (3) the application of these two points to school mental health efforts with particular groups and/or around particular problems.

The first strand of the volume, the status of research, will identify gaps in the research literature as they relate to the current status of school mental health with children and adolescents in schools. This section begins with a chapter by the coeditors that provides a rationale for culturally responsive school mental health. This introduction is followed by chapters that focus on the need for culturally responsive school mental health services in school-based behavioral health care in overseas military base schools; in rural communities; and in the growing role of school personnel.

The second strand, innovative approaches, reviews current programs and strategies that successfully focus on child and adolescent school mental health from a diverse context. Specific issues and innovations focus on working in the school context with communities that include: African American youth and their families; lesbian, gay, bisexual, and transgender youth; Asian American Pacific Islander youth; forced migrant children and their families; primary care facilities in rural communities; racially and ethnically diverse adolescents; and youth gangs.

The third strand focuses on specific problems and interventions and, as such, addresses special topics related to culturally responsive research and practice. Chapters in this section discuss training transformed school counselors; substance abuse and sex education prevention programming for middle school youth; the promotion of culturally competent assessment in schools; work/family balance; and understanding trauma through a cross-cultural lens. The concluding chapter in this section, and the *Handbook*, discusses next steps for the continued advancement of culturally responsive school-based mental health.

Endorsements

"The *Handbook of Culturally Responsive School Mental Health* is a remarkably comprehensive text addressing the needs of youth in an increasingly diverse United States society. It showcases a number of community-driven models and culturally adapted school-based mental health interventions. Several chapters include descriptions of services addressing the unique risk and protective factors of newer and fluid populations such as Asian American Pacific Islander youth and military families overseas. The lived experiences of youth in rural areas are even included. This timely and useful resource provides tools for hastening the pace of infusing cultural factors into the delivery of mental health services in 21st century schools."

Teresa LaFromboise, Ph.D., Professor of Education, Stanford University

"It is an impressive and well organized book which features an array of scholars well respected in the field and who managed to present a complex array of material in a sufficiently clear and concise manner so as to make it easier for implementation. It is a welcome book that should be very helpful to any professional working with children with a variety of educational and emotional challenges and who is determined to make a difference in these children."

Rafael Art. Javier, Ph.D. ABPP–Professor of Psychology and Director of the Postgraduate Professional Development Programs, St. John's University

"Bravo! The *Handbook of Culturally Responsive School Mental Health: Advancing Research, Training, Practice, and Policy* provides a superb source of information to teachers, administrators, practitioners, researchers, advocates, and parents. A rare combination of solid theory, research findings, and culturally appropriate psychological interventions, this excellent collection is a must read for anyone interested in children and adolescents' wellbeing."

Lillian Comas-Díaz, Ph.D., Clinical Professor, Department of Psychiatry and Behavioral Sciences, George Washington University, Washington, DC; Author, *Multicultural Care: A Clinician's Guide to Cultural Competence*

Acknowledgments

The authors are grateful to the many individuals who contributed to this *Handbook*—either through written contributions or their sheer support of this work. The paragraphs below provide personal acknowledgments followed by those we share as coeditors and colleagues.

CC—I am grateful to my husband Julian, a constant source of encouragement and support. This emotional nourishment is coupled with the many gourmet meals he has made during the organizing of these pages. Thank goodness there's a chef in the family! I am in awe of our girls, Isabel and Sabrina, who have grown leaps and bounds during the past 3 years this project has come to fruition. These three are daily sources of pride and inspiration. I thank my student mentees, Elizabeth Jensen, Kip Thompson, Keshia Harris, Laura Miller, and Lemma Taha for the wonderful collaboration they have provided throughout this project. It is truly exciting to watch them develop professionally and embark on their own careers. Many thanks to Larry Kutner for his friendship and mentoring along the way. I am grateful to the mentors who have shaped my own professional path—thank you for all that you do!

ZNS—A special thanks to my colleagues Toni Harris and Scott Graves for sharing their experiences and insight, and for making the time to brainstorm ideas. I also want to acknowledge and thank students in the Developmental Lab: Aysha Foster, Brittney Pearson, Dhymsy Vixamar-Owens, Yi Ching Lin, and Lisa Turner—each of whom was a source of inspiration and provided assistance that supported the completion of this book.

MDW—Much appreciation is extended to Melissa Dvorsky, the University of South Carolina, School Mental Health Team, and the University of Maryland, Center for School Mental Health. My work on this book is in honor of my amazing sister Dana, a wonderful person and prominent economist with the World Bank who lost a valiant 5-year battle with breast cancer in October, 2010.

We have talked a great deal about collaborating on a book. It has been wonderful to finally work together as colleagues for this project. We are grateful to Judy Jones, Senior Editor at Springer, who first reviewed our proposal and shared our excitement about constructing a handbook focused on culturally responsive school mental health. We thank Garth Haller, Assistant Editor at Springer, for his ongoing support. We appreciate the time given to work on this project by our respective universities. Having the flexibility to pull such a work together is truly a privilege offered by university life. We acknowledge the wonderful collaboration and contribution of the many authors whose ideas and words grace the pages that follow. We know that the commitment to write a book chapter is a big undertaking. We value the fact that our contributors showed their support for this work through their written word.

Contents

Part I Status of the Research on Cultural Considerations in School-Based Mental Health Interventions with Children and Adolescents

1 **Introduction: Making the Case for Culturally Responsive School Mental Health** 3
   Caroline S. Clauss-Ehlers, Zewelanji N. Serpell, and Mark D. Weist

2 **Building a "Culture of Trust": The Cultural and Practical Challenges of School-Based Behavioral Health Care in Overseas Military Base Schools** 17
   Alan R. Scheuermann and Tracey Jernigan

3 **Culturally Responsive School Mental Health in Rural Communities** 31
   Julie Sarno Owens, Yuko Watabe, and Kurt D. Michael

4 **From Guidance to School Counseling: New Models in School Mental Health** 43
   Laura Miller, Lemma Taha, and Elizabeth Jensen

Part II Innovative Approaches in Work with Diverse Children and Adolescents in Schools

5 **Culturally Competent Engagement of African American Youth and Families in School Mental Health Services** 59
   Kendra P. DeLoach, Melissa Dvorsky, and Rhonda L. White-Johnson

6 **Black Parents Strengths and Strategies (BPSS) Program: A Cultural Adaptation of the Strong-Willed Child Program** 77
   Stephanie Irby Coard, Melvin H. Herring, Monica H. Watkins, Shani A. Foy-Watson, and Shuntay Z. McCoy

7 Working with Lesbian, Gay, Bisexual, and Transgender
    Youth in Schools 89
    Nancy Bearss

8 Advancing School-Based Mental Health for Asian
    American Pacific Islander Youth 107
    Matthew R. Mock

9 Raising Consciousness: Promoting Healthy Coping
    Among African American Boys at School 121
    Keisha L. Bentley-Edwards, Duane E. Thomas,
    and Howard C. Stevenson

10 Working with Forced Migrant Children and their Families:
    Mental Health, Developmental, Legal, and Linguistic
    Considerations in the Context of School-Based Mental
    Health Services 135
    Caroline S. Clauss-Ehlers and Adeyinka M. Akinsulure-Smith

11 Mental Health and Rural Schools: An Integrated
    Approach with Primary Care 147
    Jody Lieske, Susan Swearer, and Brandi Berry

12 The Racial/Ethnic Identity Development
    of Tomorrow's Adolescent 157
    Kip V. Thompson, Keshia Harris, and Caroline S. Clauss-Ehlers

13 Culturally Responsive Strategies to Address
    Youth Gangs in Schools 177
    Nicole Evangelista Brandt, Emily Sidway,
    Melissa Dvorsky, and Mark D. Weist

Part III Specific Problems and Interventions

14 Training Transformed School Counselors 189
    Marte Ostvik-de Wilde, Denise Park, and Courtland C. Lee

15 Culturally Integrated Substance Abuse
    and Sex Education Prevention: Programming
    for Middle School Students 197
    Desi S. Hacker, Faye Z. Belgrave, Jamie Grisham,
    Jasmine Abrams, and Darlene G. Colson

16 Promoting Culturally Competent Assessment
    in Schools 209
    Toni Harris, Scott Graves, Zewelanji N. Serpell,
    and Brittney Pearson

17 Work–Family Balance: Challenges
    and Advances for Families 219
    Patricia M. Raskin

18	**Adjusting Intervention Acuity in School Mental Health: Perceiving Trauma Through the Lens of Cultural Competence** .... Leslie K. Taylor, Heather L. Lasky, and Mark D. Weist	235
19	**Next Steps: Advancing Culturally Competent School Mental Health** .... Zewelanji N. Serpell, Caroline S. Clauss-Ehlers, and Mark D. Weist	251

About the Editors 261

Index 263

Contributors

Jasmine Abrams Virginia Commonwealth University, Richmond, VA, USA

Adeyinka M. Akinsulure-Smith City University of New York, New York, NY, USA

Nancy Bearss La Red Health Center, Georgetown, DE, USA

Faye Z. Belgrave Virginia Commonwealth University, Richmond, VA, USA

Keisha L. Bentley-Edwards University of Texas at Austin, Austin, TX, USA

Brandi Berry University of Nebraska—Lincoln, Lincoln, NE, USA

Nicole Evangelista Brandt University of Maryland School of Medicine, Center for School Mental Health, Baltimore, MD, USA

Caroline S. Clauss-Ehlers Rutgers, The State University of New Jersey, New Brunswick, NJ, USA

Stephanie Irby Coard The University of North Carolina at Greensboro, Greensboro, NC, USA

Darlene G. Colson Norfolk State University, Norfolk, VA, USA

Kendra P. DeLoach University of South Carolina, Columbia, SC, USA

Melissa Dvorsky University of South Carolina, Columbia, SC, USA

Shani A. Foy-Watson The University of North Carolina at Greensboro, Greensboro, NC, USA

Scott Graves Duquesne University, Pittsburgh, PA, USA

Jamie Grisham Norfolk State University, Norfolk, VA, USA

Desi S. Hacker Norfolk State University, Norfolk, VA, USA

Keshia Harris Teachers College, Columbia University, New York, NY, USA

Toni Harris Virginia State University, Petersburg, VA, USA

Melvin H. Herring The University of North Carolina at Greensboro, Greensboro, NC, USA

Elizabeth Jensen Rutgers, The State University of New Jersey, New Brunswick, NJ, USA

Tracey Jernigan Bavaria-MEDDAC/U.S. Army Medical Command, San Antonio, TX, USA

Heather L. Lasky University of South Carolina, Columbia, SC, USA

Courtland C. Lee University of Maryland at College Park, College Park, MD, USA

Jody Lieske Children and Adolescent Clinic, P.C. Munroe Meyer Institute-UNMC, Hastings, NE, USA

Shuntay Z. McCoy The University of North Carolina at Greensboro, Greensboro, NC, USA

Kurt D. Michael Appalachian State University, Boone, NC, USA

Laura Miller Rutgers, The State University of New Jersey, New Brunswick, NJ, USA

Matthew R. Mock John F. Kennedy University, Pleasant Hill, CA, USA

Marte Ostvik-de Wilde University of Maryland at College Park, College Park, MD, USA

Julie Sarno Owens Ohio University, Athens, OH, USA

Denise Park University of Maryland at College Park, College Park, MD, USA

Brittney Pearson Virginia State University, Petersburg, VA, USA

Patricia M. Raskin Teachers College, Columbia University, New York, NY, USA

Alan R. Scheuermann Bavaria-MEDDAC/U.S. Army Medical Command, San Antonio, TX, USA

Zewelanji N. Serpell Virginia State University, Petersburg, VA, USA

Emily Sidway University of Maryland School of Medicine, Center for School Mental Health, Baltimore, MD, USA

Howard C. Stevenson University of Pennsylvania, Philadelphia, PA, USA

Susan Swearer University of Nebraska—Lincoln, Lincoln, NE, USA

Lemma Taha Pascack Valley High School, Hillsdale, NJ, USA

Leslie K. Taylor University of South Carolina, Columbia, SC, USA

Duane E. Thomas University of Virginia, Charlottesville, VA, USA

Kip V. Thompson University of South Carolina, Columbia, SC, USA

Yuko Watabe Ohio University, Athens, OH, USA

Monica H. Watkins The University of North Carolina at Greensboro, Greensboro, NC, USA

Mark D. Weist University of South Carolina, Columbia, SC, USA

Rhonda L. White-Johnson University of South Carolina, Columbia, SC, USA

Part I

Status of the Research on Cultural Considerations in School-Based Mental Health Interventions with Children and Adolescents

Introduction: Making the Case for Culturally Responsive School Mental Health

Caroline S. Clauss-Ehlers, Zewelanji N. Serpell, and Mark D. Weist

School Mental Health: Past and Present

For over two decades, the school mental health (SMH) movement has shown progressive growth in the United States (U.S.) and other countries based on some straightforward and compelling realities. First, child and adolescent mental health is among the most neglected of all health care needs, with 20% or more of children and youth presenting more concerning emotional and behavioral challenges, but less than one-third of these youth receiving any services (President's New Freedom Commission on Mental Health, 2003). Moreover, for those youth who do receive services there are serious questions about the quality of services received, with true evidence-based practice (EBP) being relatively rare, quality improvement often focused on variables such as fee-for-service productivity, and nonevidence based, even harmful services being widespread (see Evans & Weist, 2004; Weist et al., 2007).

Second, children and youth generally do not receive mental health services in traditional settings such as mental health centers and private offices, but receive them in more natural settings, with the most prominent being schools and primary care offices. However, in these settings mental health services are often very limited, under-resourced, and even marginalized. In schools, mental health services are often limited to crisis response for all students, and otherwise available only to youth in special education. Further, position constraints plague mental health services delivered by the education system. For example, too few school psychologists, counselors, and social workers (and other professionals such as school nurses and special educators with behavioral expertise) commonly work in roles that do not capitalize on their full skill sets (e.g., psychologists relegated to testing, counselors relegated to academic advisement) and they often work in isolation of their professional counterparts in other community settings (see Rappaport et al., 2003).

Connecting these themes leads to the third point—that there are compelling benefits to a shared agenda, bringing together schools, families, community mental health staff and programs, and staff and programs from other youth serving systems (e.g., child welfare, juvenile services) toward an expanded SMH approach, involving a full continuum of environmental

---

C.S. Clauss-Ehlers, Ph.D. (✉)
Rutgers, The State University of New Jersey,
New Brunswick, NJ 08901, USA
e-mail: cc@gse.rutgers.edu

Z.N. Serpell
Virginia State University, Petersburg, VA 23806, USA

M.D. Weist
University of South Carolina,
Columbia, SC 29208, USA

enhancement, mental health promotion, prevention, early identification and intervention, and treatment, for all youth, in general and special education in schools (Weist, 1997). This expanded SMH approach has been called for back to the days of John Dewey in the late nineteenth century and gained significant momentum in the late 1980s with the development and growth of the school-based health center (SBHC) movement. As SBHCs, bringing a full array of health care to schools, were being developed in pioneering locations such as Minneapolis, Dallas, and Baltimore, in the 1980s, a rapid realization was that mental health concerns were the number one or two reason for referral, and many health conditions had emotional/behavioral components. This led to advocacy and federal leadership to build more comprehensive mental health services in schools, with prominent early leadership by the Maternal and Child Health Bureau (MCHB) of the Health Resources and Services Administration, which in 1995 funded two national centers and five states to build infrastructure and work to advance SMH (see Anglin, 2003; Flaherty & Osher, 2003).

All of the above, along with a growing research base on schools as *the de facto site* for mental health services, and the advantages of effective SMH in reducing academic and nonacademic barriers to student learning, contributed to increasing federal and state investment in the field. In addition, a number of policy-focused articles and reports have been particularly influential, including Jane Knitzer's *Unclaimed Children* (1982), that documented the dire needs and neglect of the nation's children and adolescents contending with more serious emotional and behavioral challenges, the need for and advantages of a Systems of Care (SOC) approach by Stroul and Friedman (1986), and Surgeon General David Satcher's critically important reports on Mental Health (U.S. Department of Health and Human Services (DHHS), 1999) and Children's Mental Health (DHHS, 2000) calling for a paradigm change toward more proactive, preventive, flexible, and evidence-based mental health services for youth. These themes were amplified further in the historic New Freedom Commission (2003) of the Bush Administration, that called for *transformation* of the nation's mental health system, increased focus on children and adolescents, EBPs, and included as 1 of 16 specific recommendations, *to expand and improve school mental health programs* (recommendation 4.2).

The U.S. federal government has progressively increased support for SMH as reflected in research grants through the National Institute of Mental Health and the U.S. Department of Education's (DOE) Institute of Education Sciences (IES); program and infrastructure grants through U.S. DOE's Mental Health Integration into the Schools and Safe Schools/Healthy Student's grants; the Substance Abuse and Mental Health Service Administration's (SAMHSA) System of Care grants; and Capacity Building grants through the Centers for Disease Control and Prevention (CDC; *please note that some of these grant initiatives involve multiple federal sponsors, with lead sponsors indicated here). As mentioned, MCHB made an early investment in SMH in the mid-1990s and national centers for SMH funded by MCHB at the University of California in Los Angeles and at the University of Maryland Baltimore (UMB) have helped to shape the field in developing numerous helpful documents and reports, in convening meetings, in promoting dialogue and collaboration, and in purposefully helping to shape federal policy (Anglin, 2003).

Annual conferences on Advancing School Mental Health continue to be held around the nation by the UMB center with the most recent conference in Charleston, South Carolina in the fall of 2011 drawing over 900 participants from all U.S. states. In addition, in collaboration with the Individuals with Disabilities Education Act (IDEA) Partnership, funded by the U.S. DOE's Office of Special Education Programs, the UMB center is sponsoring a National Community of Practice on Collaborative School Behavioral Health, which includes over 3,000 participants and represents more than 30 professional organizations, 16 states, and 12 practice groups pursuing the development of critical themes for the field. The goal of the community is to promote *multiscale learning* or supporting schools, communities, organizations, and states in moving from discussion to collaboration and providing mutual support to escalate the pace of positive change in the field. The National Community of Practice started in 2004 with 80 stakeholders from diverse disciplines meeting and discussing key knowledge domains, also reflecting critical need areas for the field that are in need of development.

An initial group of eight theme areas/practice groups were developed and these have been refined (with some early themes dropping, some new ones surfacing) to include 12 currently. These theme areas and the work that is occurring to make progress on them in many ways reflect prominent needs of the field and work to occur in the immediate future for SMH to expand and improve. The 12 theme areas/practice groups are (with thanks to the University of Maryland, Center for School Mental Health, see http://csmh.umaryland.edu) as follows:

1. *Building a Collaborative Culture for Student Mental Health (CC).* This practice group has as its primary objective to promote the active exchange of ideas and collaboration between school employed and community employed mental health providers, educators, and families. This exchange is to support the social, emotional, and mental health and the academic success of all children and adolescents. Research suggests that the social/emotional health of children and adolescents is linked to their academic and overall success in schools. A collegial, invitational approach to working together will allow all professionals and families to effect positive systemic change resulting in better informed and skilled school personnel to address the needs of students. By working together in a collaborative and creative manner, school, family, and community resources can better serve the educational and social/emotional needs of all students and assist in ensuring good mental health.

2. *Connecting School Mental Health and Positive Behavior Supports (PBS).* This practice group is a conduit for families, researchers, administrators, and practitioners to find common interests and practices related to SMH and PBS. PBS approaches are designed to prevent problem behaviors by proactively altering the environment before problems begin and concurrently teaching appropriate behavior. School-wide PBS systems support all students along a continuum of need based on the three-tiered PBS prevention model. SMH can be thought of as a framework of approaches that promote children's mental health by emphasizing prevention programming, positive youth development, and school-wide approaches. These approaches call for collaboration among mental health providers, educators, families, related service providers, and school administrators to meet the mental health needs of all students. By working collaboratively, this practice group seeks to clarify the relationship between PBS and SMH to promote seamless practice at the local level.

3. *Connecting School Mental Health with Juvenile Justice and Dropout (JJD) Prevention.* This practice group is committed to working across stakeholder groups to advance knowledge and best practice related to effectively linking SMH with JJD prevention. For youth to be successful, effective coordination and communication across systems is needed, and resources and best practice guidelines related to this work need to be readily available. Key priority areas include advancing effective strategies for reducing truancy, unnecessary suspensions and expulsions, dropout, and delinquency; building school and community capacity to meet the needs of youth and their families; promoting successful transitions between systems; encouraging relevant professional development for school and juvenile justice staff; advancing school connectedness and family partnership; promoting best practices in diversion and early intervention for youth who are in the juvenile justice system or who are at risk of placement in juvenile detention.

4. *Education: An Essential Component of Systems of Care (EESOC).* This practice group is focused on the role of schools as significant partners with other child-serving,

community agencies/organizations and families in improving outcomes for children and youth with, or at risk of, mental, emotional, and behavioral health challenges. The EESOC practice group promotes learning as critical to social–emotional health and the adoption of effective services and supports that build and sustain community-based SOC. As a proactive, national level practice group, we will support resource sharing, cross agency training, and collaborative professional development. Our practice group is committed to looking at the multiple needs of children and families through a systemic lens. Therefore, it encourages presentations that outline or describe a system approach to service delivery and incorporating various system partners especially families and youth in any presentations.

5. *Family–School–Community Partnerships (FP)*. This practice group embodies family driven principles and is led by family members. This practice group fosters family participation in family–school–community collaboratives by supporting capacity building efforts for a shared agenda and effective infrastructure development and maintenance. In addition to advancing understanding of the value of family–school–community collaboratives, key capacity building efforts will include working with other practice groups to provide targeted information, leadership training, mentoring, coaching, and initial and ongoing family–school–community stakeholder development. Priorities are: (1) educating and informing families to help them effectively voice their needs to their school districts, in their communities and on state and national levels; (2) advocating for and supporting the participation of families across community of practice groups; (3) educating and informing schools, systems, policy groups, and others about the importance of family integration in policy work; (4) providing a place for family leaders to collaborate on discussion of needs, priorities, and opportunities; and (5) supporting the work of families.

6. *Improving School Mental Health for Youth with Disabilities (YD)*. The purpose of this practice group is to promote collaboration between schools and school systems, mental health agencies, service providers, youth, caregivers, and other key stakeholders to facilitate the delivery of quality mental health services to students with disabilities in the school setting. Enhanced collaboration will increase opportunities to deliver coordinated learning and mental health interventions, and facilitate understanding of the challenges and opportunities for youth with disabilities. Through these partnerships, this practice group seeks to ensure that students with disabilities receive appropriate programs and services in the least restrictive environment to successfully achieve targeted goals.

7. *Learning the Language: Promoting Effective Ways for Interdisciplinary Collaboration (LL)*. Creating a common language among parents, educators, pupil services personnel, and mental health providers helps to establish a strong community of understanding so students can learn, participate, and achieve. This practice group helps to promote greater understanding of the language used across interactive systems in mental health and education. In schools, a full complement of services helps to insure that students receive the necessary supports and tools for both academic and social emotional learning. This practice group recognizes that a community of multiple stakeholders is needed to address the mental health and educational needs of students. Our key priorities are: (1) to demystify the vocabulary used; (2) to add increased value to state and local educational/family/youth services agencies currently implementing expanded, SMH services/programs; (3) to promote a better understanding of how we communicate across systems/stakeholders; and (4) to build stronger relationships across SOC for families, students, and professionals involved in schools.

8. *Psychiatry and Schools (PS)*. This group focuses on issues related to psychiatric services in schools. Topics may include, but

are not limited to, the roles of psychiatrists who work in schools, and interdisciplinary collaboration among psychiatrists and other professionals working in schools, including primary health care professionals. Important issues for this practice group include the development of guidelines for appropriate medication prescribing in schools and ways to utilize psychiatric services optimally in the face of severe shortages of child and adolescent psychiatrists.

9. *Quality and Evidence-Based Practice (EBP).* The mission of the Quality and Evidence-Based Practice Group is to share information across individuals and groups interested in improving the quality of SMH programs and services and to discuss, promote, and disseminate EBPs in SMH. This practice group strives to bridge the research-practice and practice-research gaps in the field. In addition, the practice group seeks to understand and identify the best student and program-level evaluation strategies.

10. *School Mental Health for Culturally Diverse Youth (DY).* This practice group will focus on the practice, theory, and research specific to culturally diverse youth in the schools. The mission of the Culturally Diverse Youth practice group is to promote better understanding of strategies designed to enhance the success of culturally diverse youth in the school environment. Specific issues such as stigma, cultural adaptations, health disparities, disproportionality, family engagement, and linguistic and cultural competence are addressed by this practice group. The practice group will identify and disseminate information on effective treatment approaches in work with diverse communities to better inform the education, family, and youth-serving systems.

11. *Mental Health for Military Families (MF).* The vision of this practice group is to develop and implement a comprehensive array of school programs and services to support military students, family, and community. Proposed objectives include: (1) to promote a full continuum of mental health promotion and intervention programs and services to include early identification and intervention, prevention, evaluation, and treatment; (2) to remove barriers to learning and improve the academic success of students; (3) to enhance strengths and protective factors in students, families, and the school community; (4) to promote the quality of life and wellness in military families; and (5) to provide training, staff development, and research opportunities to improve children's and adolescents' mental health and education.

12. *Youth Involvement and Leadership (YIL).* This practice group is focused on advancing YIL in SMH. Priority areas include: (1) expanding youth leadership, participation, and input at local, state, and national levels, (2) advancing the development and implementation of strategies and approaches that promote greater youth leadership at all levels of the service systems that support them, (3) supporting efforts by the national community of practice and its practice groups to promote meaningful YIL, (4) organizing a dialogue around greater inclusion of youth in meaningful ways in all facets of SMH, (5) developing and promoting best practices and innovative approaches for YIL, and (6) serving as a resource for educators and involvement and leadership in schools and communities.

The Case for Cross-Cultural Competence in Today's Schools

Demographic trends. The fact that public schools are undergoing marked changes in the demographics of their student populations is increasingly evident. To date, nearly a quarter of students attending public schools are ethnic minorities. Reports from 2009 indicate that the school enrollment of Latino students has doubled and that these numbers are likely to continue increasing (National Center Education Statistics (NCES), 2011). In 2009–2010, 10%, or approximately 4.7 million students in U.S. public schools were English language learners (Aud et al. 2012). Furthermore, many students are now entering schools from households that are living well below the poverty line (Planty et al., 2009). If Census Bureau projections are accurate, an astounding growth in the diversity of the U.S. population will occur over the next 10–15 years, and the population of schools will certainly mirror these trends.

The U.S. has already seen substantial increases in demographic diversity between 2000 and 2010—both Latino and Asian populations have demonstrated a 43% growth, with the latter group demonstrating the fastest growth among all racial/ethnic groups. The latest reports indicate that in 2010, populations in at least four states—California, Hawaii, New Mexico, Texas, as well as that of the District of Columbia—were "majority minority" with over 50% of people reporting racial/ethnic minority status. Even in states that typically have not been racially/ethnically diverse, there have been dramatic increases; for example, Nevada has experienced a 46% growth in the number of racial/ethnic minorities residing in that state.

Also worthy of note is that nine million people in the 2010 Census self-identified as having more than one race (Humes, Jones, & Ramirez, 2011). This has important implications for what we conceive of as culture, as some biracial and multiracial individuals may have a unique set of cultural experiences. For example, these youth may be in appearance race-ambiguous, and may be navigating complex family networks that encompass a diverse, and possibly divergent, set of cultural values (Brown, 2009). Vast diversity is also evident within racial groups, with individuals reporting varying countries of origin, primary language, and generational status in the United States. Within the Latino population, countries of origin include Central America, South America, Mexico, and the Caribbean, thus suggesting cultural variability even within ethnic subpopulations.

Meeting the Needs of Diverse Students in Schools

The significance of the substantial growth in the diversity of students in schools cannot be underestimated and the prevailing view is that on the whole educators, counselors, and other mental health care providers are not adequately prepared to meet the needs of these students, and many will go unserved (Huang, Macbeth, Dodge, & Jacobstein, 2004). The persistence of significant disparities in service utilization by diverse communities (Diala et al., 2001; Snowden & Yamada, 2005) as well as evidence of reduced knowledge about mental health services and access in these groups (Bussing, Zima, Gary, & Garvan, 2003; dosRies et al., 2003) is of much concern. Most disturbing is the fact that access to needed services does not guarantee improved mental health outcomes among culturally diverse youth, as they are more likely than their White counterparts to receive inferior, inappropriate, and ineffective services (Alegría et al., 2002; DHHS, 1999; Oswald, Coutinho, & Best, 2002; Patton, 1998).

Schools have an important role to play in the elimination of mental health care disparities as they can afford better access. However, inequities in access and underutilization of school-based services among diverse communities underscore the need for cultural competence among service providers (DHHS, 2001). A vast majority of teachers and other school staff are economically and/or culturally different from the students they serve (Aud et al., 2010) and, many will not have had any preparation or training to effectively work with culturally diverse students and their families (Rogers, Ponterotto, Conoley, & Wiese, 1992).

Meeting the diverse needs of students in contemporary schools is far more complicated than has been the case in the past. There is a critical need to address obvious language differences (Ortiz, 2006), but also the less obvious and more intricate issues related to immigration status, acculturation, and differing cultural norms about mental health and schooling. Schools will need to contend with issues of cultural difference in all their complexity and consider the significant changes in the structural configuration of newly immigrated families, including the fact that many children will be at a different phase of adaptation to mainstream culture than their parents (Gopaul-McNicol & Armour-Thomas, 2002). Multiracial or biracial status will also warrant consideration as the experiences of these youth may entail challenges with identity development, and there is evidence that these youth may present with a greater number and earlier onset of mental health needs than their mono-racial counterparts (Choi, Harachi, Gillmore, & Catalano, 2006).

Meeting the needs of culturally diverse youth will require a framework for unpacking the factors that influence developmental outcomes of culturally and linguistically diverse children. Educators and researchers will have to shift from using a comparative lens that identifies European American middle class values and developmental processes as the norm. This framework will need to accommodate the fact that development among culturally diverse youth is influenced not just by cultural factors, but also by social position variables (e.g., race, social class, ethnicity, and gender), social stratification mechanisms (e.g., racism, discrimination, and prejudice), and segregation (García Coll, Ackerman, & Cicchetti, 2000). Meeting the needs of culturally diverse students will also require attention to how we as service providers can capitalize on the unique skill set and strengths with which these youth and their families enter schools.

Defining cross-cultural competence. A starting point to understand how service providers can be more culturally responsive to children and families is to consider how to build competence in this area. Cultural competence involves flexibility—an ability to be open to understanding the child or family's experience from their frame of reference rather than from one's own. Out of this flexibility comes an open-mindedness to being aware of one's assumptions and biases (Sue & Sue, 2008), as well as being aware of the worldview of the child/family with whom you are working (Sue & Sue). These two domains, awareness of self and awareness of other, interact dynamically so that when the helping professional is aware of his/her own biases, s/he will be better equipped to understand the child/family from their perspective. In this sense cross-cultural competence involves empathy—one looks outside oneself to see someone else from their vantage point.

Much of the cultural competence literature has defined the term with a tripartite model: awareness, knowledge, and skills (Sue, Arredondo, & McDavis, 1992; Sue et al., 1998). Within each of these domains are specific cultural competencies that further spell out specific aspects of competence. For instance, *awareness* involves having "moved from being culturally unaware to being aware and sensitive to own cultural heritage and to valuing and respecting differences" (p. 47); *knowledge* includes being "knowledgeable and informed on a number of culturally diverse groups, especially groups therapists work with" (p. 47); and *skills* encompass being "able to generate a wide variety of verbal and nonverbal helping responses" (p. 47). While these present one example for each domain, the original description includes 34 multicultural competencies (Sue & Sue, 2008; Sue et al., 1992, 1998).

Handbook co-editors view cultural competence as being systemic in nature. This philosophy is in accord with that proposed by Sue and Sue (2008) that examines the impact of cultural competence on a systemic/societal scale. For the purposes of the current volume, two systemic foci are addressed. On one level is the systemic focus on the child/family. This perspective examines the child and his/her family in the context of school, community, and the intersections among variables present in these contexts. These variables are addressed in chapters that explore the vast array of family and peer experiences faced by children and families today.

On another level is the profession itself—i.e., the researchers, mental health professionals, advocates, and policy makers who make up different constituencies. This second level presents challenges for cultural competence. One challenge concerns the lack of linkages between and among areas of research, training, practice, and policy. For instance, professional programs have a wide range of multicultural emphasis—some with cultural competence at the programs' core, others with cultural competence relegated to one course. The gap is then widened when helping professionals graduate from programs that are less culturally responsive and work in communities different from their own. In another example, while there are existing guidelines for culturally competent practice, there is less research to support the empirical use of these techniques with diverse populations. Highlighting gaps that result from a lack of interconnection is a key action item for this volume (see Chap. 19).

Goals and Objectives of the Handbook

Goals. The *Handbook* has several overarching goals that aim to tie in content and themes discussed in this chapter and those that follow. From these broad intentions come specific objectives. These are discussed below. The *Handbook's* main goal is to encourage those involved in all aspects of SMH to extend their thinking about the ways we can be responsive to the diverse youth we serve. The pages that follow discuss innovative frameworks, approaches, and strategies for cultural responsiveness in training, practice, research, and policy efforts.

This process involves acknowledging that ours is a changing landscape. Within this landscape, the role and impact of culture influences children's development and socialization. For those involved in various capacities of SMH, this acknowledgement means working to understand children within their sociocultural contexts. It also involves understanding the many variables that influence children and their families such as language, customs, culture, and historic background.

A second goal is to extend the knowledge base in the area of culturally responsive SMH. The pages that follow encourage school personnel to create linkages between innovative practice and policy that meet the needs of culturally diverse children and families. Through these linkages, schools are invited to define, discuss, and develop ways that the school climate addresses the educational, social, and emotional needs of children. SMH professionals are encouraged to consider culturally and linguistically relevant treatment. Not only does this better meet the needs of those seeking services, it also promotes access and utilization. *Handbook* co-editors articulate as a national priority, a call to action for culturally responsive advocates among the many constituencies who work with children (i.e., school personnel, administrators, policy makers, clinicians, academics, researchers).

A third goal is to address gaps and promote knowledge in culturally responsive research, training, practice, and policy. While comprehensive approaches to culturally responsive best practices have been, and are being, developed, more work is needed. For instance, ongoing efforts are needed to further refine and create an evidence base that supports comprehensive and culturally responsive practice, while also linking training and policy initiatives to these outcomes. The *Handbook's* broad focus on research, training, practice, and policy also seeks to provide readers with insights about interconnections between and among these domains.

Objectives. Concrete, specific objectives arise from these goals. Constituencies are invited to examine and identify how cultural factors play out in the each domain. In so doing, the hope is that constituencies will further refine their approach to integrate culturally relevant meanings for those with whom they work and the policies they create. This involves considering how to conceptualize teaching, training, practice, research, and policy initiatives that incorporate an understanding of cultural influences on children's development in one's day-to-day practice.

A second objective is to draw from the specific programs and frameworks presented in the *Handbook* to consider implications for best practice in one's own community. For instance, in Chap. 7, Nancy Bearss presents a comprehensive framework for working with lesbian, gay, bisexual, and transgender (LGBT) youth in schools. It is hoped that by reading this chapter, the reader will get a sense of how to promote practice and policy that promotes the well-being of LGBT youth who may feel alienated and ostracized within their school systems. Similarly, in Chap. 17, Patricia M. Raskin discusses the real pressures faced by today's families as they attempt to negotiate the demands of work and family. It is anticipated that the reader will come away from reading this chapter with a better sense of how to implement school policies that are sensitive to this tension (i.e., policy that incorporates electronic access as a way to communicate with working families).

A third objective is for the reader to turn to the *Handbook* as a much needed reference. The *Handbook* provides a base of knowledge that readers can reference when questions arise about culturally competent responsiveness in research, practice, training, and policy domains. Each chapter includes a list of contemporary references that provides readers with additional resources for their area of interest.

Overview and Objectives for Each of the Three Handbook Sections

As stated in the Preface, the rationale for the *Handbook* is to address gaps in the literature through a compilation of chapters that highlight key topics in advancing culturally responsive SMH promotion and intervention across key realms of training, practice, research, and policy. Central to this rationale is exploring connections across these domains. One question, for instance, concerns how to provide linkages between research and culturally competent practice, thus expanding culturally responsive EBP. Similarly, another question focuses on implications of training culturally responsive school personnel for the provision of culturally responsive services in the future.

The *Handbook* has three parts, each with various contributors that reflect key themes. The three critical areas are: (I) *Status of the Research on Cultural Considerations in School-Based Mental Health Interventions with Children and Adolescents*; (II) *Innovative Approaches in Work with Diverse Children and Adolescents in Schools*; and (III) *Specific Problems and Interventions*. Each area is described below.

Part I, *Status of the Research on Cultural Considerations in School-Based Mental Health Interventions with Children and Adolescents*, provides a general introduction to the text and reviews research literature as it relates to school-based interventions with children and adolescents. The section builds on previous research findings and presents an ecological approach to understanding the notion of cultural competence in school-based mental health as well as the overall school climate.

Part II, *Innovative Approaches in Work with Diverse Children and Adolescents in Schools*, focuses on innovative approaches in work with diverse children and adolescents (i.e., culture, parental involvement, role models, school setting) that promote cross-culturally competent SMH services. Specific programs are presented that provide a model for this type of work such as the Black Parents Strengths and Strategies Program. Innovative theoretical frameworks such as Phenomenological Variant of Ecological Systems Theory (PVEST) are presented as models of positive school climate.

Part III, *Specific Problems and Interventions*, is the concluding part of the text. The focus of Part III is to invite readers to consider specific issues—some illustrated with case studies—that connect science to practice. Prevention efforts associated with the healthy development of children and adolescents are also discussed. Chapters in this part address the achievement gap, advocacy, academic support, and ways to assess cultural competence in school-based interventions.

Part I: Status of the Research on Cultural Considerations in School-Based Mental Health Interventions with Children and Adolescents

Part I provides an overall framework for the *Handbook* and a foundation for Part II and III. Chapters throughout Part I make the case for culturally responsive school-based mental health. This rationale is presented through the following: a historical perspective of the SMH movement coupled with demographic trends in today's schools (Chap. 1); discussion about building a culture of trust in schools with overseas military base schools being one such example (Chap. 2); consideration of cultural responsiveness in diverse school contexts with rural schools being included among them (Chap. 3); and attention directed to the changing roles of twenty-first century school personnel against the backdrop of twenty-first century national demographic changes (Chap. 4).

In Chap. 2, Alan R. Scheuermann and Tracey Jernigan discuss the impact of military life on families and the relevance of specific cultural issues for them. The authors discuss challenges associated with providing mental health services for youth in an overseas military base located in a different culture. A key issue that results from this situation is that civilians living overseas "are subject to the civilian laws of the host nation based on a Status of Forces Agreement (SOFA)," thus there are cultural considerations housed within cultural considerations. Chapter 3 continues the conversation about the critical need for cultural responsiveness, here within a rural school context. Hence, Julie Sarno Owens and her colleagues discuss being culturally responsive in the provision of SMH services within a rural context. Definitions for the term "rural" are presented as well as how, even though different than an urban setting, rural communities "are heterogeneous with regard to demographic, economic, and cultural characteristics."

In the final chapter in this part, Laura Miller and her colleagues discuss how the school counselor's role has changed from the twentieth to the twenty-first century. The expansion of this role includes an increased focused on the social/emotional growth of the student within a sociocultural context. The importance of advocacy, cultural sensitivity, and working across professional cultures such as educational vs. counseling realms is presented. Consideration of the shift in school personnel roles has implications for the next part of the book, Part II—that examines innovative approaches in work with diverse school communities. As such, it is an appropriate segue.

Part II: Innovative Approaches in Work with Diverse Children and Adolescents in Schools

The cultural landscape of the U.S. and the world as a whole is changing. Promoting cross-culturally competent SMH services will therefore require innovation. Not only do researchers and practitioners have to consider the sociocultural, political, and historical contexts of the communities where schools are located and in which children live, but they also have to develop new conceptualizations of SMH and culture in order to address the increasingly complex needs of diverse children and adolescents.

Many of the chapters in Part II describe a re-conceptualization or broadening of what constitutes SMH. Chapters also illustrate the importance of expanding beyond the confines of the school building to reach out to families, connect with and develop a shared agenda with community partners, and incorporate flexibility into the program implementation process. Furthermore, chapters in this part of the *Handbook* highlight the importance of cultural specificity and adaptation in SMH programs.

Programs described include those that target the specific needs of a particular group and/or around particular problems. Chapters 5 and 6, by Kendra P. DeLoach and Stephanie I. Coard, and their respective colleagues, articulate key issues and effective strategies to engage and address SMH among African American youth and their families. Kendra P. DeLoach and colleagues focus on strategies to engage families, whereas Stephanie I. Coard and colleagues describe how an empirically supported parenting program can be successfully adapted to be more culturally responsive for African American families. With a similar focus on families, in Chap. 8, Matthew Mock reviews key target areas for effective practice in school settings for Asian American and Pacific Islander youth and their families—highlighting issues related to stigma, access, and service utilization.

Other chapters emphasize the need to pay attention to critical contextual factors, that is often the impetus for a strength-based approach to programming. For instance, in Chap. 9, Keisha Bentley and colleagues consider the unique experiences of African American males in school contexts and how important it is to address issues related to racial stress. In Chap. 13, Nicole Evangelista Brandt and her colleagues review the rapid escalation of gang involvement and associated problems for youth in the U.S. and present strategies for culturally competent programs and services to address this unique population of youth. In Chap. 7, Nancy Bearss discusses best practices in promoting positive school climates for LGBT youth. The author underscores the need for a positive school climate to combat alienation, suicidality, and depression experienced by LGBT youth, and discusses important cultural considerations in work with LGBT youth from diverse racial/ethnic backgrounds. In Chap. 11, Jody Lieske and her colleagues focus on SMH issues in rural school settings. These authors highlight the fact that rural communities have their own culture, and addressing mental health issues in primary care settings is an important mechanism through which to improve *school* mental health.

Remaining chapters in Part II focus on cross-cutting issues that exist within subpopulations of culturally diverse communities. For instance, Kip Thompson and colleagues discuss the role of adolescent ethnic identity development. This chapter considers theoretical frameworks of adolescent identity development as well processes associated with personal and ethnic identity development across a range of diverse communities of youth. In Chap. 10, Caroline S. Clauss-Ehlers and her colleague Adeyinka Akinsulure-Smith address specific issues faced by forced migrant children and their families. These include developmental, mental health, legal, and linguistic considerations for refugees, unaccompanied minors, and asylum seekers.

Part III: Specific Problems and Interventions

Discussion about innovation leads to a focus on specific problems and interventions, the final part of the *Handbook*. The six chapters that make up this part address a range of different issues that include: training transformed school counselors (Chap. 14); culturally responsive substance abuse and sex education prevention programming for middle school youth (Chap. 15); culturally competent assessment in schools (Chap. 16); policy implications for work/family balance issues among families (Chap. 17); understanding trauma from a culturally competent perspective (Chap. 18); and consideration of next steps to advance culturally responsive school-based mental health (Chap. 19).

The first three chapters (i.e., Chaps. 14, 15, and 16) present models of training and/or programming, In Chap. 14, Marte Ostvik-deWilde and colleagues discuss the University of Maryland's school counselor preparation program that prepares school counselors to deal with urban educational issues. School counselors learn to be advocates, to address the achievement gap, and to take a systemic, culturally competent perspective. Chapter 15 focuses on programming from another perspective, that of prevention programming for early adolescents. Desi Hacker and colleagues discuss a "culturally integrated sex education and substance prevention program" for adolescents between 11 and 14 years of age. The chapter concludes with a discussion of key variables that are central to effective culturally responsive programs. Chapter 16 provides yet another lens from which to consider culturally responsive intervention—here in the assessment arena. Toni Harris and colleagues discuss "cultural bias in school assessment" that leads to a disproportionate number of children of color and those from low-income families in special education. The chapter goes on to discuss culturally competent best practices in school-based assessment.

The remaining chapters of Part III focus on building capacity within various realms of child and family experience. In Chap. 17, for instance, Patricia M. Raskin examines trends in work/family issues over the past 30 years. Central to this discussion is consideration of the impact of race, ethnicity, and social class on work/family dilemmas. Avenues for policy are presented such as flexibility solutions. In Chap. 18, Leslie K. Taylor and colleagues make the case for the importance of "school-based interventions for traumatized youth." Taylor and her colleagues also make recommendations "for building capacities necessary for supporting and sustaining culturally competent trauma focused intervention within schools."

The *Handbook*'s concluding chapter raises overall policy and capacity building concerns. *Handbook* co-editors present current critical issues and provide an action plan to advance cross-culturally competent school-based mental health. The urgency to pursue this action plan is underscored throughout the chapter.

Conclusion

As *Handbook* co-editors we invite readers to absorb the information that follows and explore how it applies to those with whom you work. Whether as school personnel, an educator, mental health professional, policy maker, or administrator, we hope the pages that follow provide you with new perspectives about the work that you do, the impact it has, and its far-reaching implications for children and their families. Our efforts have largely focused on pulling together a comprehensive approach that creates linkages between research, training, practice, and policy. As with any project, we appreciate that there are gaps in the information provided and further work to be done. In your review of the volume, we encourage you to consider future areas of focus for these aspects of the field and the accompanying effort needed to move knowledge, practice, and policy forward.

References

Alegría, M., Canino, G., Rios, R., Vera, M., Calderon, J., Rusch, D., et al. (2002). Inequalities in use of specialty mental health services among Latinos, African Americans, and Non-Latino Whites. *Psychiatric Services, 53*, 1547–1555.

Anglin, T. M. (2003). Mental health in school: Program of the federal government. In M. Weist, S. Evans, & N. Lever (Eds.), *Handbook of school mental health programs: Advancing practice and research* (pp. 89–105). New York, NY: Kluwer Academic.

Aud, S., Hussar, W., Johnson, F., Kena, G., Roth, E., Manning, E., Wang, K., & Zhang, J. (2012). *The condition of education 2012* (NCES 2012–045). U.S. Department of Education, National Center for Education Statistics. Washington, DC. Retrieved September 28, 2012 from http.//nces.ed.gov/pubsearch

Aud, S., Hussar, W., Planty, M., Snyder, T., Bianco, K., Fox, M., et al. (2010). *The condition of education 2010*. Washington, DC: National Center for Education Statistics, Institute of Education Sciences, U.S. Department of Education.

Brown, M. R. (2009). A new multicultural population: Creating effective partnerships with multiracial families. *Intervention in School and Clinic, 45*, 124–131.

Bussing, R., Zima, B. T., Gary, F. A., & Garvan, C. W. (2003). Barriers to detection, help-seeking, and service use for children with ADHD symptoms. *The Journal of Behavioral Health Services and Research, 30*(2), 176–189.

Choi, Y., Harachi, T. W., Gillmore, M. R., & Catalano, R. F. (2006). Are multiracial adolescents at greater risk? Comparisons of rates, patterns, and correlates of substance use and violence between monoracial and multiracial adolescents. *The American Journal of Orthopsychiatry, 76*, 86–97.

Diala, C., Muntaner, C., Walrath, C., Nickerson, K. J., LaVeist, T. A., & Leaf, P. (2001). Racial/ethnic differences in attitudes toward seeking professional mental health services. *American Journal of Public Health, 91*(5), 805–807.

dosRies, S., Zito, J. M., Safer, D. J., Soeken, K. L., Mitchell, J. W., & Ellwood, L. C. (2003). Parental perceptions and satisfaction with stimulant medication for attention-deficit hyperactivity disorder. *Journal of Developmental and Behavioral Pediatrics, 24*(3), 155–162.

Evans, S. W., & Weist, M. D. (2004). Implementing empirically supported treatments in schools: What are we asking? *Child and Family Psychology Review, 7*, 263–267.

Flaherty, L. T., & Osher, D. (2003). History of school-based mental health services. In M. Weist, S. Evans, & N. Lever (Eds.), *Handbook of school mental health programs: Advancing practice and research* (pp. 11–22). New York, NY: Kluwer Academic.

García Coll, C. T., Ackerman, A., & Cicchetti, D. (2000). Cultural influences on developmental processes and outcomes: Implications for the study of development and psychopathology [Special Issue]. *Development and Psychopathology, 12*, 333–356.

Gopaul-McNicol, S., & Armour-Thomas, E. (2002). *Assessment and culture: Psychological tests with minority populations*. San Diego, CA: Academic.

Huang, L., Macbeth, G., Dodge, J., & Jacobstein, D. (2004). Transforming the workforce in children's mental health. *Administration and Policy in Mental Health, 32*(2), 167–187.

Humes, K. R., Jones, N. A., & Ramirez, R. R. (2011). *Overview of race and Hispanic origin: 2010 (C2010BR-02)*. Retrieved March 29, 2011, from U.S. Census Bureau website http://www.census.gov/prod/cen2010/briefs/c2010br-02.pdf

Knitzer, J. (1982). *Unclaimed children: The failure of public responsibility to children in need of mental health services*. Washington, DC: Children's Defense Fund.

National Center for Education Statistics. (2011). *The condition of education*. Retrieved July 2011, from http://nces.ed.gov/programs/coe/

Ortiz, S. O. (2006). Multicultural issues in school psychology practice: A critical analysis. *Journal of Applied School Psychology, 22*(2), 151–167.

Oswald, D. P., Coutinho, M. J., & Best, A. M. (2002). Community and school predictors of overrepresentation of minority children in special education. In D. J. Losen & G. Orfield (Eds.), *Racial inequity in special education* (pp. 1–14). Boston, MA: Harvard Education Press.

Patton, J. M. (1998). The disproportionate representation of African Americans in special education: Looking behind the curtain for understanding and solutions. *Journal of Special Education, 32*(1), 25–31.

Planty, M., Hussar, W., Snyder, T., Kena, G., Kewal-Ramani, A., Kemp, J., et al. (2009). *The condition of education 2009*. Washington, DC: National Center for Education Statistics, Institute of Education Sciences, U.S. Department of Education.

President's New Freedom Commission on Mental Health. (2003). *Achieving the promise: Transforming mental health care in America. Final report for the President's New Freedom Commission on Mental Health (SMA Publication No. 03-3832)*. Rockville, MD: Author.

Rappaport, N., Neugebauer, R., Stein, B., Elliott, M., Tu, W., Jaycox, L., et al. (2003). A mental health intervention for school-children exposed to violence: A randomized controlled trial. *Journal of the American Medical Association, 290*(19), 2541–2542.

Rogers, M. R., Ponterotto, J. G., Conoley, J. C., & Wiese, M. J. (1992). Multicultural training in school psychology: A national survey. *School Psychology Review, 21*, 603–616.

Snowden, L. R., & Yamada, A. M. (2005). Cultural differences in access to care. *Annual Review of Clinical Psychology, 1*, 143–166.

Stroul, B. A., & Friedman, R. M. (1986). *A system of care for children and youth with severe emotional disturbances*. Washington, DC: Grorgetown University Child Development Center, CASSP Technical Assistance Center.

Sue, D. W., Arredondo, P., & McDavis, R. J. (1992). Multicultural competencies/standards: A call to the profession. *Journal of Counseling and Development, 70*(4), 477–486.

Sue, D. W., Carter, R. T., Casas, J. M., Fouad, N. A., Ivey, A. E., Jensen, M., et al. (1998). *Multicultural counseling competencies: Individual and organizational development*. Thousand Oaks, CA: Sage.

Sue, D. W., & Sue, D. (2008). *Counseling and culturally diverse: Theory and practice* (5th ed.). Hoboken, NJ: Wiley.

U.S. Department of Health and Human Services. (1999). *Mental health: A report of the surgeon general—Executive summary*. Rockville, MD: U. S. Department of Health and Human Services, Substance Abuse and Mental Health Services Administration, Center for Mental Health Services, National Institute of Health, National Institute of Mental Health.

U.S. Department of Health and Human Services. (2000). *Report of the surgeon general's conference on children's mental health: A national action agenda*. Rockville, MD: U.S. Department of Health and Human Services, Substance Abuse and Mental Health Services Administration, Center for Mental Health Services, National Institute of Health, National Institute of Mental Health.

United States Department of Health and Human Services. (2001). *Mental health: A report of the Surgeon General*. Rockville, MD: United States Department of Health and Human Services, Substance Abuse and Mental Health Services Administration, Center for Mental Health Services.

Weist, M. D. (1997). Expanded school mental health services: A national movement in progress. In T. H. Ollendick & R. J. Prinz (Eds.), *Advances in clinical child psychology* (Vol. 19, pp. 319–352). New York, NY: Plenum.

Weist, M. D., Stephan, S., Lever, N., Moore, E., Flaspohler, P., Maras, M., et al. (2007). Quality and school mental health. In S. Evans, M. Weist, & Z. Serpell (Eds.), *Advances in school-based mental health interventions* (pp. 4:1–4:14). New York, NY: Civic Research Institute.

Building a "Culture of Trust": The Cultural and Practical Challenges of School-Based Behavioral Health Care in Overseas Military Base Schools

Alan R. Scheuermann and Tracey Jernigan

Zeke and his parents were in the Senior Counselor's office of a high school on a military base overseas. Zeke's father was preparing to deploy to a combat zone within 3 weeks. Zeke was facing a risk of not graduating. When the counselor informed Zeke and his parents of the likelihood of not graduating based on current performance, Zeke, a stoic 18 year old who liked to read fantasy novels, play video games and his guitar, began to cry. He said he didn't want to disappoint his parents but was unsure if he could make up the work he had missed. He was particularly upset that his dad would be worried and distracted about Zeke when he needed to be more focused on his dangerous upcoming mission. He had also been struggling the past year to adjust to being in Germany after having lived his entire life in the United States. His family moved overseas for his father's final assignment, but this required Zeke to move away from his friends and the high school he had attended for the three previous years just outside an army base in the Southeastern United States. With this information and the family in tears in her office, the Senior Counselor contacted the School-Based Behavioral Health provider on-site. An intake evaluation was conducted and treatment plan initiated the same day. Seven weeks later, after a course of cognitive-behavioral therapy to address a long-standing anxiety disorder and solution-focused therapy to improve his academic production, Zeke completed his coursework successfully and graduated on time. His father, down-range in the Middle East, was able to watch his son graduate via satellite broadcast. Zeke had accomplished his goal and his father was able to continue his mission without distraction.

Introduction

This case vignette illustrates the benefit of having mental health professionals serving military adolescents in Department of Defense secondary schools overseas. The U.S. Army Medical Command (Army MEDCOM) has begun emphasizing the value of community embedded clinical service, following the lead of established practice in the civilian sector. In fact, school-based behavioral health (SBBH) is a central pillar of the U.S. Army Surgeon General's Comprehensive Behavioral Health System of Care-Campaign Plan (CBHSOC-CP). The CBHSOC-CP is an organized and unified plan to address the growing behavioral health needs in today's U.S. Army. This is based on the challenges facing the military due to 10 years of significant involvement in the War on Terror. This plan involves organizing effective and efficient behavioral health support for soldiers and their families based on the Army Family Covenant. This value-driven commitment to army families

A.R. Scheuermann, Ph.D. (✉) • T. Jernigan, LCSW
Bavaria-MEDDAC/U.S. Army Medical Command,
San Antonio, TX, USA
e-mail: alan.scheuermann@us.army.mil

focuses on providing comprehensive health care support throughout the life span due to the risks and sacrifices that soldiers and their families make when serving. These support structures include a broad range of services for soldiers and families. The most prominent service line for the purposes of this chapter is SBBH. The CBHSOC-CP identifies SBBH as the preferred way to provide routine behavioral health services for children and adolescents. The foundational goal of the Army Family Covenant is to build of "culture of trust" between army families and the army itself. Providing SBBH services is an effort to improve upon the culture of trust by being more accessible and more effective than clinic-based care.

This chapter is a review of issues that one SBBH program has faced in entering into secondary schools in military bases overseas. First, a brief review of the impact of military life on dependents is presented followed by a brief review of the SBBH model in the U.S. Army. Specific issues that the SBBH program in Bavaria, Germany have encountered will be presented to review the cultural challenges of SBBH service delivery to military dependents overseas. Additionally, program structures that support cultural sensitivity will be presented.

Impact of Military Life on Adolescents and Families

That SBBH care has become the preferred method for service delivery for children and adolescents is a direct result of many studies that have identified the negative impact of a high tempo of cycles of deployment on military members and their families (Chandra, Burns, Tanielian, Jaycox, & Scott, 2008; Tanielian et al., 2008). Studies have found that adolescents in military families suffer higher rates of emotional and behavioral difficulties when compared to their civilian counterparts, particularly higher rates of anxiety and behavioral problems (Chandra et al., 2008). Gorman, Eide, and Hisle-Gorman (2010) found higher rates of outpatient mental health visits among children and adolescents of military families. Millean (2011) even found that military dependent youth in one community (Hawaii) experienced greater rates of psychiatric hospitalizations. It is speculated that the military culture within which these children live is not necessarily the cause of problems. Hypotheses regarding the reasons for increases in anxiety and behavioral problems include impact of deployment separations on family and individual functioning and multiple transitions due to frequent moves (Chandra et al., 2008; Military Child Education Coalition, 2007; Tanielian et al., 2008).

Serving in the military necessarily means that one may be deployed or otherwise absent from one's family for lengthy periods of time. In recent history, U.S. Army soldiers could expect to be deployed for half of their career with multiple deployments to war zones. These deployments remove parents from their children's day-to-day life for 12 months at a time. For a period of time, these absences could have been as long at 15 or more months during the Iraq war surge of 2007–2008. In addition to the specific length of deployments, service members are often away from their family while training for deployment or attending intensive training schools. Regular and ongoing training, the daily life of a soldier when not deployed, often requires the soldiers to be away from home for physical training early in the morning (often well before dawn) and completion of training or other tasks well into the evening. This can keep a soldier from being present with their children for much of the workweek. Ideal child development that minimizes emotional or behavioral difficulties is based on consistency of care and on consistency of attachment figures present in a child's life (Cummings & Davies, 1994; Gottman, 1997). Without that "secure base" (Bowlby, 1988), there is significant risk for the development of greater emotional and behavioral difficulties (Weinfield, Ogawa, & Sroufe, 1997; Weinfield, Sroufe, & Egeland, 2000).

The fact that one's parent may be absent is one level of stress. However, the absences of parents for lengthy periods of time due to military deployment can add additional stress. Many children are acutely aware of the risk of potential loss of their parent when deployed (Military Child Education Coalition, 2007). This awareness can increase the intensity of personally felt distress based on their parent's absence. In the civilian world, when one's father or mother is away for a long period of time for work their life is generally not at risk. For military adolescents, it is a real risk. Given that the core concept of anxiety is vulnerability, growing formal operational/abstract thinking allows the teen to consider the loss of their parent with greater realism, and with it an increase in anxiety (Beck & Emery, 1985; Yalom, 1980). This can impact the youth's understanding of relative meaning of her actions within the context of her life, for example, "if my dad could die, what does homework matter?"

For these reasons, it is likely that military youth will require significant behavioral health support. The increase in anxiety and behavioral problems alone suggest an increased need for this type of support. Therefore, the U.S. Army has been working to address the need identified in recent experience and studies.

SBBH in the U.S. Army

In the U.S. Army MEDCOM a specific model of SBBH care has been developed. Originally conceived at Tripler Army Medical Center, Michael Faran, M.D., Albert Saito, M.D. and their team developed a SBBH program model that emphasizes the ongoing collaboration between school personnel, behavioral health personnel, and families when providing behavioral health services in school districts that have large military dependent populations (Faran et al., 2002). This model is based on public health assumptions. These assumptions include the following: delivering services where the population is located rather than having them come to a specialty clinic; focusing on prevention in addition to intervention, and being engaged fully in supporting the whole educational system vs. a more limited "co-located" model of service delivery (Faran, 2010a). This model also supports increased access to care, increased focus on resiliency and wellness rather than deficiency, and helping to create systems and environments that support better functioning overall for military children and families.

In order to accomplish these goals, the Army MEDCOM Child and Family Behavioral Health Office (CAF-BHO) has emphasized a set of structural program elements for SBBH that support collaborative program development, continuous improvement, and maintenance. These structural program elements are triage teams (TRIAGE), building-level advisory (BLA) teams, and community-level advisory (CLA) teams. Of course, the central activities of SBBH programs include a wide range of clinical services such as evaluation and evidence-based treatment of behavioral, emotional, and mental disorders.

In order to effectively support the clinical needs of students in concert with school needs, the Army SBBH model encourages a regular inter-disciplinary and multiagency TRIAGE team meeting that engages in case coordination and staffing. It is at this meeting that much of the clinical collaboration among staff occurs.

Additionally, SBBH program providers engage their partner schools in prevention activities and faculty support. In order to accomplish these activities effectively, the Army SBBH model encourages the development of what are called BLA teams in each school. The purpose of a building advisory group is to have a team that can coordinate general services, identify emerging needs among students and faculty, and address concerns that are related to how the various agencies are working together. Given that coordination among various agencies can be difficult, it is the U.S. Army MEDCOM's conclusion that putting BLA teams in place in each school allows for the regular management of issues that could otherwise develop into problems in the delivery of services. Staff and administrators meet regularly and proactively to address mental health and agency coordination concerns rather than reactively meeting only when there are problems.

One last structure that is a part of the Army MEDCOM SBBH model is a CLA team. This team is comprised of leadership from the community within which SBBH programs are located in order to provide advice and consultative/collaborative oversight regarding how the SBBH program is being implemented in the schools in that locality. This allows for accountability to the leadership in each community so that the SBBH program is tailoring their provision of services in a coordinated manner that fits the needs of that particular community.

While SBBH is the preferred model moving forward in the U.S. Army MEDCOM vision for behavioral health services, only a handful of bases currently have SBBH programs in place. Two of those programs are located outside of the U.S. in Germany, serving military dependents of soldiers stationed in support of European allies. The Bavaria-SBBH program will be described below.

Bavaria-SBBH Program

The Bavaria School-Based Behavioral Health Program has been in operation for 3 school years. The U.S. Army MEDCOM granted funding for this program in the Spring of 2009 to provide behavioral health services in five schools serving military dependents living at the two military communities that support the largest ground force training area outside of the U.S. as well as two regularly deploying brigade-size (approximately 4,000 soldiers) units. These schools include three elementary schools (K-5), one middle school (6–8), and one high school (9–12). The proposed and funded program was based directly on the U.S. Army MEDCOM model that included an emphasis on treatment and prevention services with the goal of including the recommended structures of coordination (TRIAGE, BLA, and CLA). The team is comprised of four clinical staff members (three licensed clinical social workers with specific child training and one child clinical psychologist who also serves as assistant director) serving a student population of approximately 2,600.

Within 2 months of inception, the average case load within the program had risen to above 20 for each provider. By the end of the first school year, average case loads were over 40 with only the assistant director of the program having a case load lower than 30. A quote from the movie *Field of Dreams* is an apt description, "Build it and they will come." The viability of the program was demonstrated early based on provider productivity.

Clinical services were provided and providers were integrated into a number of different school committees, including student success teams, crisis management teams, and even being included in the school improvement process in one school. Use of outcome measures demonstrated that effective care was being delivered based on significant improvement of pre- and posttreatment measurement of ratings of overall distress.

It was also found that the need was greater than projected. The program served approximately 12 % of the student population, but many referrals continued to be made to local clinic-based behavioral health providers and many students referred to B-SBBH were seen less frequently than might have been clinically indicated due to time pressure on the staff's schedule. During deployment cycles, deployment-related cases (cases in which the presenting problem is directly due to deployment or, if already existing, exacerbated by deployment) averaged 50 % in the schools and were as high as 82 % in one. The projected rate of military children requiring some form of mental health services approaches 25 % (Faran, 2010b). Therefore, our staffing along with the local school personnel has not been able to fully meet the referral demands in the military community from which the units deploy frequently.

In seeking consultation regarding the development of the program and addressing issues that arose in the secondary schools, many issues were identified that had not been addressed in specific training for U.S. Army SBBH program development. The following sets of issues confronted are included: the role of the SBBH provider and practical issues of providing clinically sound and ethical services for teens within the social context of a single school and small community; addressing adolescent cultural issues as behavioral health providers in a school and on a military base overseas; and being culturally sensitive in delivering services on a military base overseas. As a caveat, many aspects of the issues discussed are anecdotal. However, empirical literature on the development of SBBH for military families is still very limited (Faran, 2010a), so anecdotal observations such as those provided here should help build effective practices and research on them.

Issues in Serving Adolescents of Military Families in the Bavaria-SBBH Program

Challenges of Multiple Roles for the Overseas Military SBBH Provider

The nature of living and working on a military base overseas is that it functions like a small community, and the American community is socially isolated even in populated areas. Additionally, the role of an SBBH provider in secondary schools on an overseas military base is complicated due to the multiple professional relationships that they must maintain. Providers are clinical therapists to many individual children and their families; consultants to teachers, faculty, and staff; and provide educational or prevention presentations in the classrooms, making them appear to youth as part of the faculty. They are perceived differently with different roles by many people in a single setting, and in some cases friendships develop in the small communities often found in military bases overseas. Managing these multiple layers of relationships and associated role strain is critical to the success of a school-based provider in order to reduce the likelihood of dual-relationship difficulties (Bennett et al., 2006).

Given that SBBH providers work fully as a team, many functions that would never fall to a clinic-based behavioral health provider may fall to a school-based behavioral health provider. For example, clinic-based providers are rarely consulted when a student is facing some form of disciplinary action at school. School-based providers are often consulted in these cases and this can create a confusion regarding the definition of who is the client (child/family or the school administrator). With teens, in particular, a provider can risk their credibility (e.g., with the family) by being aligned with the school administration. Alternatively, each provider will necessarily work with multiple clients who know each other. Therefore, each provider may have information about a student from other students that they see or be told a story from a parent regarding another parent or student. In these types of situations, managing roles is a necessary skill for each provider to develop so that they can clearly communicate and collaborate with others in the system and maintain therapeutic credibility with teens in the school. Therefore, the provider is placed in a "political" role in the community of the school with various constituencies. The provider must work to maintain their positive relationship with the various constituencies in order to be positioned to have the greatest positive influence.

Clearly, there are positive aspects of being a behavioral health provider in the school as well. The students, faculty, and staff all develop relationships with the provider outside of a therapy referral. Many of the referrals that one gets in a school are due to being known in the school where the children and teens become familiar with the provider's presence and see them as someone to turn to for assistance.

The issue of multiple role management may, however, limit the types of interventions one may choose because a part of any attempted intervention is to limit any unintentional harm (Bennett et al., 2006). When delivering behavioral health services to adolescents, in addition to individual and family modalities, group-based interventions are often recommended. However, confidentiality concerns regarding adolescents within the same school often arise when group interventions are attempted. For instance, when SBBH providers in the middle and high school began developing groups within their schools, in every possible case of group composition they found likely conflicts among the group members that would keep the group from being initially successful. Since the group member client pool was approximately 500–600 (the population each of the middle and high schools) and all were in the same environment, most youth are acquainted with each other and have ongoing relationships. In this environment, the providers could identify enough students for a variety of sustainable groups reflecting critical themes (emotion management, anxiety, social skills, etc.). It was often found that in trying to identify a group of teens to work with each other, they often came from socially conflicting groups (e.g., reflecting different "classes" of soldiers), making the engagement in therapy tenuous due to initial mistrust of other members. An alternative approach could be to work with teen groups that already exist (naturally formed peer groups). The problem is that for many in existing peer groups, treatment may not be appropriate, even if one or a few of a group would be candidates. Therefore, the SBBH program has tended to err on the side of more individual approaches in order to protect confidentiality and treatment integrity but this decision comes with the downside of potentially limiting the number of students who can be reached.

Adolescent Culture and the SBBH Provider

Please note that most of the Army SBBH programs at the present time operate mostly with students and families in elementary schools (Faran, 2010a), giving the Bavaria program a unique opportunity to explore service delivery with adolescents and their families in the middle and high school in the program. Here we describe some of the unique issues encountered in working with adolescents from military families.

Adolescence is often described as a "subculture" in which there are separate rules, power relationships, and values as well as different ways of communicating (Murphy, 1997; Selekman, 1993). Adults in a school often do not have awareness of much of what is communicated among teens. SBBH providers, however, often have access to that information. When information, such as trends regarding risky behavior, various cliques and bullying, etc. becomes available through the clinical contact, there are more options available to a SBBH provider than a clinic-based provider. With that information, consultation can occur with the rest of the school team toward the development and implementation of interventions that might address the risky behaviors in question. Additionally, staff may be educated in the ways that adolescents are communicating with each in order to raise their "adolescent IQ" and become more aware themselves of the trends that are occurring. For instance, one day at the high school, a number of students had used face paint to apply "NO H8" to their left cheek. An SBBH provider and an Adolescent Substance Abuse Counselor (ASACS; another outside agency) both found out in separate clinical sessions that this was a way of supporting lesbian/gay/bisexual/transsexual (LGBT) peers. With this information, the SBBH and ASACS counselor addressed the working BLA group to discuss whether there was a problem with LGBT bullying/acceptance. This has led to a needs assessment to determine what response may be required. Our role as SBBH providers allows us to be a "humint" or human intelligence asset for the adult system (school/community) in order to more effectively address concerns that arise from within the subculture of adolescence.

Another issue within the adolescent subculture is that of confidentiality and protection of information about them as well as their peers (Jacob & Feinberg, 2002). The SBBH provider may work with youth who have relationships with other youth on their case load. A provider may become aware of information from one teen regarding another teen's behavior. This has implications for the therapeutic relationship with each teen in question, but also for the limits of confidentiality. For instance, when a girl describes what happened at a party over the weekend and in the story information regarding another client's behavior is disclosed the provider now must consider how to manage that information. For most disclosures, there are few problems with considering the information hearsay and not introducing that information into a session. The provider then only has to ensure that the information she heard does not obviously inform her approach so that the other client is identified, which would constitute a breach of confidentiality (Bennett et al., 2006).

Greater consideration of the information is required when the information includes risky behavior and safety issues. One must address safety issues when there is information regarding reasonable risk of harm to self or others. If the information that the teen discloses includes, for example, that a friend was cutting herself over the weekend, then additional steps must be considered.

However, the teen who disclosed the information must be cared for during the process of disclosure and the insuring of safety of all involved. Therefore, a good informed consent process includes informing each client about the program's responsibilities for ensuring safety when information about someone else, as well as themselves, is made known. The risks and benefits of disclosure and how each provider might handle the disclosure are reviewed generally at the beginning of therapy and more specifically when students make a disclosure regarding a peer (Jacob & Feinberg, 2002). Having teens understand in advance what may happen goes a long way to keeping therapeutic relationships intact when forced to disclose or support the disclosure of concerns for safety regarding others. In the above circumstance, it is often desirable to encourage the teen to meet with the school counselor (often accompanied by the SBBH provider) to disclose their safety concerns directly. The SBBH provider, then, as part of the larger mental health team in the school, has activated the other resources available within the school system to follow up with safety assessments based on the facilitated disclosure by the peer. This approach also allows for the ongoing confidentiality of the student's relationship to the SBBH provider outside of the school's counselors and administrators.

The SBBH Provider and Military/German Cultural Considerations

One of the significant issues when providing behavioral health services for youth on a military base overseas is the placement of that base in a different culture. The U.S. Army and other military bases that are located overseas often support more than just the military members. Many military members have the option of having their whole family stationed with them when based overseas. Therefore, the family can follow their military parent and continue to live together during lengthier assignments (typically 2–3 years). Many of these overseas bases have existed for decades. Two more prominent cultural issues arise from this situation. The first is that civilians who live overseas are subject to the civilian laws of the host nation based on a Status of Forces Agreement (SOFA), essentially a treaty that governs how the U.S. Army and its members and dependents are to operate within a foreign country. The second is that there are many bi-cultural families who are members of the military, making the cross-cultural implications of understanding and working overseas directly related to clinical work.

The SOFA rules govern how military civilians are treated in the host nation. In Germany, SOFA regulations stipulate that civilians working for the U.S. Military are governed by German laws. The implications for this in working with teenagers in secondary schools are that one must consider the differences in typical American laws regarding such things as age of consent and the legal age for alcohol and tobacco consumption. For example, in Germany, the drinking age for beer is 16 years old, while for wine and hard alcohol it is 18 years old. Understanding that many of the secondary school students can legally have access to alcohol may impact the possible clinical responses to its use among whom Americans might consider minors. While it is clear that the program would never support children under the age of 21 drinking, how the therapist addresses this issue to maintain clinical credibility with the teen is likely to be impacted. In the U.S., it is easy to say that alcohol use is illegal for one's age, therefore if it is used, then illegal actions are being taken and that must be considered as one of the potential consequences of youth substance use. But in Germany, that argument is less clear and often clinicians and parents have more difficulty convincing their American children of the dangers of use when the host nation supports its use by its laws.

Insuring that teens understand their legal responsibilities is also a critical aspect of clinical care within this cross-cultural setting. Another consideration regarding age of consent is how one applies that to decisions regarding provision of services (Bennett et al., 2006). When providing behavioral health services as an American organization serving American dependents subject to the laws of a foreign country, competing regulations may apply. When providing services to military children on bases in the U.S., the age of consent for entering into a professional relationship without parental consent is governed by the state in which the military base is located. This varies from state to state. Overseas, however, federal regulations governing provision of services may be inconsistent with the foreign laws and SOFA status.

The SBBH program had to consider how to address consent for services particularly for children 15 years and older. The program could have provided services to them if they sought out services without their parents' knowledge as federal regulation allows for medical care, substance abuse care, and care for reproductive decisions. However, there were additional considerations. One was regarding maintenance of confidentiality of the youth's access to services due to billing procedures. The SBBH services are paid for through the military members' health care coverage which does not typically incur a cost that the parent experiences. Not all students who could access care are military dependents. In the cases of military civilian employees or contractors, the parents' private insurance is billed when services are provided. Therefore, it was possible for parents to become aware of their child's involvement in SBBH services through receiving a bill in the mail or through access to their medical records. This is not the most desirable means for informing parents of their children's involvement in behavioral health services (even though students may have the legal right to access this care independent of their parents' authorization).

The ethical consideration of being able to protect a client's confidentiality as well as appropriately address informed consent with the potential risks of involvement with behavioral health led us to consider requiring parental permission for all students served by the program regardless of age (including students in high school aged 16–18). This was made easier knowing that a number of other services in the school allow students to access them without parental permission, including school counselors and school psychologists and the ASACS counselor, all of which are funded differently than a fee-for-service model.

While SOFA status and federal regulations could have allowed for some youth to be able to have access to SBBH care without parental knowledge or permission, it is the value of our program that parents in the military overseas should be intimately involved in the mental health care of the children, particularly if we are addressing not just the individual student's functioning, but how that impacts the family and vice versa. The program concluded in this instance that requiring parental permission for all students regardless of age would be appropriate.

Surrounding military bases overseas, the local population is integrated into the structure of service as many are employed on the base. Due to this close relationship, many military members meet and marry people from the local population. Often military members return to an overseas tour in a country from which their spouse originates. This leads to having bi-cultural families. While any generalizations regarding German and American cultural differences are suspect, understanding that differences exist must be taken into account when addressing family functioning issues that are often present when supporting teens with behavioral health services. Being sensitive to the possibility of cultural differences or historical contexts that differ is important. One must have an ear for different perceptions based on cultural heritage/experience (Sue & Sue, 2007).

One example of having to consider cultural issues came up when one SBBH provider spoke with a German mother (whose daughter was struggling with issues of depression and self-harm). The mother discussed her parents' history, relating that her father and mother were significantly impacted by the aftermath of World War II. Apparently they had been born just before the war, and their earliest memories were of deprivation, maltreatment by their own government and by occupying forces, and self-hatred they saw in their parents and others due to the history of participation in Hitler's regime. This led to a life of silence and interpersonal remoteness that then translated into significant criticism of their daughter. This story of trans-generational emotional abuse opened the door for increased compassion and insight into the experience of the client and her mother along with a cultural exploration of the impact of historical experiences on current functioning. Significant criticism that the mother made of the daughter was framed as a continuation of the cultural "self-hatred" stemming from the aftermath of World War II. The case led to a resolution involving "re-writing" the history of the family (that had a split between the American optimism of the father and the German pessimism of the mother) into a set of realistic values and judgments. The daughter appreciated hearing the historical context (to which she had not been privy due to a cultural and family value of silence regarding emotional issues) and this helped to allow herself to give up her self-injury. She was able to see the self-injury as a continuation of self-hatred within a historical/cultural context. This layer of meaning-centered work, coupled with specific behavioral interventions, led to an elimination of self-injury and the development of greater self-compassion. This was particularly possible as the mother began to reduce her criticisms and increased her compassionate statements to others in the family as well as increasing her self-compassion.

Outcomes Management, Feedback Informed Treatment, and Cultural Sensitivity in SBBH

No matter what type of clinical work is done, the focus of psychotherapy and behavioral health services in recent years has been its value; does it actually do anything to improve the functioning of those it serves? SBBH is no different. Funders are interested in supporting programs that provide value in terms of impact on functioning of those served. Of course, the key consideration in determining value is what type of outcome is desired. Levison-Johnson, Dewey, and Wandersman (2009) described a process of determining outcomes in collaboration with stakeholders in any social service endeavor that they coined "Getting To Outcomes (GTO)." While the Bavaria-SBBH program has not specifically used this 10-point process to determine the outcomes sought, the GTO framework has informed our thinking regarding improving outcomes management when looking to the future.

Targeting and achieving improvement in clinical outcomes are necessary for any behavioral health program. Levison-Johnson et al. (2009) suggest considering the impact of the service provision by an agency not only on the individuals served by the program, but the impact of the services on the functioning of the partner agencies that support the service being provided. In the case of the Bavaria-SBBH program, it is important to consider how behavioral health services impact the larger mission of the schools served. Questions to consider beyond clinical improvement in identified behavioral health problems include the following: How is the service impacting students' academic functioning, behavior, and attendance? Are there impacts on overall school atmosphere? Are there impacts on families, soldiers, and soldier readiness? These questions are more difficult to answer as the lines of causality are more difficult to determine. It is the goal of the program to continue to engage in a collaborative effort to identify the larger community impact of our program in these schools.

The initial focus of the Bavaria-SBBH program on outcomes, however, has been in determining the clinical impact of our therapeutic efforts. This should be an established practice for any behavioral health service as there is quite a large literature on tracking clinical outcomes (Hubble, Duncan, Miller, & Wampold, 2010). The central task is to identify which measures to use for determining clinical effect. While it may be desirable to use diagnosis-specific measures to determine impact of clinical work for individual clients, these types of scales are more difficult to use to aggregate program effectiveness. Therefore, scales that track changes in overall distress of the youth or parent regarding the presenting concerns that can be used regardless of the identified diagnosis are desirable. Additionally, client ratings of change are more reliable than clinician ratings of change in determining impact, therefore client ratings are desirable (Hubble et al., 2010).

Beyond reliability and validity, feasibility for a rating scale is an important consideration.

Brown, Dreis, and Nace (1999) concluded after surveying practicing therapists that any measure taking longer than 5 minutes to administer, score, and interpret is not likely to be regularly used. This results in incomplete program outcome data if many clients are not included in the evaluation. Unfortunately, most measures of outcome are designed for research rather than clinical purposes and result in a much longer time for administration, scoring, and interpreting and then not used in a collaborative manner with the client (Brown et al., 1999).

Statistically, all measures used to track therapeutic change load primarily on the factor of client's subjective distress (Duncan, Miller, & Sparks, 2004) and this subjective distress is a primary factor in leading clients to seek services. In our experience, one set of outcome measures focuses primarily on subjective distress and appears to be the most feasible in respect to the amount of time involved in administration, scoring, and interpretation; the Outcome Rating Scale (ORS) and Child Outcome Rating Scale (CORS) (Miller & Duncan, 2004). Internal consistency of this ultra-brief measure (takes about a minute to complete, and an additional minute to score and interpret) is high at 0.93 and concurrent validity of the ORS has been demonstrated by high correlations with the Outcome Questionnaire (Campbell & Hemsley, 2009; Miller, Duncan, Brown, Sorrell, & Chalk, 2006). The Outcome Questionnaire is a 45-item scale that provides overall ratings of distress as well as identifying levels of distress in different areas of a person's life (Lambert, 2010). The ORS (for ages 12 and up) and CORS (for ages 6–11) are 4 item scales that provide distress ratings of individual, relationship, academic/school functioning along with a rating of overall distress (Miller & Duncan, 2004). Therefore, the ORS/CORS provides much of the same information that the Outcome Questionnaire provides but in a much briefer format. This allows for clinicians to feasibly track outcome of every session. In doing so, the clinician can track change from intake to any future point and determine whether individual distress has been positively affected. A more complete picture of clinical effectiveness can be seen with this approach than with one that focuses on just pre- and postmeasure data points due to a data from a larger proportion of clients enrolled in the program (Hubble et al., 2010).

An additional advantage to assessing outcomes every session is that it creates an opportunity to utilize an awareness of measurable progress (or lack thereof) to inform a collaboration with the client in choices about the direction of treatment in service to the goal of positive and meaningful change (Lambert, 2010). A growing literature supporting the use of outcome measures to track change every session and include that information in the therapeutic conversation has developed in the past decade (Hubble et al., 2010; Lambert, 2010). The American Psychological Association's task force on Evidence Based Practice (2006) concluded that evidenced-based practice is not reflected just in the application of specific therapies for specific diagnoses as is often the interpretation, but the application of treatment efforts made in collaboration with the client based on information regarding the individual preferences of the client as well as relative progress toward treatment goals. This approach has been come to be known as Feedback Informed Treatment, or FIT. Lambert's (2010) research over the past decade has suggested that a significant positive impact on clinical outcomes is obtained not only when therapists have access to real-time information regarding clients' ratings of distress relative to their intake scores, but also when this information is shared in real time with the clients so that the therapeutic endeavor is informed by whether progress is being made. Direct discussions regarding progress can then happen, creating a collaborative relationship with a focus on the outcome.

One of the primary factors that contribute to overall outcome in therapy is the therapeutic alliance (Hubble et al., 2010; Asay & Lambert, 1999; Norcross, 2010; Wampold, 2001). Therefore, if one is to assess what to change if progress is not being made in therapy the therapeutic alliance is one factor that cannot be overlooked. The therapeutic alliance can be measured, and client ratings of therapeutic alliance are found to be more directly related to outcome than therapist ratings

(Norcross, 2010). One set of measures that are a companion to the ORS are the Session Rating Scale (SRS) and Child Session Rating Scale (CSRS) (Miller & Duncan, 2004). The SRS/CSRS are similar in that they are ultra-brief; can be administered, scored, and interpreted in under a few minutes; and has the advantage of allowing for a direct conversation regarding the feedback from a client about the therapeutic alliance in real time. This conversation allows for the therapist to solicit feedback from the client about three central factors contributing to overall alliance: the *relationship* or the degree to which the client felt heard, understood, and respected; the *goals and topics* of the session or the degree to which the therapist focused on issues of pertinence to the client; and the *approach or method* or the degree to which the therapist's approach is a good fit for the client. An additional factor is also assessed; an *overall* rating of the degree to which the session was "right" or there was "something missing" for the client. These factors allow for a collaborative discussion with the client regarding their experience of each session. If positive progress is being made, then this information, while valuable, may have little bearing on the ultimate outcome, but if the client is reporting little progress or is worsening, then it is extremely important to address alliance problems. Changing what one does based on negative feedback regarding the perception of the therapeutic approach with an individual client can have a significant impact on the ultimate outcome of therapy (Anker, Duncan, & Sparks, 2009; Lambert, 2010).

Changing or clarifying how one relates to the client, the approach or method used, the goals identified, or some other aspect of therapy delivery that the client identifies are specific options arising from the unique context of the therapy with that individual or family for response with the goal of improving outcomes. Many only focus on the approach or method ("Does Cognitive Behavioral, or Solution-Focused, or Multi-Systemic Therapy work best for this diagnosis/client?") and do not directly consider the other aspects of service delivery. Certainly, there is quite a bit of evidence to suggest that many approaches, techniques, or aspects of models are more likely to work for various types of problems/diagnoses for youth (Chorpita, Daleiden, & Weisz, 2005; Kazdin, 2004). This probabilistic approach is important to include in decision-making regarding treatment options. The literature regarding evidenced-supported therapies suggests, however, that no approach or method, no matter how much evidence regarding relative efficacy in particular circumstances exists, will work with every single client (Kelley, Bickman, & Norwood, 2010). Making a decision to apply evidenced-supported therapies tied to specific populations and diagnoses based on probabilistic inferences will still result in some treatment failures. Some authors even suggest that there is relative equivalency of the effectiveness of many approaches of therapy for many disorders in youth (Kelley et al., 2010; Miller, Wampold, & Varhely, 2008). FIT essentially ties choices for treatment model, method, and approach to feedback from the client regarding outcome and alliance. The questions FIT-informed therapists ask in every case are the following: "Is the treatment working for this client, in this circumstance, within the context of this specific therapeutic relationship?" And "If not, what should I change; the what (model/technique/modality) of treatment, the how (alliance) of treatment, the how often (frequency) of treatment, or the 'who' (therapist) of treatment?"

The Bavaria-SBBH has chosen to utilize the ORS/CORS and SRS/CSRS for the above reasons. The use of these scales to engage in FIT also has an impact on cultural responsiveness. The impact is seen when addressing those within the culture of teens. FIT is necessarily a transparent process. This transparency is often novel when experienced by teens. Teens and children, in general, typically experience adults as exerting control from their legitimate position as holding greater power. This often leaves the teen in a position of passive acceptance of the direction of therapy, letting the adult lead the process. The teen, then, is not fully engaged in the therapy. When a Feedback Informed therapist solicits feedback from the teen not only about progress toward goals, but also about their criticisms regarding the delivery of the service, then the therapist is reducing the power differential in a direct way and inviting the youth to more actively participate in their own therapy. This collaboration enhances the ownership of the therapy by the teen. It engages the teen in a cooperative effort that allows for the teen to not only be more involved in the treatment, but to encourage them to "lead the way" to change by allowing them greater decision-making power in the process (Duncan, 2011; Murphy, 2008). In this way, the teen's strengths and capabilities are identified and capitalized upon through the exploration of what the teen likes, doesn't like, and finds effective or not in the therapeutic experience. These discussions can lead to identifying the processes of change that will fit for the teen. The therapist also models for the teen an appreciation of "mistakes" in service of improvement.

Seeking feedback from not just the teen, but from parents as well, can increase the cultural sensitivity of the therapist. If a therapist follows up with the administration of the SRS and CSRS with questions for the clients about how their approach fits with their cultural backgrounds, then the client can inform the therapist directly about how they wish to work and what approaches do or do not fit for them. Ultimately, the research has suggested that the use of client ratings of outcome and alliance enhance outcomes (Lambert, 2010). When therapists and clients work collaboratively and transparently, cultural differences can be addressed directly rather than guessed at and the outcomes are likely to be better (Lambert, 2010).

Review and Conclusions

> Zeke reported at the end of treatment that he appreciated that the SBBH provider 'respected me enough' to ask his thoughts regarding how change would happen. He stated that he had been in therapy before, in middle school, to address the very same issue of academic production, but that the therapist 'had all the ideas' and 'none of them worked for me.' He also said that leaving school to go to an office in the clinic 'made me feel like something was really messed up with me,' but that stopping in an office just down the hall from his Language Arts class for a talk every couple of weeks made therapy 'like a drive-up window' during his school day. He also liked that he could 'see' his progress in the scores on the ORS, showing that he felt differently about himself than he had on the first day. He said he felt most proud of the fact that he knew his father, while in Afghanistan, was watching him walk across the stage and receive his diploma.

The U.S. Army leadership is committed to making sure stories like Zeke's occur more often when it could have ended up in failure with greater complications for those who serve. It is a part of the Army Family Covenant to provide services that support the best functioning of the soldier and their families throughout their life span. With this case and many others the U.S. Army's SBBH Program initiative has been helping to build the *culture of trust* with the families and soldiers who make so many sacrifices in their service. This *culture of trust* is the central cultural consideration in serving the military and their members. It is the intent of Bavaria-SBBH to continue to develop a culture of trust and collaboration with the military community in service of their youth, and by extension, their soldiers. For a culture of trust to develop among the soldiers and families and the behavioral health institutions, these institutions must be positioned to maximize their benefit, must be responsive to their needs, and must be open to adopting a mindset that the stakeholders have significant input in the delivery of these services (Tanielian et al., 2008). In providing for care in the schools, SBBH is positioned to maximize the benefit of behavioral health services. In adopting structures for success such as CLA and BLA groups, and adopting a FIT approach, SBBH is developing a stance that is responsive to needs and holds a mind-set that stakeholders should have significant input in the delivery of services. In fact, these structures form the basis of SBBH programs engaging in culturally sensitive practice. Advisory groups and FIT approaches advocate for and support collaborative discussion of all issues pertinent to the successful implementation of SBBH programs and individual treatment. In this manner, the programs and providers can be sensitive to the stated needs of the community, as well as individual clients.

This review has the goal of identifying some of the practice issues that face SBBH providers and programs in secondary schools on military bases overseas. These issues are not presented from a perspective of having settled them completely, rather that the thought processes regarding addressing them are highlighted so that others may learn as we have learned from other's real-world struggles in implementing best practice. Building a *culture of trust* is based on establishing collaborative relationships that value the sharing and learning from successes and mistakes that all are bound to make when important issues are addressed (Wenger et al., 2002).

References

American Psychological Association Presidential Task Force on Evidence-Based Practice. (2006). Evidence-based practice in psychology. *The American Psychologist, 61*(4), 271–283.

Anker, M., Duncan, B., & Sparks, J. (2009). Using client feedback to improve couples therapy outcomes: A randomized clinical trial in a naturalistic setting. *Journal of Consulting and Clinical Psychology, 77*, 693–704.

Asay, T. P. and Lambert, M. J. (1999). The Empirical Case for the Common Factors in Therapy: Quantitative Findings. In Hubble, M. A., Duncan, B. L. & Miller, S., D. (Eds.), The Heart and Soul of Change: What Works in Therapy. Washington, D.C.: American Psychological Association.

Beck, A. T., & Emery, G. (1985). *Anxiety disorders and phobias: A cognitive perspective*. New York, NY: Basic Books.

Bennett, B. E., Bricklin, P. M., Harris, E., Knapp, S., VandeCreek, L., & Younggren, J. N. (2006). *Assessing and managing risk in psychological practice: An individualized approach*. Rockville, MD: The Trust.

Bowlby, J. (1988). *A secure base: Parent-child attachment and healthy human development*. New York, NY: Basic Books.

Brown, J., Dreis, S., & Nace, D. (1999). What really makes a difference in psychotherapy outcome? Why does managed care want to know? In M. Hubble, B. Duncan, & S. Miller (Eds.), *The heart and soul of change: What works in therapy*. Washington, DC: American Psychological Association.

Campbell, A., & Hemsley, S. (2009). Outcome rating scale and session rating scale in psychological practice: Clinical utility of ultra-brief measures. *Clinical Psychologist, 13*(1), 1–9.

Chandra, A., Burns, R., Tanielian, T., Jaycox, L., & Scott, M. (2008). *Understanding the impact of deployment on children and families: Findings from a pilot study of Operation Purple Camp participants*. Santa Monica, CA: RAND Corporation.

Chorpita, B., Daleiden, E., & Weisz, J. (2005). Identifying and selecting the common elements of evidence based interventions: A distillation and matching model. *Mental Health Services Research, 7*, 5–20.

Cummings, E. M., & Davies, P. (1994). *Children in marital conflict: The impact of family dispute and resolution*. London: Guilford.

Duncan, B. (2011). *On becoming a better therapist*. Washington, DC: American Psychological Association.

Duncan, B., Miller, S., & Sparks, J. (2004). *The heroic client: A revolutionary way to improve effectiveness through client-directed, outcome-informed therapy (revised edition)*. San Francisco, CA: Jossey-Bass.

Faran, M. (2010a, October). *Behavioral health support for army children, adolescents, and families*. Presentation at 15th annual conference for advancing school mental health, Albuquerque, NM.

Faran, M. (2010b). Personal communication.

Faran, M., Weist, M., Saito, A., Yoshikami, L., Weiser, J., & Kaer, B. (2002). School-based mental health on a United States army installation. In M. D. Weist, S. W. Evans, & N. A. Lever (Eds.), *Handbook of school mental health: Advancing practice and research* (pp. 191–202). New York, NY: Springer.

Gorman, G., Eide, M., & Hisle-Gorman, E. (2010). Wartime military deployment and increased pediatric mental and behavioral health complaints. *Pediatrics, 126*(6), 1058–1066.

Gottman, J. (1997). *Raising and emotionally intelligent child: The heart of parenting*. New York, NY: Simon and Shuster Paperbacks.

Hubble, M., Duncan, B., Miller, S., & Wampold, B. (2010). Introduction. In B. Duncan, S. Miller, B. Wampold, & M. Hubble (Eds.), *The heart and soul of change: Delivering what works in therapy* (2nd ed.). Washington, DC: American Psychological Association.

Jacob, S., & Feinberg, T. (2002). Administrative considerations in preventing and responding to crisis. In S. E. Brock, P. J. Lazarus, & S. R. Jimerson (Eds.), *Best practices in school crisis prevention and intervention*. Bethesda, MD: National Association of School Psychologists.

Kazdin, A. (2004). Psychotherapy for children and adolescents. In M. J. Lambert (Ed.), *Bergin and Garfield's handbook of psychotherapy and behavior change* (5th ed., pp. 543–589). New York, NY: Wiley.

Kelley, S., Bickman, L., & Norwood, E. (2010). Evidenced-based treatment and common factors in youth psychotherapy. In B. Duncan, S. Miller, B. Wampold, & M. Hubble (Eds.), *The heart and soul of change: Delivering what works in therapy* (2nd ed.). Washington, DC: American Psychological Association.

Lambert, M. (2010). Yes, it is time for clinicians to routinely monitor treatment outcome. In B. Duncan, S. Miller, B. Wampold, & M. Hubble (Eds.), *The heart and soul of change: Delivering what works in therapy* (2nd ed.). Washington, DC: American Psychological Association.

Levison-Johnson, J., Dewey, J., & Wandersman, A. (2009). *Getting To Outcomes®: In systems of care: 10 steps for achieving results-based accountability.* Atlanta, GA: ICF Macro.

Military Child Education Coalition. (2007). *Living in the new normal.* Retrieved from 10-August-2008 http://www.militarychild.org

Millean, J. (2011, May 16). *Deployment linked to child psychiatric hospitalizations.* Presented at the American Psychiatric Association (APA) 2011 annual meeting: Poster NR07-15, Honolulu, HI.

Miller, S., & Duncan, B. (2004). *The outcome and session rating scales: Administration and scoring manual.* Ft. Lauderdale, FL: Authors.

Miller, S., Duncan, B., Brown, J., Sorrell, R., & Chalk, M. (2006). Using outcome to inform and improve treatment outcomes. *Journal of Brief Therapy, 5,* 5–22.

Miller, S., Wampold, B., & Varhely, K. (2008). Direct comparisons of treatments for youth disorders: A meta-analysis. *Psychotherapy Research, 18,* 5–14.

Murphy, J. (1997). *Solution-focused counseling in middle and high schools.* Alexandria, VA: American Counseling Association.

Murphy, J. (2008). Solution-Focused Counseling in Schools (2nd Edition). Alexandria, VA: American Counseling Association.

Norcross, J. (2010). The therapeutic relationship. In B. Duncan, S. Miller, B. Wampold, & M. Hubble (Eds.), *The heart and soul of change: Delivering what works in therapy* (2nd ed.). Washington, DC: American Psychological Association.

Selekman, M. (1993). *Pathways to change: Brief therapy solutions with difficult adolescents.* New York, NY: Guilford.

Sue, D. W., & Sue, D. (2007). *Counseling the culturally diverse: Theory and practice* (5th ed.). New York, NY: Wiley.

Tanielian, T., Jaycox, L., Schell, T., Marshall, G., Burnam, M. B., Eibneer, C., et al. (2008). *Invisible wounds of war: Summary recommendation for addressing psychological and cognitive injuries.* Santa Monica, CA: RAND Corporation.

Wampold, B. (2001). *The great psychotherapy debate: Models, methods, and findings.* Mahwah, NJ: Lawrence Erlbaum Associates.

Weinfield, N. S., Ogawa, J. R., & Sroufe, L. A. (1997). Early attachment as a pathway to adolescent peer competence. *Journal of Research on Adolescence, 7*(3), 241–265.

Weinfield, N. S., Sroufe, L. A., & Egeland, B. (2000). Attachment from infancy to early adulthood in a high-risk sample: Continuity, discontinuity, and their correlates. *Child Development, 71*(3), 695–702.

Wenger, E., McDermott, R. A., & Snyder, W. (2002). *Cultivating communities of practice: A guide to managing knowledge.* Cambridge, MA: Harvard Business Press.

Yalom, I. (1980). *Existential psychotherapy.* New York, NY: Basic Books.

Culturally Responsive School Mental Health in Rural Communities

Julie Sarno Owens, Yuko Watabe, and Kurt D. Michael

When a reader selects a book about cultural competence or responsiveness, the characteristics that typically come to mind are race and ethnicity. The saliency of race and ethnicity is understandable given that by the year 2050 nearly 50 % of the population of the United States will be comprised of racial and ethnic minority populations (U.S. Census Bureau, 2010). However, in recent years, culture is being conceptualized more broadly to include the culture of gender, age, economic status, location (e.g., urban, rural), and community (e.g., military). Thus, it is important that school mental health (SMH) services are sensitive to these diverse cultures and contexts. The goals of this chapter are to highlight some of the unique challenges associated with SMH service provision in rural contexts and to discuss strategies for advancing culturally responsive care in rural SMH. In particular, we focus on issues related to limited access to services, interpersonal connections, and ethical challenges specific to rural contexts (i.e., competence and dual relationships). We also develop a vignette throughout the chapter to help these issues come to life. We begin with a few contextual comments.

The first challenge in describing issues relevant to rural communities is defining "rural." The definition of rural has been debated in multiple scientific fields for decades (Halfacree, 1993; Hart, Larson, & Lishner, 2005; Philo, Parr, & Burns, 2003). In addition, the connotations ascribed to rural contexts have ranged from positive and desirable (e.g., serene, picturesque, family-based) to neutral (e.g., slower paced, remote, rustic), and to negative and derogatory (e.g., redneck, backwoods). There are a variety of methods for defining rural in the literature. For example, the U.S. Census Bureau utilizes several geographic and population-based indices, including persons per square mile and distance from urban centers. There is evidence within the sociological literature that urban and rural communities can be distinguished from each other based on the social networks within each context (Beggs, Hains, & Hurlbert, 1996). Namely, the personal networks of rural constituents are more intense (e.g., frequency and longevity of contacts), more complex (multiple roles), more dense (interconnectedness), and include a greater number of kin-based interconnections than those of their urban counterparts.

The second challenge is that, although rural communities can be distinguished from urban communities, as a group, rural communities are heterogeneous with regard to demographic, economic, and cultural characteristics. Whenever a group of people is being defined (e.g., based on race, location, or community), it is important to

J.S. Owens, Ph.D. (✉) • Y. Watabe, M.A.
Ohio University, Athens, OH, USA
e-mail: owensj@ohio.edu

K.D. Michael, Ph.D.
Appalachian State University, Boone, NC, USA

remember that often times there are as many within-group differences as between-group differences. Thus, when approaching a new client or community, a culturally responsive SMH provider must take responsibility for obtaining accurate information about the culture (beyond labels and stereotypes) and for exploring (rather than assuming) the extent to which the characteristics of that culture are relevant and meaningful to the client or group being served. For example, there may be clients whose family has lived in a given rural region for multiple generations, yet these individuals may not necessarily hold the stereotypic values of the region. Thus, assuming that these values apply to this client would be erroneous and possibly harmful.

Given that each rural context may have unique characteristics that affect mental health utilization and outcomes (e.g., Hauenstein et al., 2007; U.S. Department of Health & Human Services (DHHS), 2005), and given that some of the challenges present in rural contexts are also present in some urban contexts, understanding the local culture can be a powerful guide in determining the most appropriate strategy for achieving culturally responsive SMH services. The authors' SMH research, training, and practice activities are conducted with the Appalachian region (Southeastern Ohio and Western North Carolina). Because our commentary on challenges and strategies is derived from this setting, we offer a brief description of our local rural context.

Mental Health Correlates and Outcomes in Rural Communities

Broadly speaking, there are three primary challenges associated with mental health in rural areas. First, although the prevalence rates of most mental disorders do not differ greatly between children living in rural and nonrural communities (Gamm, Stone, & Pittman, 2008), there is evidence that some mental health outcomes (i.e., suicide rates among males and nonprescription drugs use among teenagers) may be worse for rural constituents (Eberhardt, Ingram, Makuc, et al., 2001; Havens, Young, & Havens, 2010). Second, mental health services utilization is lower in rural than nonrural contexts (Fischer, Owen, & Cuffel, 1996; Hauenstein et al., 2007; Rost, Fortney, Fischer, & Smith, 2002). This lower rate may be related to the lack of availability and accessibility of general mental health services and specialty services. For example, 95 % of rural counties with populations below 20,000 lack a child psychiatrist (Gamm et al., 2008). Lastly, the stigma associated with mental disorders and seeking mental health services is more likely to be reported by rural than nonrural constituents (Hoyt, Conger, & Valde, 1997).

All of these characteristics are representative of the Appalachian region (see http://www.arc.gov) where the authors work. While some communities in the region have successful, growing economies, others still lack that basic infrastructure. The counties in which the authors conduct their work have high school completion rates, per capita income, and median household income that fall below state averages, as well as poverty rates that exceed state and national averages (U.S. Census Bureau, 2010), and suicide rates that exceed state rates. Further, most of these counties are Mental Health Professional Shortage Areas and are Medically Underserved (U.S. DHHS, 2011). As a result, many families in the region fail to receive mental health care, receive care at more impairing stages of the problem, or receive substandard care.

Notably, there are only a few empirical studies examining mental health issues for children and families in the Appalachian region (Costello et al., 1996). Much of the work in this area is qualitative and focused on describing the socioeconomic and political history of the region (e.g., the exploitation of natural resources from outsiders) that, in turn, has been associated with particular values (e.g., mistrust of outsiders, focus on kinship ties) (see Keefe, 2005). However, given that the Appalachian region spans 13 states with diverse histories and cultures, we encourage readers to obtain accurate information about the specific culture within any given rural community, rather than assuming that these purported values are applicable and meaningful to the client or group being served. This information can be obtained by speaking with persons from the community (both community leaders and clients whose families have lived in the region for multiple generations) and by exploring the community through local museums, monuments, festivals, and documents that chronicle the history of the community.

Strategies for Responding to Common Challenges in Rural School Mental Health

The above-described statistics that characterize many rural communities create a unique context for SMH service delivery. We now introduce a vignette that will unfold as we discuss challenges related to limited access to services, interpersonal connections, and ethical issues specific to rural contexts. Following each challenge, we discuss implications for practice and offer culturally sensitive strategies for navigating this challenge.

> Meet Janet: She is a professional school counselor at a rural high school. She arrives at work on a Monday. Over the course of this day, she conducts a check-in with several students who have a history of tardiness and truancy. Later in the day, she meets with a freshman who is struggling to maintain grade-level performance in the context of her parents' recent divorce. Janet also consults with the nurse about a student who is suspected of purging behaviors, but who denies such behaviors and refuses to meet with the school counselor. On Tuesday, Janet receives two requests. The first is from the special education teacher who has a large proportion of students who have been diagnosed with ADHD and are struggling with peer relationships. The teacher is requesting that the Janet conduct a social skills group to help students navigate specific issues (e.g., romantic relationships, online social networking). The second request comes from the Algebra teacher who asks Janet to begin counseling sessions with a student who is showing severe anxiety. Janet would like to refer the student with suspected eating disorder and the student with severe anxiety to the local mental health clinic. However, she is doubtful that either the teen or their family would pursue such services.

Limited Access to Quality Services

Challenges. The requests made of Janet are not uncommon to SMH staff in the schools that we serve. However, these schools are located nearly 100 miles from an urban center that commonly provides specialty health and mental health services. Thus, access to quality mental health care for students is limited in multiple ways. First, the rural communities we serve lack full-time child psychiatry services, board certified pediatricians, and child psychology specialty clinics (e.g., specific to a disorder, age range, or therapy orientation). As a result, school professionals (like Janet) have few high quality options for referring children to receive mental health services or for developing partnerships that could offer services within the school. Second, the schools with which we collaborate have student-to-mental health staff ratios that exceed state averages and recommended ratios (U.S. Department of Education, 2010). Such high ratios limit the resources available to the total population of students, as well as the quality of services provided to any given individual student. For example, given all the demands placed on Janet, she may have limited time and resources for mental health promotion and screening activities. Similarly, she may implement an evidence-based intervention protocol for a student with depression or anxiety, but may have to reduce the duration and frequency of sessions to 30 minutes on a biweekly basis. These modifications may reduce the possibility of positive student outcomes and may leave Janet feeling less effective or professionally burned out.

Implications and strategies. The primary implication of the lack of access to other mental services is that SMH providers in rural contexts often find themselves adopting a generalist approach to service delivery, primarily out of necessity (Jameson & Blank, 2007; Jones & Parlour, 1985). Indeed, a culturally responsive rural SMH provider must be comfortable providing services across the continuum of care, including prevention programming, screening, assessment, and intervention. However, achieving this comfort can difficult and the generalist approach can leave the provider feeling like a "Jack of all trades, but master of none." The solution to such a challenge is not clear-cut, but rather an ongoing struggle with which the authors, and many others, are grappling. Below are strategies for delivering culturally responsive SMH within the generalist framework.

First, rural SMH providers are encouraged to periodically conduct a needs assessment and resource mapping (Chinmann, Imm, & Wandersman, 2004) for their local area to prioritize student needs for prevention and treatment and to identify areas of expertise in the community. The data resulting from these processes can highlight areas for potential partnerships, guide a SMH provider's pursuit of additional professional development, and serve to reduce redundancies across limited resources. For example, in the vignette, a needs assessment may reveal that someone in the region (e.g., private practice psychologist) has expertise in evidence-based treatments for anxiety and is willing to conduct a group at the high school. Yet, given the lack of expertise in the community on evidence-based behavioral screening and treatment for teenage depression, Janet could focus her next professional development hours on obtaining such training.

Second, in the context of their professional development, rural SMH providers are encouraged to obtain trainings that highlight core features that are common across multiple evidence-based intervention strategies. Because evidence-based services produce outcomes that are superior to standard care (Weisz, Jensen-Doss, & Hawley, 2006), by integrating evidence-based services into school, we maximize the impact of the limited personnel resources that are available in rural contexts. The distillation and matching model presented by Chorpita and colleagues (Chorpita & Daleiden, 2009; Chorpita, Daleiden, & Weisz, 2005) offers a potentially viable mechanism for identifying core practice elements that may be best matched to each referred student and for developing efficiencies within services delivered. Research is currently underway (see http://www.childsteps.org/index.html) to examine the effectiveness and feasibility of this approach; however, because this work is being conducted in clinic settings, additional research will be needed to determine effectiveness and feasibility within rural SMH delivery models.

Third, rural providers are encouraged to develop a network of colleagues from other rural contexts and from nearby urban contexts for consultation and/or supervision. In our experience, providers benefit the most from seeking out targeted consultation in the context of experiences that present themselves (e.g., contacting an Amish community leader to understand relevant terminology and challenges expressed by an adolescent coping with the stress of seeking independence from or within his religious community). We also recommended that providers include university faculty within this network. Collaborative partnerships with universities offer a mechanism for enhancing resources in the school, such as supervised graduate student trainees for service delivery, professional development for teachers and SMH providers, and consultation for developing an infrastructure for data-driven decisions (Owens, Andrews, Collins, Griffeth, & Mahoney, 2011).

Finally, the generalist is likely to be asked to help out with more basic tasks (e.g., class scheduling, lice checks, test proctoring) that, in more resourced schools, might be taken care of by other entities (e.g., substitute teacher, parent volunteer). However, while it is culturally responsive to "pitch in" and help out with these tasks, it is also important for SMH providers to protect their time, as the energy and time devoted to these tasks significantly compromise the quality of the mental health services they provide. More specifically, proportional to the resources available in rural schools, even a loss of 2–3 hours/week to such tasks could be a waste of a valuable and limited resource.

There are several steps that a SMH provider could take to protect their service delivery time and to demonstrate the value of these services to school district administrators. Namely, providers are encouraged to develop a system for documenting the outcomes of the services that they provide. First, providers may obtain brief ratings scales from youth, their parents, and/or their teacher at the start of a given service (e.g., prior enrolling a student in a group or program) and at a meaningful later date (e.g., on a monthly basis, at the conclusion of the group). This would follow the procedures of progress monitoring and evaluation of response to intervention at the individual level, but also would allow the provider to demonstrate the impact of the service on a group of students. Such data, when combined with anecdotal evidence (e.g., testimonials, success cases) documents the value of SMH services and provides a compelling rationale to administrators and school boards for protecting such services.

Another approach is to partner with other professionals (e.g., Directors of Special Education, School Psychologists, the school improvement planning team) to take leadership in developing and defining the mental health agenda within the school district. This agenda could include an initial needs assessment, recommendations or requests for specific types of professional development, and the development of initiatives that address a specific need along the continuum of services (e.g., reducing high school dropout, screening for suicide potential). In our experience, school districts have been most willing to adopt such an agenda when it is well aligned with existing educational systems, such as a three-tiered model of Positive Behavior Intervention and Support (see http://www.pbis.org) or the district's special education procedures.

Interpersonal Connections

> We return to the vignette: On Wednesday, Janet gets a phone call from her husband's cousin Betty. In addition to being distant relatives, Janet and Betty attend church together. Betty is concerned about her teenage son, Dustin who has been "acting differently." His grades have slipped, he spends most of his time alone in his room, and he no longer plays his guitar, an activity he has long enjoyed. Betty described her unsuccessful efforts at encouraging Dustin to speak to his physician or a therapist at the local mental health clinic. He refused, saying "I'm not crazy" and "they won't understand." He has expressed concerns to Betty about "what the guys would say" (referring to his father, brother, and male cousins). Betty believes that because Janet is a familiar face at Dustin's school and "from around here," Dustin would talk to her.

Challenges. Family relationships and values play a significant role in health behaviors (e.g., nutrition, sleep and exercise patterns, risk behaviors) and in the help-seeking process. There is some evidence that this role may be stronger in rural than nonrural communities (Conger, Elder, Lorenz, Simons, & Whitbeck, 1994). As described previously, people from rural communities tend to have a greater number of kin-based relationships in which extended family members are closely linked to one another (Beggs et al., 1996). On one hand, these kin-based communities may offer significant social support and a psychological resource, so much that a given family member may not feel a need to seek support outside of this network (e.g., Lohmann, 1990). On the other hand, the strength of this network may prohibit family members from seeking needed professional services for fear that others would be offended or would disapprove (e.g., family secrets are shared with others, help seeking is a sign of weakness).

Other barriers to help seeking in rural contexts include difficulty trusting mental health providers, unfamiliarity with service options, and concerns for confidentiality (Owens, Richerson, Murphy, Jageleweski, & Rossi, 2007; Starr, Campbell, & Herrick, 2002). When community members recognize each other through the cars they drive and the routines in which they engage, privacy about appointments at a mental health clinic may be difficult to maintain. In the vignette, Dustin's expressed concerns reflect several of these barriers.

Implications and strategies. These interpersonal barriers to mental health service seeking provide a strong rationale for embedding support services within schools, as school-based service delivery can reduce some of these barriers. Indeed, data from one of our SMH programs indicate that some parents (22 %) preferred school-based services to clinic-based services because attending school meetings was less embarrassing than clinic meetings (Owens, Murphy, Richerson, Girio, & Himawan, 2008). The above interpersonal barriers also highlight the importance of developing procedures for understanding roles and expectations within each family so that SMH providers can frame their assessments, recommendations, and interventions in a way that is palatable and inviting of trust. Below are strategies for enhancing cultural sensitivity with regard to these procedures.

First, when approaching a parent to communicate about a child's problem, it is important to ask the parent if they would like other family members to join the meeting. This invitation acknowledges the importance of their extended family support network. It also offers the opportunity for a parent who has difficulty asserting her help-seeking desires to her family to gain support from the school in communicating with these family members. Gaining support from extended family members could reduce distress for the help-seeking parent, as well as help to prevent possible sabotage by the extended family member. Thus, even if a parent initially declines to invite other members, it would be culturally responsive to repeat the invitation at other junctures (e.g., at the time of assessment, feedback, treatment planning, progress monitoring), as the client's trust in you and the treatment process may have grown over time.

Second, with regard to developing trust with families, providers are encouraged to consider the constructs of ascribed credibility (i.e., the status that one is assigned by others) and achieved credibility (i.e., that which is earned through therapeutic actions; Sue & Zane, 1987). Aside from education credentials, in rural communities, SMH providers who grew up in the local region may have more ascribed credibility than those who did not. This nuance is true within the vignette, as Betty believes that Dustin would be more willing to talk with a "familiar face" and "someone from around here." Thus, to help students and families feel more connected, SMH providers are encouraged to share relevant information about the area in which they grew up and to communicate knowledge about common places and activities. There is some empirical evidence that for men in rural environments, one factor that promotes an alliance with persons who are not within their immediate social network (e.g., a SMH professional) is identification of similarity with that person (Haines & Hurlbert, 1992). Thus, those not from the region may be able to earn credibility by showing genuine interest in that which is important to families. For example, we have found that fathers grant more credibility to clinicians when they take time to informally inquire about and make connections with their interests (e.g., trucks, Harley Davidson motorcycles, hunting, fishing) than when the clinician remains formal and focused solely on clinical tasks.

Finally, although some rural communities are affluent, greater rurality is often associated with higher levels of poverty (see Wagenfeld, 2003). In order to develop trust and a meaningful alliance with clients in low-income rural communities, culturally responsive SMH providers must understand the impact that poverty has on child and parent language, belief systems, and resources. As an example of how a provider's choice of language may unintentionally convey assumptions based on a culture of privilege, a provider may ask a child to describe their house and may ask questions that include references to "upstairs," "your bedroom," or "the garage." Similarly, providers may ask mothers questions that refer to "when you are at work," or "when you discipline your child." These may not be culturally sensitive terms for a child living in a one-bedroom trailer, a mother who does not work, or a family who believes that discipline is solely in the hands of the father. In addition, it is recommended that SMH providers become familiar with the empirical literature that documents the negative impact of low SES on treatment outcomes. For example, SMH providers should anticipate that families in economic hardship may attend appointments less consistently, that session content may need to be modified to match a lower level of education (e.g., more concrete, visual handouts), and that treatment outcomes may be more modest and may take longer to achieve when compared to families with greater resources (Chronis, Chacko, Fabiano, Wymbs, & Pelham, 2004; Owens et al., 2008). Further, it is important to acknowledge that clients of low SES have been grossly underrepresented in most studies designed to document the efficacy of empirically supported treatments (e.g., MTA Cooperative Group, 1999; Walkup et al., 2008). This highlights the need for additional research in rural, low-income contexts. As noted earlier, partnerships between schools and universities can facilitate such research (e.g., Michael, Renkert, Wandler, & Stamey, 2010; Owens et al., 2011).

Ethical Challenges

We return to the vignette: Janet and Betty (the cousin of Janet's husband) are speaking on the phone about her son, Dustin. Janet would like to help Dustin, but explains to Betty that being his therapist would really not be appropriate given that they also see each other at monthly family functions and church. Betty expresses her disappointment and reluctantly accepts Janet's rationale for not being able to see Dustin. Janet informs Betty that she could arrange for Dustin to see a graduate student therapist, Jeff, who has started providing services at the high school, under the supervision of a university faculty member who has developed a partnership with the school district. Upon hearing the name, Betty's says "I think I recognize his name." He was friends with my baby brother (who is 10 years younger than Betty). Yea, let's try that. Dustin might connect with him since he's "from around here." After a brief conversation with Dustin, Janet receives consent for him to begin speaking with Jeff. Jeff soon discovers that Dustin is showing significant signs of depression. He does not have an extensive background in treating depressed male teenagers, but is currently in a graduate level child therapy course where he is learning the techniques. Given the lack of alternative options in the community, coupled with Dustin's reluctance to seek help elsewhere, Jeff begins a course of cognitive-behavioral treatment under the supervision of the university-based faculty.

Challenges. As indicated in the above vignette, SMH practitioners encounter ethical challenges involving scope of practice, competence, and the management of professional and personal boundaries. Below we describe challenges related to the ethics of competence and dual relationships, followed by strategies for navigating these challenges.

The first ethical dilemma is maintaining high standards of competence in professional work while meeting the demands of a broad array of problems within the school community. The ethical standards set forth by most professional organizations require that the professional provide only those services and techniques for which that they are qualified by education, training, or experience (e.g., American Psychological Association (APA), 2002; American School Counselor Association (ASCA), 2010). As described in the vignette, the graduate student clinician, Jeff, faces the challenge of providing evidence-based therapy to the client while simultaneously learning the techniques in his graduate course. Janet, the SMH provider, faces the challenge of providing high quality services for a broad array of problems (depression, anxiety, eating disorders, social skills interventions, and consultation to education professionals). Further, for some of the requests (e.g., social skills interventions for youth with ADHD), there is a very limited empirical base from which to glean guidelines or strategies. Janet must decide whether these domains are within the boundaries of her professional competence. And if they are not, where does she send these referrals? Rural providers are often faced with the question "is the limited service that I can provide (i.e., limited by frequency of contact, intensity of the intervention, or provider education and experience) better than no service or a service that is likely too distant for the family to access?" These are challenges often faced by other rural health care providers as well, including pediatricians and primary care physicians, who, in the absence of adequate mental or behavioral healthcare, often provide some form of mental health treatment, even if it is insufficient or exceeds the knowledge, skills, and abilities of the physician (e.g., Kelleher & Long, 1994).

The second ethical challenge is that of managing multiple relationships, often cited as the most difficult ethical dilemmas for rural providers (Campbell & Gordon, 2003; Harowski, Turner, LeVine, Schank, & Leichter, 2006). In rural communities, it is inevitable that the boundaries of one's personal and professional life overlap. For example, as described in the vignette, it is common for relatives of rural SMH providers to leverage this family relationship to seek opinions and/or assistance about their child's challenging behavior. Similarly, as a function of their own family's interests, a rural SMH provider may be in a leadership role in the community (e.g., soccer or little league coach, church group leader) that may place them in contact with past, current, or future clients. Further, even if the potential for a dual relationship does not exist, the potential for public interface with clients is virtually unavoidable (e.g., at the grocery store) in small communities. With each of the examples above, the SMH provider must decide how to prevent and/or manage these informal requests and interactions.

Given the geographic isolation of rural communities (e.g., often 100 miles from an urban center), in combination with the above-described ethical challenges, rural SMH providers are at risk for feeling isolated, both professionally and personally. Professionally, they have less physical access to colleagues as consultants for training, collaborative case conceptualization, and ethical decision making than do their nonrural counterparts. They also likely have to travel greater distances to obtain training on state-of-the-science therapies. This isolation has the potential to reduce work stimulation, interfere with ongoing competency development, and increase anxiety when handling challenging situations. On the personal side, SMH providers may grow weary of being constantly vigilant about their behaviors and interpersonal interactions in public and may even choose to restrict some personal activities to reduce contact with clients. If not managed appropriately, such restriction can result in feelings of isolation, reduced quality of life, and even resentment on the part of the provider (Campbell & Gordon, 2003).

Implications and strategies. First and foremost, rural SMH providers must be knowledgeable of the ethical standards within their profession, as well as the subsections of the code (albeit few) that offer guidelines for rural providers (e.g., APA, 2002, code Section 2.01(d)). Second, the above challenges are best managed by taking a proactive and early detection approach using the limited guidelines available (e.g., Schank & Skovholt, 2006; Werth, Hastings, & Riding-Malon, 2010).

The challenge of practicing within the bounds of competence requires continued vigilance to the relative risks of harm vs. the benefits of the services that the provider could offer. Given that education colleagues may not be familiar with such principles, SMH providers can feel pressed by teachers or principals to accept referrals and even persuaded that "something is better than nothing." However, as Werth et al. (2010) aptly noted, the principle of "first, do no harm" (i.e., nonmaleficence) trumps any desire on the psychologist's part to be helpful. Thus, we encourage rural SMH providers to develop a network of colleagues, both in the nearest urban area and within other rural regions who can be contacted to consult about the decision to accept the case, to provide the services via video or teleconference, or to provide consultation and supervision for the services that the SMH provider has decided to provide. Such networks can be developed and cultivated at conferences focused on rural mental health and on school-based mental health. Once developed, this network can also serve to reduce the risk of professional and/or personal isolation described earlier. As described earlier, it is recommended that rural providers seek out professional development trainings that maximize their ability to address a broad array of problems, such as trainings focused on needs assessments, resource mapping (Chinmann et al., 2004) techniques, and core intervention elements that are common across multiple evidence-based protocols (Chorpita et al., 2005). Similarly, if providers engage in data-based evaluation of services provided, they may obtain feedback about positive outcomes (a possible reflection of competence), as well as areas that may benefit from additional training or partnerships.

With regard to dual relationships, we have found that the most successful outcomes emerge when rural SMH providers proactively inform clients, early in the relationship, that public encounters are likely to happen, and develop a plan for navigating such encounters that take into account the client's and the provider's desires and concerns. In fact, having this discussion can serve to facilitate trust between the client and provider, and can offer important insights about the client's view of therapy and his/her perceptions of others' reactions to their pursuit of services. Beyond the chance public encounters, rural SMH providers may also need to make alternative arrangements, establish specific boundary guidelines, or decline a case if a dual relationship situation arises. For example, in the vignette, if Janet were supervising Jeff's work with Dustin,

Janet, Betty, and Dustin she would need to establish clear guidelines for when and how to discuss Dustin's needs and progress (e.g., only in designated sessions and not informal meetings at church). Similarly, there may be situations where the provider asks a parent to have their child placed on a different recreational sports team because the provider is the coach of the team, or scenarios where the provider requests that their own child be placed in a given classroom to avoid the potential for a dual relationship with the teacher or other students. It is important to note, however, that the mere presence of a dual relationship does not constitute unethical behavior, as the standard is based on relationships that cause impairment in the psychologist or create risk of exploitation or harm for the client (APA, 2002; ASCA, 2010). Providers must remain vigilant of these potential risks and make decisions accordingly.

One strategy that SMH providers can incorporate in light of these ethical challenges is to include a discussion of them in the context of a standard comprehensive informed consent procedure (Werth et al., 2010). During this procedure, providers can discuss a plan for informal encounters, the known and unknown limits of confidentiality, as well as the possible need for future consultation with other specialty providers (with written informed consent to exchange information obtained as necessary) in the event that their child's challenges exceed the services that can be offered in the current setting. By incorporating this into a standard procedure, as opposed to addressing it on a case-by-case basis, providers are more likely to maintain alignment with ethical standards and aspirations of their professions.

Summary

As described by Bourke et al. (2004) "rural health is not just health in a rural setting, but health in a complex web of social relations, cultural history, and socio-political networks" (p. 184). Thus, providing culturally responsive SMH in rural contexts requires an awareness of and sensitivity to several challenges, including lower rates of utilization, limited access to high quality evidence-based services, interpersonal barriers to help seeking, and ethical dilemmas unique to this context. Our discussion and clinical vignette were designed to highlight these challenges and to provide the reader with some practical approaches for providing culturally responsive SMH services in this context. Our recommendations are summarized as follows:

- SMH providers must be aware of documented contextual factors that are common among, and often unique to rural communities, including poverty, kin-based communities, lack of access to health and mental health services. In addition, SMH providers should take responsibility for getting to know the values and dynamics within any specific local community and its constituents, as some of these commonalities may not be applicable. It is important to remain cognizant of the power and importance of the local context in shaping the behavior and beliefs of client and colleagues.
- As a culturally responsive provider, it is important to be aware of your own assumptions and biases, refrain from acting on these assumptions, and remain open to solutions and ideas that may differ from your own experiences. Assuming that group-level stereotypes are applicable to an individual client or family is imprudent, and possibly harmful. Thus, SMH practitioners should be committed to learning more about those who present to them for evaluation and treatment, monitor privately, potentially biased personal reactions, and making adjustments accordingly.
- Given that rural SMH providers are likely to be practicing within a generalist model, they must be strategic in the professional development activities that they seek. Efficiency in one's work may be best achieved if providers develop skills in implementing core intervention components that are common across multiple, evidence-based intervention strategies (Chorpita & Daleiden, 2009).
- Providers should engage in data-driven assessment and evaluation to guide decisions related to resource allocation, professional

development needs, and service provision (Chinmann et al., 2004) and to advocate for the value of a school mental health agenda within the district.

- We recommend that rural SMH providers develop a network of colleagues for consultation, supervision, and referral both within other rural contexts and within nearby urban contexts. Within this network, it behooves providers to develop partnerships with university faculty, as they can assist with data collection, evaluation, and dissemination of data from rural contexts (Owens et al., 2011; Owens & Murphy, 2004).
- It is incumbent on rural providers to know the ethical guidelines pertinent to rural practice and to respond appropriately when ethical challenges emerge. Some of the most common ethical challenges include practicing within the bounds of our professional competencies, managing professional boundaries amid the ever-present dynamic of dual relationships in small communities, and defending against personal and professional burnout that result from geographic isolation. Rural SMH providers are encouraged to be proactive by anticipating such challenges and consulting regularly with colleagues in preparing and executing appropriate responses.

While the above recommendations are grounded in the experiences of the authors and in the empirical literature, the literature on which these recommendations are based is quite limited. Research conducted in schools across a variety of rural contexts stands to better represent and inform the strategies offered in this chapter. For example, such research could begin to substantiate which issues are unique to rural contexts and which are shared with urban and suburban contexts. Research in rural contexts could also document the potential benefits and cost savings of evidence-based services provided by school-employed mental health professionals relative to clinic-based employees, as well as the feasibility and effectiveness of core practice elements relative to disorder-specific, evidence-based treatment manuals. Finally, qualitative and quantitative are needed to help formulate evidence-based guidelines for navigating challenges related to the ethics of competence and dual relationships in rural communities. University–school partnerships similar to those described in this chapter can facilitate such research (Owens et al., 2011).

We recognize that in isolation, many of these recommendations may be applicable to providers in nonrural contexts. However, we hope that we have highlighted the importance and uniqueness of these recommendations for the rural provider through our commentary and contextualized vignette. We also recognize that many of our recommendations may be addressed through innovations in graduate level training programs (Jameson & Blank, 2007). However, recommendations specific to training and macro-level systems change are beyond the scope of this chapter and addressed elsewhere in this handbook.

In closing, we hope that our commentary on common challenges does not dissuade others from pursuing a career in rural SMH health. Indeed, we find SMH research, training, and service in rural communities to be a personally and professionally fulfilling endeavor that addresses an important need for many children and families.

References

American Psychological Association. (2002). *Ethical principles of psychologists and code of conduct*. Washington, DC: Author.

American School Counselor Association. (2010). *Ethical standards for school counselors*. Alexandria, VA: Author.

Beggs, J. J., Hains, V. A., & Hurlbert, J. S. (1996). Revisiting the rural-urban contrast: Personal networks in nonmetropolitan and metropolitan settings. *Rural Sociology, 61*(2), 306–325. doi:10.1111/j.1549-0831.1996.tb00622.x.

Bourke, L., Sheridan, E., Russell, U., Jones, G., DeWitt, D., & Liaw, S. T. (2004). Developing a conceptual understanding of rural health practice. *The Australian Journal of Rural Health, 12*(5), 181–186. doi:10.1111/j.1440-1854.2004.00601.x.

Campbell, C. D., & Gordon, M. C. (2003). Acknowledging the inevitable: Understanding multiple relationships in rural practice. *Professional Psychology: Research and Practice, 34*(4), 430–434. doi:10.1037/0735-7028.34.4.430.

Chinmann, M., Imm, P., & Wandersman, A. (2004). *Getting to outcomes 2004: Promoting accountability through methods and tools for planning, implementation, and evaluation.* Santa Monica, CA: Rand Corporation.

Chorpita, B. F., & Daleiden, E. L. (2009). Mapping evidence-based treatments for children and adolescents: Application of the distillation and matching model to 615 treatments from 322 randomized trials. *Journal of Consulting and Clinical Psychology, 77*(3), 566–579. doi:10.1037/a0014565.

Chorpita, B. F., Daleiden, E., & Weisz, J. R. (2005). Identifying and selecting the common elements of evidence based interventions: A distillation and matching model. *Mental Health Services Research, 7*(1), 5–20. doi:10.1007/s11020-005-1962-6.

Chronis, A. M., Chacko, A., Fabiano, G. A., Wymbs, B. T., & Pelham, W. E. (2004). Enhancements to the behavioral parent training paradigm for families of children with ADHD: Review and future directions. *Clinical Child and Family Psychology Review, 7*(1), 1–27. doi:10.1023/B:CCFP.0000020190.60808.a4.

Conger, R., Elder, G. H., Lorenz, F. O., Simons, R. L., & Whitbeck, L. B. (1994). *Families in troubled times: Adapting to change in rural America.* Hawthorne, NY: Aldine de Gruyter.

Costello, E. J., Angold, A., Burns, B. J., Stangl, D. K., Tweed, D. L., Erkanli, A., et al. (1996). The Great Smoky Mountains Study of youth: Goals, design, methods, and the prevalence of DSM-III-R disorders. *Archives of General Psychiatry, 53*(12), 1129–1136.

Eberhardt, M., Ingram, D., Makuc, D., et al. (2001). *Urban and rural health chartbook. Health, United States.* Hyattsville, MD: National Center for Health Statistics.

Fischer, E. P., Owen, R. R., & Cuffel, B. J. (1996). Substance abuse, community service use, and symptom severity of urban and rural residents with schizophrenia. *Psychiatric Services, 47*(9), 980–984.

Gamm, L., Stone, S., & Pittman, S. (2008). *Mental health and mental disorders: A rural challenge: A literature review. Rural healthy people 2010: A companion document to healthy people 2010* (Vol. 2). College Station, TX: The Texas A & M University System Health Science Center, School of Rural Public Health, Southwest rural Health Research Center.

Haines, V. A., & Hurlbert, J. S. (1992). Network range and health. *Journal of Health and Social Behavior, 33*(3), 254–266. doi:10.2307/2137355.

Halfacree, K. H. (1993). Locality and social representation: Space, discourse and alternative definitions of the rural. *Journal of Rural Studies, 9*(1), 23–37. doi:10.1016/0743-0167(93)90003-3.

Harowski, K., Turner, A. L., LeVine, E., Schank, J. A., & Leichter, J. (2006). From our community to yours: Rural best perspectives on psychology practice, training, and advocacy. *Professional Psychology: Research and Practice, 37*(2), 158–164. doi:10.1037/0735-7028.37.2.158.

Hart, L. G., Larson, E. H., & Lishner, D. M. (2005). Rural definitions for health policy and research. *American Journal of Public Health, 95*(7), 1149–1155. doi:10.2105/AJPH.2004.042432.

Hauenstein, E. J., Petterson, S., Rovnyak, V., Merwin, E., Heise, B., & Wagner, D. (2007). Rurality and mental health treatment. *Administration and Policy in Mental Health and Mental Health Services Research, 34*(3), 255–267. doi:10.1007/s10488-006-0105-8.

Havens, J. R., Young, A. M., & Havens, C. E. (2010). Nonmedical prescription drug use in a nationally representative sample of adolescents: Evidence of greater use among rural adolescents. *Archives of Pediatric & Adolescent Medicine.* Published online November 1, 2010. doi:10.1001/archpediatrics.2010.217.

Hoyt, D. R., Conger, R. D., & Valde, J. G. (1997). Psychological distress and help seeking in rural America. *American Journal of Community Psychology, 24*(4), 449–470. doi:10.1023/A:1024655521619.

Jameson, J. P., & Blank, M. B. (2007). The role of psychology in rural mental health services: Defining problems and developing solutions. *Clinical Psychology: Science and Practice, 14*(3), 283–298. doi:10.1111/j.1468-2850.2007.00089.x.

Jones, L. R., & Parlour, R. R. (1985). The psychiatric role of the rural primary care practitioner. In L. R. Jones & R. R. Parlour (Eds.), *Psychiatric services for underserved rural populations* (pp. 92–102). New York: Brunner/Mazel.

Keefe, S. E. (2005). *Appalachian cultural competency: A guide for medical, mental health and social service professionals.* Knoxville, TN: University of Tennessee Press.

Kelleher, K., & Long, N. (1994). Barriers and new directions in mental health services research in the primary care setting. *Journal of Clinical Child Psychology, 23*, 133–142.

Lohmann, R. A. (1990). Four perspectives on Appalachian culture and poverty. *Journal of the Appalachian Studies Association, 2*, 76–88.

Michael, K. D., Renkert, L. E., Wandler, J., & Stamey, T. (2009). Cultivating a new harvest: Rationale and preliminary results from a growing interdisciplinary rural school mental health program. *Advances in School Mental Health Promotion, 2*, 40–50.

MTA Cooperative Group. (1999). A 14-month randomized clinical trial of treatment strategies for attention-deficit/hyperactivity disorder. *Archives of General Psychiatry, 50*(12), 1073–1080. doi:10.1001/archpsyc.56.12.1073.

Owens, J. S., Andrews, N., Collins, J., Griffeth, J. C., & Mahoney, M. (2011). Finding Common Ground: University research guided by community needs for elementary school-aged youth. In L. Harter, J. Hamel-Lambert, & J. Millesen (Eds.), *Participatory partnerships for social action and research* (pp. 49–71). Kendall Hunt Publishers.

Owens, J. S., & Murphy, C. E. (2004). Effectiveness research in the context of school-based mental health. *Clinical Child and Family Psychology Review, 7*(4), 195–209. doi:10.1007/s10567-004-6085-x.

Owens, J. S., Murphy, C. E., Richerson, L., Girio, E. L., & Himawan, L. K. (2008). Science to practice in underserved communities: The effectiveness of school mental health programming. *Journal of Clinical Child and Adolescent Psychology, 37*(2), 434–447. doi:10.1080/15374410801955912.

Owens, J. S., Richerson, L., Murphy, C. E., Jageleweski, A., & Rossi, L. (2007). The parent perspective: Informing the cultural sensitivity of parenting programs in rural communities. *Child & Youth Care Forum, 36*(5–6), 179–194. doi:10.1007/s10566-007-9041-3.

Philo, C., Parr, H., & Burns, N. (2003). Rural madness: A geographical reading and critique of the rural mental health literature. *Journal of Rural Studies, 19*(3), 259–281. doi:10.1016/S0743-0167(03)00005-6.

Rost, K., Fortney, J., Fischer, E., & Smith, J. (2002). Use, quality, and outcomes of care for mental health: The rural perspective. *Medical Care Research and Review, 59*(3), 231–265. doi:10.1177/1077558702059003001.

Schank, J. A., & Skovholt, T. M. (2006). *Ethical practices in small communities: Challenges and rewards for psychologists*. Washington, DC: APA Press.

Starr, S., Campbell, L. R., & Herrick, C. A. (2002). Factors affecting use of the mental health system by rural children. *Issues in Mental Health Nursing, 23*(3), 291–304. doi:10.1080/016128402753543027.

Sue, S., & Zane, N. (1987). The role of culture and cultural techniques in psychotherapy: A critique and reformulation. *The American Psychologist, 42*(1), 37–45. doi:10.1037/0003-066X.42.1.37.

U.S. Census Bureau. (2010). *Population profile of the United States. National population projections*. Retrieved November 8, 2010, from http://www.census.gov/population/www/pop-profile/natproj.html

U.S. Department of Education National Center for Education Statistics. (2010). *United States student-to-counselor ratios by elementary and secondary schools*. Retrieved December 1, 2010, from http://www.counseling.org/PublicPolicy/ACA_Ratio_Chart_2010_Overall.pdf

U.S. Department of Health and Human Services. (2011). *Shortage areas: HPSA by state & county*. Retrieved January 5, 2011, from http://hpsafind.hrsa.gov/

U.S. Department of Health and Human Services, Health Resources and Services Administration, Maternal and Child Health Bureau. (2005). *The national survey of children's health 2003*. Rockville, MD: Author.

Wagenfeld, M. O. (2003). A snapshot of rural and frontier America. In B. H. Stamm (Ed.), *Rural behavioral health care: An interdisciplinary guide* (pp. 33–40). Washington, DC: American Psychological Association. doi:10.1037/10489-002.

Walkup, J. T., Albano, A. M., Piacentini, J., Birmaher, B., Compton, S. N., Sherrill, J. T., et al. (2008). Cognitive behavioral therapy, sertraline, or a combination in childhood anxiety. *The New England Journal of Medicine, 359*(26), 2753–2766. doi:10.1056/NEJMoa0804633.

Weisz, J. R., Jensen-Doss, A., & Hawley, K. M. (2006). Evidence-based youth psychotherapies versus usual clinical care: A meta-analysis of direct comparisons. *The American Psychologist, 61*(7), 671–689. doi:10.1037/0003-066X.61.7.671.

Werth, J. L., Hastings, S. L., & Riding-Malon, R. (2010). Ethical challenges of practicing in rural areas. *Journal of Clinical Psychology, 66*(5), 537–548.

From Guidance to School Counseling: New Models in School Mental Health

Laura Miller, Lemma Taha, and Elizabeth Jensen

Introduction

A variety of professionals work in conjunction with one another to encourage the successful academic and personal development of students within an educational environment. Teachers, principals, and school counselors work collaboratively to support the student body and encourage the personal achievement of those with whom they work. The role of the school counselor, however, has changed considerably between the twentieth and twenty-first centuries. As student needs began to change over time, the responsibilities and roles of the school counselor have also shifted to address them. The expansion of the school counselor's role does not just include a new focus on social and supportive counseling, but also encompasses a new responsiveness to student issues. Former models of counseling within the school environment often involved a "quick fix" mentality, meaning that students' needs were addressed expeditiously so they could promptly return to the classroom setting.

Twenty-first century models of school counseling encourage counselors to closely consider the underlying concerns that influence the student experience. This effort involves training school counselors to be responsive to student needs within the educational culture, while consistently exercising sensitivity towards social and emotional development as well as racial/cultural background (Reicher, 2010). Being responsive to students in contemporary schools also involves work across generations of counselors as the profession continues to transition from one that is guidance based to one that is attentive to a new school counseling focus. This chapter will describe both models of school mental health, the merging of the two models, transition of the school counselor identity, and relationships between school counselors and other educational professionals.

Work Across Generations: Guidance Counseling in the Twentieth Century vs. School Counseling in the Twenty-First Century

The changes between guidance counseling of the twentieth century and school counseling in the twenty-first century may not be evident to many. However, the transition from guidance to school counseling is influential in terms of the role in which counselors within the educational setting work with their students. Originally, school guidance began in 1889 when a guidance program was introduced to address vocational concern;

L. Miller (✉) • E. Jensen
Rutgers, The State University of New Jersey, New Brunswick, NJ, USA
e-mail: lem1222@gmail.com

L. Taha
Pascack Valley High School, Hillsdale, NJ, USA

this initiative was delivered to students while in English class. This concept of vocational guidance entailed educational or academic guidance and *counseling* was first perceived as merely a tool to assist this vocational guidance program (Bauman et al., 2003). As early as 1949, Robert Mathewson argued that teachers alone could not provide all the necessary experiences which students must obtain. This was a prominent stance for developing guidance programs and enhancing the educational experience (Bauman et al., 2003). Portman (2009) emphasized the importance of recognizing the shift in the counseling profession and how awareness to this continually changing process is a necessary component for counselors to effectively assist students. By recognizing these changes, counselors who work under either model (guidance or school counseling) are more inclined to work collaboratively to improve the quality of the educational experience for their students. This section discusses the history of such changes and differing roles in the profession that have resulted from them.

To fully understand the role of the school counselor, it is important to examine the transition from the twentieth century model of guidance counseling to the twenty-first century model of school counseling. The main function of guidance counselors was to assist students in determining the vocational field they would like to pursue in the future. In 1905, the chairman of the Students' Aid Committee of the High School Teachers' Association of New York, Eli Weaver, concluded that before students enter the workforce, they were in need of advice and counsel. With no funds from school administration, he was able to secure the volunteer services of teachers to work with students discussing such plans postgraduation. By 1910, he was able to witness teachers actively assisting young people in discovering what they could do best and how to secure a job in which "their abilities could be used to the fullest advantage" (Glosoff, 2009, p. 7). Vocation, as defined during the twentieth century, referred to the counselors and the expectation that they were to assist students in determining what type of career for which they were most suited. The Strong Vocational Interest Inventory was first published (1928) and used by counselors in discovering appropriate career options (Glosoff, 2009). The evolution of the definition of the term vocation as well as the field is discussed further below.

Guidance counselors worked with students primarily to identify careers and professions that might be of interest to them and to assist them in identifying the appropriate steps to acquire their chosen fields. The general process of vocational placement was achieved by focusing on the transition from school to work, thereby emphasizing an appropriate match between the client's aptitude and abilities and the occupational requirements (Lambie & Williamson, 2004). Vocational guidance was originated to enhance the postschool vocational transition from student status to work force employee. As a result, guidance counselors did minimum to no work regarding student emotions or personal and social development of the student because origination of this field began as a support to those entering the workforce; a major variant when comparing the guidance counseling model vs. the school counseling model (Lambie & Williamson).

Training requirements also differed under the twentieth century model. For instance, guidance counselors were required to have teaching experience prior to receiving counselor licensure. This requirement is no longer in place in some states.

A brief history of the transition from guidance counseling to school counseling would not be complete without recognizing the key individuals who influenced changes that have taken place over time, as well as acknowledging the need for counselors within the school setting. Counseling was initially introduced in education during the early twentieth century to address students' growing need for vocational guidance and advice. In 1908, Frank Parsons established the Bureau of Vocational Guidance, which was designed to assist students in successfully transitioning from the school environment of which they were familiar to the work world of which they were not. Development of career counseling continued during the 1930s in the face of the Great Depression, at which time the loss of employment demonstrated a need for counseling to assist adults and youth in identifying and developing new vocational skills (Glosoff, 2009). To further help students choose careers that were best suited for their personality, the publication of the *Dictionary of Occupational Titles* in 1938 provided counselors with a basic resource to match people with "occupations for which they were theoretically well suited" (Glosoff, 2009, p. 11). The economic and social occurrences of the 1940s and 1950s "reinforced counselors' emphasis on educational guidance because, following World War II, the GI bill made educational guidance popular as veterans exercised their right to counseling" (Minkoff & Terres, 1985, p. 424). Over the next several decades, the role of the guidance counselor was used to identify students who would perform well as scientists, mathematicians, or military personnel, depending on the needs of the nation at the time (Minkoff & Terres, 1985).

The Russian launching of Sputnik led to the U.S. Government taking particular interest in developing vocational/career guidance and the National Defense Education Act (NDEA) was passed in 1958. The legislation was intended to support and guide those students with high aptitudes in the areas of math and science so that they might become future members in the technological fields. NDEA funded the training of guidance counselors at both the elementary and secondary levels, as well as establishing programs to produce counselors suitable for public schools (Glosoff, 2009).

By the 1970s, Dr. Norm Gysbers shifted the profession from being unilaterally focused on career placement to a comprehensive developmental school counseling program for all grades (American School Counselor Association (ASCA), Hatch, & Bowers, 2005). Rising concerns regarding social justice and civil rights movements began to influence the lives of students. Gysber's realization of these social changes prompted the shift in school counseling from a main focus in vocational development to addressing the needs of students as whole, including their social, personal, and emotional growth. This change in professional expectations no longer left counselors as ancillary, expendable members of the school community, but rather integral individuals who would play an active role in promoting successful student development (Gysbers, 2001).

The comprehensive school counseling program was further shaped in the 1990s when Dr. Carol Dahir, on behalf of the American School Counselor Association (ASCA), began reviewing school counseling literature, consulting with other experts, and conducted a nationwide survey of 2,000 practitioners to get their opinions and suggestions (Mariani, 1998). As Dr. Dahir and her co-author, Dr. Chari Campbell, obtained results, the drafting of the national standards began. After review and various rounds of revisions, the national standards became final in August 1997 and appear in their entirety in Sharing the Vision: *The National Standards for School Counseling Programs* (Mariani, 1998). These standards laid out the competencies which students should gain as a result of participating in a comprehensive school counseling program. Such competencies belong to three areas which resonate with student development: academic, career, and personal/social (Mariani, 1998). With the creation of such standards, this was the first time that counselors and administrators would have a national model that could be used to implement future school counseling programs. With the changing needs of American students since the early twentieth century, the role of the counselor was amended appropriately, leading to what is now considered the profession of School Counseling (ASCA et al., 2005).

Furthermore, the ASCA created a national model in 2003, meant to assist school counseling professionals in developing and delivering comprehensive services to students (ASCA, 2003). Additionally, "the national model clarifies school counselor roles and expands the vision of the profession by clearly framing the work that counselors do" (Wilkerson, 2007, p. 421). The model addresses four main components (program foundation, delivery of services, program management, and accountability) and promotes collaboration between school counselors and other education professionals (ASCA et al., 2005). Essentially, this means that school counselors aim to deliver programs and then measure the impact those programs have on student learning outcomes (Wilkerson, 2007).

Over time, the needs of students began to change due to differences in societal and cultural influences on personal development. Instead of a strong emphasis on just vocational counseling, school personnel increasingly recognized that students also benefited from assistance in the three critical developmental domains previously mentioned—academic, career, and personal/social development. Additionally, these domains carved out specific areas in which the identity of the school counselor was strengthened, specifically within the educational context, therefore further defining the need for school counseling programs and that of the counselor. The role of the counselor dramatically changed as students began utilizing counselors within the school for a plethora of reasons expanding beyond vocational decision making. School counselors began to emphasize growth in a variety of different areas of student development. Counseling programs administered by school counselors now incorporated character education, bullying, prevention effort and education about drug and alcohol abuse, and multiculturalism. These programs may be delivered to small groups of students in a group counseling setting or through regular classroom sessions depending on the needs of each school (Portman, 2009).

Advocacy. School counselors need to be able to advocate for their students in a variety of ways and as a result, it is vital that counselors stay current on changes not only within the profession but also within the culture of the students around them. According to the ASCA National Model (2005), "Counselors consult with parents or guardians, teachers, other educators, and community agencies regarding strategies to help students and families. School counselors serve as student advocates" (p. 42). Moreover, school counselors also serve to identify school system practices that have an impact on student success. As they identify such systemic changes, school counselors work to replicate or eradicate practices that enhance or inhibit student opportunities (ASCA et al., 2005). To be an advocate for students, societal changes that have an impact on the school environment need to be considered by school counselors.

Cross-cultural awareness and skill. The field also recognizes that an awareness of societal changes coupled with a sensitivity towards working with diverse cultural groups will assist counselors in their work with diverse populations, leading counselors to understand how societal changes affect differing cultural groups. Moreover, school counselors can play a significant role in a students' life by being responsive to the needs of diverse cultural groups. An essential component of the school counselor's role is to deliver culturally competent services that improve student academic performance, as well as to identify barriers that impede student achievement and success (Schellenberg & Grothaus, 2011). Identifying and addressing barriers accordingly can have a positive impact on student adjustment to the school environment, as well as building positive and supportive relationships with school counselors (Goh, Wahl, McDonald, Brissett, & Yoon, 2007).

Ongoing professional development. The learning and educational experience of school counselors should not cease upon completion of the educational requirements to enter the profession. School counselors will be better able to advocate for their students by staying current on the latest research and exploring and employing new interventions and coping strategies with their students as trends change and develop over time. School counselors are also charged with being aware of changes in school policy, both at the national and local level. Attendance at professional development sessions such as those provided by national conferences promotes ongoing awareness of resources and new trends in the field.

The goal of school counselors, regardless of the century in which they were trained, is to improve the educational experience of students and act in ways that encourage successful student development across social, emotional, and academic realms. This can only be achieved by recognizing all aspects of student life and how various facets of student life intertwine with the academic setting to encourage or deter successful development. In addition, recognition of how cultural and societal changes affect student development are to be considered so that school counselors can better advocate for the students with whom they work.

Bridging the Counselor Culture with the Educational Culture

There is no doubt that bridging the gap between twentieth century and twenty-first century school counselors is essential for students to receive the types of services that promote successful development and promotion from grade to grade. The twenty-first century student needs attention in various areas like vocational and college advisement, as well as having their emotional and personal needs met. Without merging the twentieth and twenty-first century models of counseling, being able to comprehensively meet student needs would be a challenge. The differences between guidance counseling and school counseling are not the only shifts to be considered. To appropriately address student needs within the school setting, it is also necessary to bridge the gap between the counseling culture and the educational culture. Before this bridge can be established, it is important to understand and acknowledge the perspective of each cultural domain (Clauss-Ehlers, 2008).

The counseling culture differs from the educational culture in a variety of ways. Counseling generally focuses on the individual or small group dynamics. Counselors are interested in how circumstances affect individuals' feelings, emotions, and coping strategies. Also, the counseling culture examines how members of small groups interact with one another, support each other, and develop through the counseling or therapeutic process. In working with individuals and groups of students, the counselor is able to model and coach students in areas such as self-management, navigating peer relationships, appropriate decision making, and organizational skills which will aid in positive changes (Clark & Breman, 2009).

Additionally, the process within this culture encourages students or counselees to explore various areas of uncertainty and introspection as they develop socially and personally (Clauss-Ehlers, 2008). This culture emphasizes the uniqueness of each counselee, or student; with the goal of helping the client make positive changes in "coping, adapting, or specific behaviors that are problematic" (Clark & Breman, 2009, p. 9). This aspect of the culture involves highlighting the strengths of each student and encouraging students to continue engaging in positive behaviors. Most students will exhibit areas of weakness. The counseling culture encourages working with students to develop problem-solving strategies and appropriate goal setting. Perhaps of most importance, the counseling culture is dependent on the therapeutic relationship that is shared between counselors and their counselees. This relationship provides counselors with a platform to work with students regarding academic, career, and personal development, addressing the specific and individualized needs of each student with reasonable measures taken to protect student privacy (Clauss-Ehlers, 2008).

The educational culture, as compared to the counseling culture, varies greatly in terms of the way students interact with one another and education professionals. As opposed to the counseling culture where the focus is on the individual or small groups of students, the focus within the educational culture is on classes and the school as a whole (Clauss-Ehlers, 2008).

Emphasis is placed on common aspects of students. This includes grouping large numbers of students by age and shared grade level. This also includes grouping students by similar learning styles and speed at which they learn. This may mean placing students who are considered to be high achieving in the same classes or grouping students with special needs or learning disorders together through each grade level. Once classroom assignments have been composed, the nature of learning is restricted to classroom instruction by an adult/teacher to the group as a whole. In the counseling culture, a major focal point is acknowledging uncertainty and working towards resolution. In contrast, the educational culture involves knowledge of clear concepts and the learning of facts and concepts. Lesson plans and measurable results are used to determine the progress of students throughout the school year and to determine whether students progress from one grade to the next (Clauss-Ehlers, 2008).

A final comparison to the counseling culture deals with the issue of privacy within the educational culture. The relationship between students and educators occurs in a classroom with other students, limiting the amount of privacy that is possible. For students to feel a sense of trust, school counselors must create a safe haven where information discussed is kept private and confidential. It is the school counselor's respect for confidentiality that is critical for successful student–counselor relationships. According to the American Counseling Association's Code of Ethics (2005), counselors must recognize that trust is a cornerstone for the counseling relationship. It is apparent that a student's relationship with an educator, as opposed to a counselor, varies tremendously. While educators use an approach or technique that suits the student body as a whole, counselors delve into the individual needs and focus on building a relationship that fosters social and emotional development. Without a sense of privacy, students may feel the need to withhold certain thoughts or emotions because of fear, embarrassment, or shame in front of peers. A confidential environment furthers the development of a working professional relationship that provides the context for personal and academic growth.

Addressing Shifting Trends

Shifts in trends that face professional school counselors in the twenty-first century undoubtedly play a substantial role in their daily schedules and meeting the demands that accompany the school counselor title. Some professionals routinely feel besieged and overworked, finding it nearly impossible to keep up with the demands and expectations placed on them (Johnson, Rochkind, & Ott, 2010). ASCA recommends a student–counselor ratio of 100 to 1. Yet, on average, it has been found that in public schools across the United States, the ratio is closer to 265 students for every one counselor; more than double the ASCA recommendation (Clinedinst & Hawkins, 2009).

Furthermore, many of the tasks that consume the school counselor's daily schedule are composed of administrative responsibilities, addressing disciplinary concerns, and aiding students with scheduling predicaments (Johnson et al., 2010). Other duties that encompass a daily schedule may entail: overseeing testing programs, lunch duty, attendance monitoring, and even substitute teaching (Johnson et al., 2010). The mindset held by many within the public school systems "often seem to assume that counselors can juggle a whole roster of duties and still effectively assist hundreds of students in planning their futures" (Johnson et al., 2010, p. 76).

This assumption, however, is impractical, creating an impossible scope of job duties and expectations that cannot be practically met. At a time when guidance counselors only saw a small number of students, few students went to college, and a high school diploma was all that graduates needed to obtain jobs and various professions, this kind of system may have been the cornerstone of the guidance counseling profession (Johnson et al., 2010). Presently, however, given the rising number of students pursuing postsecondary education and an economy in which many jobs require some college or certification, school counselors are required to meet with more students based on academic need alone. As a result, for the school counseling profession to forge through the twenty-first century, education professionals and various stakeholders are called upon to acknowledge and understand the current scope of job duties faced by school counselors.

With the variations between the counseling culture and the educational culture, it is not surprising to find that differences have led to barriers that may prevent or interfere with effective partnerships (Clauss-Ehlers, 2008). Collaboration between the two cultures would likely cause a more comprehensive learning and educational experience for students, with benefits that would outnumber detriments. However, misconceptions regarding each culture and several obstacles can prove to be barriers in developing this successful, comprehensive partnership (Clauss-Ehlers, 2008).

Within the school day, teachers are provided with a regimented schedule of classes they teach. The times when they teach each class have been prescribed and there is little to no variation in their schedules on a day-to-day basis. Although teachers are aware of this fact when entering the profession, they may view their schedules as more rigid than those of counselors working within the same school setting. For most school counselors, the task of scheduling appointments and meetings is often under their control, an opportunity not afforded to teachers. As a result teachers might view counselor schedules to be less structured than their own and may view counselors as having too much free time (Clauss-Ehlers, 2008). They may also feel that because counselors, in most cases, design their own schedules, they are able to assign themselves breaks during the day that teachers are not given. This sense of unfairness between counselor and teacher schedules may lead to an increased resentment by teachers towards the counselors that they should be working collaboratively with for the betterment of their students (Clauss-Ehlers, 2008). One way to mitigate the potential for these misconceptions is to foster greater communication between educators and school counselors so that each group is more aware of the role and function of the other.

The manner in which space is used and constructed also differs for teachers and school counselors. Teachers are given a space in which to teach their class(es). The classroom is a vehicle to promote this learning environment. For some counselors, however, finding adequate space to counsel students in a confidential manner can be an obstacle. Confidentiality, for instance, necessitates a private room where the student and school counselor can discuss concerns privately. Depending on the size of the school, the number of school counselors employed, and the amount of space designated as a school counseling office, it is possible that private office space is a scarce resource.

This dilemma can present issues associated with having to respond to multiple crises simultaneously. For instance, two counselors who share an office may be presented with differing crisis situations at the same time, in which case one counselor will have to locate to a different location in which to address the crisis at hand. Having to search for private office space when a student is in crisis takes away from the ability to be responsive during this critical moment.

These challenges are in contrast to teachers who are scheduled by school administration to a classroom for each period of the day, preventing the overlapping of classes being taught in one classroom at any given time. Despite this organizational element for teachers, they too, however, may experience space issues such as feeling the classroom space is too small for increasingly larger classrooms. Students may also have different learning needs and the classroom may feel too small to adequately respond to varied student experiences. Clearly the role of space and implications for learning and counseling is an ongoing question to be addressed by school personnel.

A key role of the school is to educate children on a variety of subjects. In addition to supporting students in their successful completion of coursework and to develop skills appropriate for each grade level, schools are increasingly recognizing the important link between healthy social and emotional development and personal/academic success. Social and emotional learning (SEL) can be defined as "the process of socialization and education related to personal, interpersonal and problem-solving skills and competencies" (Reicher, 2010, p. 213). This concept offers teachers, educators, school counselors, and others a background for attending to the social and emotional needs in a systematic way, while still focusing on the academic front (Reicher).

The SEL concept refers to a safe, caring, supportive, cooperative, and well-managed learning environment for students (Reicher, 2010). Student needs within the school setting, however, are not limited to only learning the necessary information to be promoted from grade to grade. Rather, students must also be encouraged to successfully develop both personally and socially. As a result, "SEL refers to the knowledge and skills children acquire through social and emotional related education, instruction, activities, or promotions efforts that help them to recognize and manage emotions, engage in responsible decision-making, and establish positive relationships" (Reicher, 2010, p. 214). School counselors today play a major role in being responsive to the social and emotional needs of students. This may include counseling students on various topics such as: school phobia, anxiety, peer relations, bullying, peer relationships, family issues, self-awareness, self-management, and social awareness, among others. Educators and school counselors are encouraged to recognize all aspects of the child's development.

SEL theory presents important implications for connections between social/emotional development and academic success (Clark & Breman, 2009). For instance, a number of school reforms and instructional modifications can be used to promote school achievement such as: curricular-based SEL programs; infusion of SEL into the regular curriculum; altering and optimizing the instructional process; service learning that engages students actively and "experientially in the learning process in community life; and attention to informal learning process in community life" (Reicher, 2010, p. 223). Implementing such reforms can target SEL as a protective mechanism that fosters academic learning and works to prevent youth problematic behaviors (Reicher, 2010).

School-based mental health programs that have been specifically initiated to attend to youths' emotional, behavioral, or social functioning have been found to show evidence of impact across a multitude of behavioral and emotional problems (Reicher, 2010). If school counselors can promote school success skills (i.e., organization, listening, and being responsive) students may very well show academic gains. For instance, cooperating with peers and completing homework assignments in a timely fashion contribute to academic success and can reinforce the reoccurrence of such new behaviors as a result (Clark & Breman, 2009). These findings demonstrate the importance of investing in the counseling work done by school mental health professionals.

An issue may arise, however, when counselors need to use classroom instructional time to work with and counsel students. Removing students from classes for counseling sessions may be deemed as disruptive to the educational process. Teachers may opt out of sending students to the school counselor for support services during scheduled visits if it means that the student will miss a portion of their classes. This lack of communication increases the cultural divide between educational and counseling worlds. Additionally, this may mean that students who are in need of regular counseling may not receive it on a consistent basis. Ongoing communication between teachers and school mental health personnel about the importance of both educational and counseling needs is critical here. Teachers and school mental health personnel are encouraged to work together to jointly determine the schedule that best suits student needs.

Extended school breaks are another scheduling concern faced by school mental health professionals. The summer vacation typically spans over 2–3 months. This extended time period can be disruptive to the counseling process between school counselor and student. Summer vacations, as well as other extended school breaks, interfere with school counselors maintaining ongoing counseling relationships with the students who would benefit from one-to-one and/or group sessions on a regular and frequent basis (Clauss-Ehlers, 2008).

While summer vacations provide students with an opportunity for growth and maturation, the summer break may hinder the counseling process as well. Upon returning to school in the fall, some of the progress achieved between the school counselor and student may be negated by the 2- to 3-month vacation (Clauss-Ehlers, 2008). In some cases, school counselors may need to return to previous themes before working with a student on new issues that have developed over the extended break. For others, issues and concerns that were unresolved prior to summer vacation may need extra attention, depending on how the student is coping after not having counseling support during the summer holiday.

While school is out of session and school-based counseling services are not available to students, school counselors need to recognize those students in need of additional help and work with their families to find community-based supports as needed. School counselors must also recognize the sense of abandonment certain students may feel when the school year ends and counseling opportunities decrease. These can be addressed with the student and family through communication and the exploration of a referral for support services during the summer months. When making a referral, school counselors must sit down with both the family to discuss why the referral has been made and how the referral can help the student's present situation (Clauss-Ehlers, 2006).

Addressing the social, emotional, developmental, and academic needs of students requires collaboration between teachers, administrators, and school counselors. This collaboration can be achieved more effectively if the aforementioned barriers between the counseling culture and the education culture are addressed. When the obstacles mentioned are resolved, teachers and counselors will work better together to address student needs. Teachers may learn new approaches from working with school counselors, and counselors can observe and interact with students in the "real world" of the classroom (Clark & Breman, 2009).

The collaborative effort results in greater movement towards providing students with a healthy learning environment where their academic and personal needs are met simultaneously (Clark & Breman, 2009). The common goal between all types of educators is to provide students with an opportunity to learn and grow as individuals, and ultimately, to promote student success. Yet, if a clash exists between the two cultures, collaboration and accomplishing student goals may be stunted. When issues between the cultures become apparent, it is especially important for school personnel professionals to remember the purpose of their role within the school system—the student—and to encourage collaboration that acts in the best interest of all students.

Forging a Twenty-First Century Professional School Counselor Identity: A Five-Step Model

Institutional systems and schools are notorious for resisting change and remaining stagnant in their everyday tasks, skills, and goals (Lambie & Williamson, 2004). As a result, resistance to change must be confronted if counselors are to break out of the potential for limiting roles and explore more effective practices (Lambie & Williamson). To ensure that counselors remain active in their professional development and stay current with societal changes, Lambie and Williamson recommend a four-step approach to promote the modern school counselor's identity: educating principals, abolishing teaching requirements for counseling licensure, providing supervision in schools, and reassigning inappropriate duties. In addition to the four steps, being responsive to student needs in a multicultural context is a crucial facet to any model being used in the twenty-first century. As a result, it is recommended that a multicultural component be added.

According to the first component of Lambie and Williamson's (2004) approach, *principals who are educated* about professional school counseling and who support the ASCA National Model have a clearer understanding of the appropriate role for school counselors. With greater understanding, principals work to ensure that every day tasks and assignments represent effective helping skills that promote overall student success (Finkelstein, 2009). For instance, in a survey conducted by The College Board and the ASCA, principals and counselors agreed that an understanding of counselor roles is established through equal communication between school counselors and principals (Finkelstein, 2009). Not only does communication assist principals and other school administrators in understanding the role of the counselor, it also promotes a strong sense of respect between the two parties (Finkelstein, 2009). Principals who support the ASCA National Model recommend that counselors develop trust and maintain frequent communication with their students, establish a clear understanding of their role as a counselor, view staff as a team rather than individual entities, and stay visible throughout the course of the day to ensure easily accessible and reliable services (Lambie & Williamson, 2004). A principal with an accurate perception of the school counselor's role is more likely to support counselors in their role and function within the school. This perception is established through open dialogue and communication, as well as shared decision making regarding matters that influence student success (Finkelstein, 2009).

According to Lambie and Williamson (2004), the second step to promote the professional school counselor's identity involves *removing teacher certification as a requirement for endorsement as a school counselor*. For many years, teaching experience has been a requirement to entering into a program to receive school counseling licensure. Reasoning behind this theory implied that the school counselor must have a strong knowledge base of classroom discipline, management, and teaching methods to be effective as a school counselor.

Over the past few years, some state legislation eradicated teaching as a requirement indicating that teaching is not necessarily related to school counselor effectiveness. While some states have abolished teaching as a prerequisite for entering into a school counseling program, there are a few states that make teaching experience mandatory. According to the ASCA, each state has different requirements for their applicants. For example, while states such as New Jersey and California do not make teaching experience a requirement, Alabama and North Dakota require 2 years of successful professional experience in teaching. Illinois applicants must also hold or be qualified to hold a teaching certificate. Each state has varying beliefs about whether or not teaching experience is what makes an effective school counselor. Lambie and Williamson (2004) argue that counselor education programs can equip counselors with the knowledge pertinent to working in a school environment and administrators can provide induction and orientation support to new counselors to assist them in becoming familiar with school policies, procedures, and protocols.

Characteristics, maturity level, clinical supervision, and quality of training are key characteristics that foster the *identity development of a professionally competent and effective school counselor*. Even though teaching requirements for counseling licensure have been abolished in certain states, some school personnel continue to believe that the teaching requirement is an indicator of school counselor effectiveness and skill. To ensure that school counselors are appropriately equipped and prepared to guide and counsel students in various educational settings and within diverse communities, this component of the model contends that effectiveness should be determined by a high quality educational background, on-site training, and constant supervision from an on-site school counselor with excellent experience and who follows the ASCA National Model and ethical standards.

The fourth step in the model involves *reassigning inappropriate duties*. To effectively serve the diverse students that make up our educational system, school counselors should devote a majority of their time and energy to appropriate counselor-related assignments (i.e., providing direct service with students, parents, and guardians). Appropriate counseling services, such as individual and group counseling, classroom guidance lessons, career counseling, and parent conferences are but a few examples of the direct services school counselors can implement on a day-to-day basis. It is a culmination of these services that allows school counselors the opportunity to be effective, while also offering a comprehensive developmental counseling program where students are valued and guided towards becoming productive members of society. Non-counselor-related jobs such as lunch duty, substitute teaching, filing, and many other jobs that some educational systems still require of their school counselors, diminish the time that counselors can use to directly work with students. It is imperative that non-counselor-related assignments are eliminated with. This change will support a shift from counseling programs that are guidance based to those that are comprehensive and developmental in design (Lambie & Williamson, 2004).

To ensure that school counselors utilize their time appropriately and fulfill ASCA guidelines, educational systems are to become knowledgeable of what duties and services counselors are to provide throughout the course of the school day. This focus aims to avoid unproductive routines and amplify direct service opportunities (i.e., the provision of counseling) to students and members of the school community. The ASCA National Model proposes that counselors spend approximately 80% of their time providing direct service to students (Clark & Breman, 2009).

The fifth step that the current authors add to this model involves *being responsive to student needs in a multicultural context*. Being multiculturally responsive to students consists of understanding the developmental needs and stages of adolescence, while also remaining sensitive and cognizant of diverse groups (Ivey, D'Andrea, Ivey, & Simek-Morgan, 2007). Key components of any culturally competent counselor consist of being: "aware and sensitive to [one's] own cultural issues"; "aware of [one's] own values and biases and how they affect minority clients"; "comfortable with differences that exist between oneself and clients in terms of race and beliefs"; and "knowledgeable and informed about the particular group with whom the counselor is working" (Yeh & Arora, 2003, p. 82).

When working with various groups, Goh et al. (2007) suggest utilizing experiential activities that allow participants to engage in multicultural issues in a safe, monitored, and enjoyable, yet effective way. The role of the school counselors is enhanced and becomes "builders of cross-cultural bridges" (Goh et al., p. 67). Additionally, facilitation of these activities can build positive cross-cultural understanding and insight among students, teachers, school administrators, and staff. Another mechanism includes staff training workshops that focus on specific objectives such as building faculty support for "classroom guidance lessons on diversity; to provide lessons for the teachers that support and enhance the guidance lessons on personnel diversity" (Goh et al., p. 68).

Acknowledging multicultural competency involves a fundamental ability to recognize similarities and differences among oneself and others (Yeh & Arora, 2003). The counselor who is culturally sensitive contributes to an empathic environment where effective helping relationships can develop. When working within an educational system, school counselors are encouraged to understand the ways in which every student is unique, while also inviting students to bridge commonalities with their peers (Clauss-Ehlers, 2006). Multicultural competence on the part of the school counselor is essential.

A Twenty-First Century Perspective: The Multifaceted School Counselor

This chapter has discussed the professional trajectory in which school counselors engage to be effective advocates, helpers, and leaders within a diverse educational system. A key component to the chapter is that counselors are responsive to the diverse needs of students within a multicultural context. As United States (U.S.) school districts evolve at a rapid pace, schools are experiencing demographic changes. Currently public school enrollment is up to 48.7 million (consisting of pre-kindergarten through 12th grade) and is projected to reach 51.2 million by 2015 (Clark & Breman, 2009). From 1972 to 2004, the percentage of White students enrolled in schools has dropped from 78 to 57%, while the percentage of Latino students has increased from 6 to 19% during this time (National Center for Education Statistics (NCES), 2006). There has also been an increase in the number of students identified with disabilities, such that 6.6 million students received special education services in 2004 in comparison to the 3.7 million in 1972 (NCES).

Given the increase in students identified with disabilities, school counselors provide a key role in connecting these students with disabilities to appropriate services that can be utilized. Often times, these students are provided with a personalized educational plan that outlines course work, goals, variations in classroom participation, and any other specific considerations or recommendations pertaining to an educational, physical, medical, or safety stand point. Being involved in the students' Individualized Education Program (IEP) process allows the school counselor to collaborate with IEP teams and others that are dedicated to helping students with disabilities (Milsom, Goodnough, & Akos, 2007). ASCA supports school counselor involvement with students who have disabilities as cited in their handbook that outlines practitioner guidelines. These guidelines spell out appropriate roles and responsibilities regarding school counselor's work with students who have special needs (ASCA, 2010).

School counselors are equipped to work with special needs students as direct service providers through individualized and group counseling sessions. Working with students in this capacity allows school counselors the opportunity to address social and emotional concerns as well as assist with postsecondary planning. Postsecondary planning may include discussing future goals and types of services needed, in addition to determining course requirements that further future endeavors (Milsom et al., 2007). ASCA recommends that counselors get involved in multidisciplinary teams (MDTs) to serve as advocates for students with disabilities and function as a multifaceted counselor for the student body.

Given these changes in the United States' educational system, the role of the multicultural school counselor becomes even more pivotal. To maintain multicultural competence within schools and respond effectively and ethically to culturally diverse individuals, Ivey et al. (2007) recommends that three goals are met. First, counselors must be aware of their own cultural values and beliefs so they can experience a genuine sense of empathic understanding for people of various backgrounds. Second, counselors must be aware of their client's worldviews by making a commitment to learn about culturally diverse groups. This includes reading about and engaging with individuals within culturally diverse populations. Third, counselors must also seek out and adapt to culturally appropriate intervention strategies to effectively work within a multicultural population (Ivey et al., 2007). The multicultural school counselor recognizes that one approach may not work as well for one student as it does for another. Multicultural counselors identify differences and use personal knowledge, understanding, and experience to determine best practices and approaches in work with diverse students and their families.

Effective communication between counselors and parents, teachers, and administration can create positive relationships that benefit all students. Demonstrating effective communication skills entails remaining cognizant of one's own verbal and nonverbal messages and how others may receive them. The tone of one's voice or a body gesture can influence how a message is perceived. As a result, when working with students and parents, school counselors are encouraged to consider effective verbal and nonverbal communication skills to promote consistently positive relationships with members of the school system. Nonverbal communication is also influenced by cultural context so understanding the meaning of a nonverbal cue in one context vs. another is critical. For example, Western culture promotes direct eye to eye gaze. In fact, children are encouraged to look adults in the eye while speaking, for this develops positive communication and conversation etiquette. Yet, in other cultures such as Japan, avoiding eye contact depicts respect. As a result, if a school counselor was unaware of this difference, building rapport with the client or their family may be adversely affected if the school counselor viewed this interaction negatively.

On the other hand, more advanced approaches in communication such as paraphrasing (rephrasing in one's own words), reflecting (restating back to the client what they have communicated to you/mirroring), and clarifying (finding the meaning of what the client is thinking or feeling by asking questions) can ensure effective verbal communication between counselors and counselees. Communication skills are the fundamental foundation of the counselor–client relationship. They are key aspects of building rapport.

The charge of school counselors is to: respond to students when they have difficulty with school work; provide guidance with social issues so that positive relationships may be maintained; offer an outlet for students to express their emotions in a judgment-free environment; work with students to plan for their future; and help them to achieve a better understanding of who they are and how to relate to others and the world around them. To effectively address these needs, the multicultural school counselor is familiar with the varying cultures of those with whom they work. Understanding cultural norms and beliefs is essential in respectfully and effectively assisting the student, and his or her family, with the current issue at hand. Seeking consultation or supervision when unsure about cultural best practices within a specific cultural group can aid in ensuring effective helping practice. A counselor who is proactive in developing an understanding of various cultures, who takes initiative in staying up-to-date with research and best practices, and who recognizes change and how to adapt appropriately will be a more effective leader and advocate for all students within the educational environment.

References

American School Counselor Association. (2003). *The ASCA National Model: A framework for school counseling programs*. Alexandria, VA: Author.

American School Counselor Association. (2010). *The professional school counselor and students with special needs*. Retrieved June 5, 2011, from http://www.schoolcounselor.org/files/PositionStatements.pdf.

American School Counselor Association, Hatch, T., & Bowers, J. (2005). *The ASCA National Model: A framework for school counseling programs* (2nd ed.). Alexandria, VA: Author.

Bauman, S., Siegel, J., Falco, L., Szymanski, G., Davis, A., & Seabolt, K. (2003). Trends in school counseling journals: The first fifty years. *Professional School Counseling, 7*, 79–90.

Clark, M. A., & Breman, J. C. (2009). School counselor inclusion: A collaborative model to provide academic and social-emotional support in the classroom setting. *Journal of Counseling and Development, 87*, 6–11.

Clauss-Ehlers, C. S. (2006). *Diversity training for classroom teaching: A manual for students and educators*. New York, NY: Springer.

Clauss-Ehlers, C. S. (2008). Creative arts counseling in schools: Toward a more comprehensive approach. In H. L. K. Coleman & C. Yeh (Eds.), *Handbook on school counseling* (pp. 517–530). Newbury Park, CA: Sage.

Clinedinst, M., & Hawkins, D. (2009). *State of college admission*. Alexandria, VA: National Association for College Admission Counseling.

Finkelstein, D. (2009). *A closer look at the principal-counselor relationship: A survey of principals and counselors*. New York: National Office for School Counselor Advocacy, American School Counselor Association, and National Association of Secondary School Principals. Retrieved June 5, 2011, from http://www.schoolcounselor.org/files/CloserLook.pdf.

Glosoff, H. (2009). The counseling profession: Historical perspectives and current issues and trends. In D. Capuzzi & D. Gross (Eds.), *Introduction to the counseling profession* (pp. 3–56). Columbus, OH: Pearson/Merrill.

Goh, M., Wahl, K., McDonald, J., Brissett, A., & Yoon, E. (2007). Working with immigrant students in schools: The role of school counselors in building cross-cultural bridges. *Journal of Multicultural Counseling and Development, 35*, 66–79.

Gysbers, N. C. (2001). School guidance and counseling in the 21st century: Remember the past into the future. *Professional School Counseling, 5*, 96–105.

Ivey, A., D'Andrea, M., Ivey, M. D., & Simek-Morgan, L. (2007). *Theories of counseling and psychotherapy from a multicultural perspective* (6th ed.). Boston, MA: Allyn & Bacon.

Johnson, J., Rochkind, J., & Ott, A. (2010). Why guidance counseling needs to change. *Educational Leadership, 67*, 74–79.

Lambie, G. W., & Williamson, L. L. (2004). The challenge to change from guidance counseling to professional school counseling: A historical proposition. *Professional School Counseling, 8*(2), 124–131.

Mariani, M. (1998). National standards for school counseling programs: New direction, new promise. *Occupational Outlook Quarterly, 42*, 41–43.

Milsom, A., Goodnough, G., & Akos, R. (2007). School counselor contributions to the Individualized Education Program (IEP) process. *Preventing School Failure, 52*, 19–24.

Minkoff, H., & Terres, C. (1985). ASCA perspectives: Past, present, and future. *Journal of Counseling and Development, 63*, 424–427.

National Center for Education Statistics. (2006). *Condition of education*. Washington, DC: Author.

Portman, T. A. A. (2009). Faces of the future: School counselors as cultural mediators. *Journal of Counseling and Development, 87*, 21–27.

Reicher, H. (2010). Building inclusive education on social and emotional learning: Challenges and perspectives—A review. *International Journal of Inclusive Education, 14*, 213–246.

Schellenberg, R., & Grothaus, T. (2011). Using culturally competent responsive services to improve student achievement and behavior. *Professional School Counseling, 14*, 222–230.

Wilkerson, K. (2007). School counselor reform and principals' priorities: A preliminary content analysis of the National Association for Secondary School Principals (NASSP) Bulletin (1997-2007) informed by guiding documents of the American School Counselor Association (ASCA). *Education, 131*, 419–436.

Yeh, C., & Arora, A. (2003). Multicultural training and interdependent and independent self-construal as predictors of universal-diverse orientation among school counselors. *Journal of Counseling and Development, 81*, 78–83.

Part II

Innovative Approaches in Work with Diverse Children and Adolescents in Schools

Culturally Competent Engagement of African American Youth and Families in School Mental Health Services

Kendra P. DeLoach, Melissa Dvorsky, and Rhonda L. White-Johnson

African American adults and youth are more likely to drop out of mental health treatment compared to other racial/ethnic groups (Austin & Wagner, 2010; McMiller & Weiz, 1996). The reasons contributing to their premature dropping out are varied and complex. Studies suggest that African American youth typically engage in only two to three treatment sessions (Cuffe, Waller, Cuccaro, Pumariega, & Garrison, 1995; McMiller & Weiz, 1996). Premature dropout is especially concerning because African American youth are diagnosed as experiencing depression, anxiety, and disruptive behaviors more than youth from other racial/ethnic groups (Roberts et al., 1999; Wu et al., 2001), yet they are not remaining in treatment long enough to receive optimal benefits. It has been speculated that sociocultural dynamics in the engagement of African American youth play a major role in their premature dropout. Based on the chronic nature and magnitude of the issues facing African American youth and families, culturally sensitive and culturally specific engagement strategies may be most effective in resolving this problem.

K.P. DeLoach, Ph.D., L.M.S.W. (✉) • M. Dvorsky, B.A.
R.L. White-Johnson, Ph.D.
University of South Carolina,
Columbia, SC 29208, USA
e-mail: deloackp@mailbox.sc.edu

Chapter Overview

Engaging African American families and youth in school mental health (SMH) programs involves SMH professionals employing culturally specific, pragmatic, and task-oriented strategies, while simultaneously enhancing their own worldview of African Americans through culturally specific conscious raising activities. This twofold process of engaging African Americans involves interpersonal work between SMH professionals and clients and among professionals of different disciplines and cultural/ethnic/personal backgrounds. Professionals must evaluate the effectiveness, extent, and cultural specificity of their engagement strategies with African American youth and their families (Thomas & Weinrach, 2004).

It should be mentioned that this chapter does not aim to use generalizations about African Americans to present a cookie-cutter approach to engaging them, which occasionally occurs in discussions on specific groups of color. There seems to be a tendency to present generalized information about specific racial/ethnic groups with little attention or mention of the individual-level differences that exist within the specific group (Vera, Buhin, Montgomery, Shin, & Carter, 2005). Given this, the chapter aims to present background information about African Americans under the caveat that it is used to build a general framework. However, this framework should be specified for each individual youth and their family.

Thus, this chapter will present a brief historical overview on the relationship between African Americans and the mental health profession; present straightforward culturally specific and culturally sensitive engagement strategies that should be employed throughout the therapeutic process; and discuss the implications for research, practice/training, and policy on engaging African American youth and families in SMH programs.

Historical and Contemporary Overview of African Americans and Mental Health

Within American society, people of African descent have occupied a unique niche because they were forcibly brought into the country and experienced humiliating systems of control over their behavior through slavery. Upon emancipation from slavery, they have been left to deal with the residuals stemming from it (Gibson & Denby, 2007). Consequently, the understanding of their mental health needs must be examined through both a historical and contemporary lens (Logan, 2007). The extant literature on African and African American studies has documented how the enslavement of Africans and the legacy left behind from it has continued to haunt the minds, bodies, and spirits of African Americans (Sanders & Bradley, 2002). Although slavery ended more than a century ago, the residuals of ideas, behaviors, attitudes, and stories resulting from it still negatively affect the social, environmental, political, economic, physical, and mental functioning of African Americans (Logan, 2007). Thus, the mental health experiences of African Americans is challenging and continues to be impacted by the legacy of slavery because of the ongoing experiences of racism, intolerance, minimization, exclusion, and limited economic resources (Gibson & Denby, 2007).

Much has been written about how the stress of oppression (e.g., racism, classism, sexism, discrimination) affects the mental health of African Americans (Hines-Martin, Brown-Piper, Kin, & Malone, 2002), but little has been written about how mental health professionals can identify and incorporate the strengths of African American in addressing their mental health needs and services. Sanders and Bradley (2002) asserted that this paucity within the mental health profession "reinforces the stereotypical and deficit-ridden information" taught to professionals in the past (p. ix). This silence allows discriminatory or prejudicial racial schemas that mental health professionals have about African Americans to go unchallenged, which can have deleterious effects on the mental health services that African Americans receive.

The Surgeon General David Satcher's landmark report (1999) on Mental Health addressed the state of mental health needs of African Americans as a high priority. In this seminal document, the emphasis was on addressing the state of mental health services—the type and quality of services provided to African American consumers for community-based and school-based mental health services. To engage African Americans, mental health professionals need to actualize multicultural competencies put forth by many professions (American Psychological Association, Association for Multicultural Counseling and Development, National Association of Social Workers, and so forth) into culturally specific and culturally relevant interventions. Sanders and Bradley (2002) noted that the mental health profession has been slow to engage in scholarship that provides pragmatic, culturally responsive strategies for engaging African American children and families.

Although the history of mental health includes very limited references to the experiences of people of African descent, prevailing ideologies and social policies that guided their mental health treatment reflect contention between African Americans and their attainment of services (Logan, 2007). Reflected in the pejorative terms and theories on the mental health of African descendants, mental health leaders have historically embodied disparaging perceptions and ideas about this group. Carl Jung (1930), a psychiatrist, proposed the theory of racial infection, a condition that occurred when Whites were outnumbered by a primitive race (i.e., Blacks) and became infected by them. Although this theory was proposed to explain the mental and moral peculiarities of Whites, it identified African Americans as the contagious and diseased source. Carothers (1947), a psychiatrist, asserted that Blacks experienced low levels of depression because they lacked a sense of responsibility. Today's mental health professionals may disagree with these beliefs. However, racism in its covert form is so incendiary that without intentional introspection of one's own beliefs, attitudes, ideas, behaviors, and values toward African Americans, professionals may be unaware of how inculcated these disparaging perceptions and ideas are within their own worldview and practices. As noted, African American clients have reported feeling that their mental health professional did not understand their life (Garretson, 1993). Furthermore, they reported feeling that cultural biases and stereotypes undergirded the communication between them and the professional (Thomspon, Bazile, & Akbar, 2004).

Barriers Experienced by African Americans Seeking Mental Health Treatment

Not all African American youth and families share a common heritage because of the variety of ancestry within this racial/ethnic group. There is a long history of people from different backgrounds mixing with others; thus, the construct of race is believed to be a social construct not inherently rooted in any biological processes (Coleman, 2011). Among youth who self-identify as African American, their racial identity may not necessarily be a true composite of their heritage. These individuals may also assume other racial identities, symbolizing a multicultural identity (e.g., Latin America, Europe, Asia, or Caribbean) (Stevenson & Arrington, 2009). Multiple identities present unique differences and complexities of cultural expressions and realizations, making agreement about cultural competence challenging (Cunningham, Foster, & Henggeler, 2004). Given all of the diversity and complexities of culture, Black youth hold a variety of perceptions, values, ideas, and behaviors.

Adopting culturally responsive and sensitive ways of speaking (e.g., avoiding jargon, using culturally understood terms), different strategies for partnering (e.g., finding out what interests the youth and including those interests into therapeutic relationship), and different techniques for working with individual-level youth (e.g., client-centered techniques) may help SMH professionals engage African American youth (Vera et al., 2005). Professionals should avoid using jargon or language that is specific to the trained professional and confusing to families and youth. Instead, professionals should use plain language and periodically have the youth and family summarize the conversation to create a shared understanding (Stevenson & Renard, 1993).

Sociocontextual issues (economic, cultural, social, environmental, political, and spiritual factors) may affect the use of mental health treatment in community-based facilities. However, school-based mental health programs offer a different and unique opportunity. SMH services are uniquely situated to treat a population that may otherwise forgo treatment in community-based mental health facilities. These facilities may offer unaffordable, subpar, and inaccessible mental health treatment deterring some African American youth and families from receiving services (Stepanikova & Cook, 2008). However, these youth and family may be more inclined to receive services at school. Though this opportunity is great for increasing the likelihood of youth and families receiving services, professionals need to use screening measures, diagnostic procedures, or treatment interventions that account for the history, characteristics, experiences, needs, and behaviors as their foundation (Jones, 1996) more likely to connect and engage African American youth (Rainey & Nowak, 2005). Wade and Bernstein (1991) discovered that the perceptions formed by African American clients during the first treatment session were predictive of premature dropout. At the first session, the lack of cultural specificity and cultural relevance tended to deter some African Americans from receiving ongoing treatment (Sellars, Garza, Fryer, & Thomas, 2010).

Consistently, the stigma of mental health diagnosis and treatment has been a cultural barrier which has invoked fear in many African Americans (Bradford, Newkirk, & Holden, 2009). This fear may stem from consequences, either perceived or real, that occur if anyone learns that they have received a diagnosis or treatment for mental illness (Alvidrez, Snowden, & Patel, 2010). Specifically, they may fear the identification of "being crazy" or being treated as if they "were crazy" (Smith, Friedman, & Nevid, 1999). Some of this fear has been associated with the misuse and abuse of particularly rural, poor, low educated African Americans who participated in medical experiments (e.g., Tuskeegee Syphilis Experiment [1940–1973], New York HIV/AIDS Foster Care Experiment [1995]). SMH professionals may be able to offer services to African American youth and families in a neutral setting, evading some of the stigma attached to receiving mental health treatment in community-based mental health facilities. Using the language of the youth and family to describe their concerns and issues, instead of relying on psychopathology labels decreases the families' perceptions and association with being labeled "crazy" (Alvidrez et al., 2010). By adopting culturally responsive language and avoiding problematic labels of mental illness, SMH professionals may be able to effectively encourage and engage African American youth and families in receiving mental health services (see Baker-Sinclair, Weist, & Petroff, 1996).

Within mental health services and the extant literature, spirituality, religious affiliation, and attendance in religious services have been documented as protective mechanisms that buffer the hardships of oppression many African Americans endure (Bierman, 2006; Hunter & Lewis, 2010; Owens et al., 2004). Nevertheless, fewer studies have identified these factors as barriers in attaining mental health treatment by some African Americans (Goldston et al., 2008). These youth and families may be reluctant to seek mental health services, opting instead to rely mainly on prayer and faith (Stanford, 2007) or counseling from faith-based leaders whose training in mental health varies (Ryan, 2011; Spriggs & Sloter, 2005). SMH professionals may improve upon their connection and engagement with spiritually and religiously expressive African American youth and families by affirming their religiosity and spirituality. Professionals can assess the degree of religiosity and spirituality of youth and families and ask them the extent to which they would prefer incorporating spiritual or religious literature, adages, or resources into their engagement (Bishop, 1992; Boyd-Franklin, 2010). For example, youth and families may rely heavily on prayer to mitigate daily stressors. Instead of discounting this practice, professionals would affirm it by providing other suggestions in behaviors, thoughts, and practices to accompany it.

Strategies for Working with African American Youth

Racial Socialization

In light of the historical injustices and social inequities that continue to disproportionately impact African Americans, members of the racial group have developed strategies to successfully adapt and function in society. Generally, these strategies are learned during childhood and adolescence using a practice called racial socialization. Racial socialization is defined as a transactional process by which explicit and implicit messages about the significance and meaning of race and ethnicity are communicated (Coard & Sellers, 2005). While racial socialization processes are present among members of all racial and ethnic groups, this practice is particularly common among African American families. Racial socialization is a vital practice within the racial group, as race-related messages provide contextual and meaningful guidance in a society where African American youth encounter racism and discrimination. This is critical, as previous literature indicates a majority of African American children have had at least one encounter with unfair treatment based on their race, which has negatively affected their psychosocial functioning (Fisher, Wallace, & Fenton, 2000; Harris-Britt, Valrie, Kurtz-Costes, & Rowley, 2007; Neblett et al., 2008; Neblett, Philip, Cogburn, & Sellers, 2006; Sellers, Copeland-Linder, Martin, & Lewis, 2006). According to a growing body of research, youth who receive messages instilling pride in their racial group or messages warning of racism and discrimination fare better when encountering such treatment (2008; Harris-Britt et al., 2007, Neblett et al., 2006). With this in mind, African American families have historically used racial socialization as a means to provide youth with the information and skills necessary to negotiate racially hostile contexts.

While one of the primary goals of racial socialization is to provide African American youth with the strategies and information necessary to manage racism and discrimination, it also serves a number of other functions. For instance, racial socialization processes inform individual's engagement with and perceptions of intra- and intergroup relations. This is especially important considering the increase in diversity within the nation's population (Humes, Jones, & Ramirez, 2011). African American youth also receive messages about race that are designed to instill a sense of pride in the culture and history of the racial group (Coard & Sellers, 2005; Hughes et al., 2006). These messages inform youth of cultural customs and traditions within the racial group, as well as instill more positive affective feelings about being African American. This is critical as African American culture is devalued and youth often face stigma regarding their racial group membership. The fundamental goal of racial socialization is to ensure the healthy development of African American youth, despite the challenges they face in society.

Research suggests receipt of racial socialization messages is associated with a host of positive child outcomes. For instance, African American adolescents who received racial socialization communications that emphasized racial pride and awareness of cultural history also reported less engagement in problem behaviors (Bennett, 2007). Similarly, findings by Hughes and colleagues indicated that African American adolescents who received messages from their parents emphasizing culture and heritage reported better academic outcomes compared to adolescents who did not receive such messages (Hughes, Witherspoon, Rivas-Drake, & West-Bey, 2009).

Research also indicates that receiving combinations of certain racial socialization messages (e.g., racial pride, racial barrier) is related to higher levels of self-esteem among youth (Neblett et al., 2008).

Clearly, there is sufficient evidence to indicate racial socialization is a vital cultural practice used to encourage the healthy development of African American youth. Unfortunately, there have been few efforts to examine racial socialization outside of the family domain, particularly as it relates to mental health service use (Rodriguez, Cavaleri, Bannon, & McKay, 2008). This would be an important avenue for research and practice, as African American youth do not receive messages about race exclusively from the family unit; they also take in information about the meaning and significance of race from clinical settings, schools, and other community settings (Nasir, McLaughlin, & Jones, 2009). Considering research that supports the utility of racial socialization in ensuring positive outcomes among African American youth, SMH professionals and school staff may be missing a prime opportunity to address the needs of African American youth.

Traditionally, African American youth have been less likely than youth of other racial and ethnic backgrounds to seek help from mental health professionals (U.S. National Institute of Mental Health, 2001; also compare to previously cited studies on premature drop out—Austin & Wagner, 2010; McMiller & Weiz, 1996). While research suggests lack of mental health service use is impacted by feelings of mistrust (Terrell, Taylor, Menzise, & Barrett, 2009), research also indicates that as a community, African Americans feel mental health professionals are not in tune with their cultural needs and will not understand their struggles with racism and discrimination (Mock, 2003; Trivedi, 2002). This presents a clear unmet clinical need for African American youth and their families, who would benefit from the integration of racial socialization into SMH settings. Though this area of practice and research is in its infancy, Stevenson (1994) has provided a framework to begin implementing racial socialization practices in schools and SMH settings. First, school counselors, faculty, and staff must take steps to identify youth and families who are struggling with issues of race and discrimination. Stevenson recommends utilizing reliable and validated scales (i.e., the Scale of Racial Socialization, Stevenson, 1994) to elicit information about race and culture from youth and families. It is expected that utilization of reliable and valid scales will stimulate more in-depth conversations about issues of race and cultural strengths in the therapeutic setting. Second, SMH professionals must provide a therapeutic setting where youth can openly discuss and explore their racial identity, as well as question where and how they fit into the larger school context. Third, SMH professionals must become more familiar with the racial worldviews and ideologies of youth and families of color by incorporating a more culturally competent curriculum in training programs focusing on oppression, multiculturalism, and racial socialization. Finally, this framework asserts that SMH professionals be careful not to stigmatize or label African American youth and families who demonstrate pro-Black attitudes or engage in behaviors that are outside of mainstream cultural awareness. Instead, SMH professionals and other school staff must create settings that are more culturally relevant to African American youth and families.

Assessing School Climate

School climate is another critical influence that should be considered when assessing the engagement of African American youth and families. School climate refers to the quality and totality of the individual and group experience of school life. It includes the norms, goals, values, interpersonal relationships, intrapersonal processes, educational opportunities, and organizational and environmental structures (Cohen, McCabe, Michelli, & Pickeral, 2009). Creating positive school climate depends heavily on the relationship among school staff and students. When the school climate is positive, the school becomes more conducive to learning and for students to begin exhibiting positive behaviors (Brookover & Schneider, 1975; Purkey & Smith, 1985).

While all racial groups are affected by school climate, African American families and youth may be especially sensitive to school climates that have either been hostile or dismissive of them altogether (Serpell, Hayling, Stevenson, & Kern, 2009). Research suggests that poor school climate has decreased African American families' engagement in schools (Harry, 1992). These families encounter negative school climate experiences such as poor interactions with school personnel and feeling intimidated (Anderson, 1994), lacking a clear understanding of the educational system and policies (Roa, 2000), and being unable to attend school meetings because meetings were held at inconvenient times (Trotman, 2002; Weitock, 1991).

It would be advantageous for school personnel to use discussions, curricula, and environmental stimuli to engage African American youth and families. School personnel would reflect that they care for these youth and families by showing interest in their needs, wants, and goals. Before school policies have been broken, school personnel could hold meetings at convenient times for families to explain the main school policies. During the explanation of the policies, personnel should use plain language that is positive, empowering, and respectful and free of professional jargon, contention, or condescension. School personnel should present as if they care about youth and families because caring has been associated with African American students achieving higher grades and exhibiting fewer disruptive behaviors (Wiggan, 2008). Caring school personnel demonstrate a commitment to their students and to developing professional relationships with them by promoting teamwork, self-direction, student involvement, and critical thinking.

A Culturally Diverse Framework for Engaging African American Youth in SMH

In terms of SMH programs, school counselors, staff, and administrators should engage African American youth and families through a continual process of establishing and sustaining an interpersonal relationship through a logical step-by-step order of behaviors. Lum (2004) proposed a culturally diverse practice framework for working with culturally diverse populations. The five process stages of the framework include (1) contact, (2) problem identification, (3) assessment and diagnosis, (4) intervention, and (5) service closure.

Stage 1: Contact

During the contact stage, relationships are established between school personnel, youth, and families. At the initial contact, school personnel need to work towards establishing a mutually trusting relationship. This is especially important for African American youth and families who have a healthy cultural mistrust of institutions that have been historically hostile towards them (Terrell et al., 2009). School personnel would express respect towards families by speaking positively about the strengths and resources African American youth and families possess and empathizing with families about the challenges they endure (Thompson & Alexander, 2006). For instance, school personnel would encourage youth and families to talk about their family strengths, identify what youth and families view as problematic their psychosocial functioning, and seek solutions from them. School personnel who do this, then, assume the role of learner (not expert) and achieve a culturally responsive, client-specific, and client-centered approach.

Another culturally responsive approach is identifying the cultural characteristics that are unique to African American youth and families and the characteristics that are unique to the professional (Morris, 2001). For example, SMH professionals may believe that the youth's family needs to be more involved in the therapeutic process. Instead of SMH professionals assuming that only the parents should be involved, SMH professionals should ask the youth and parents if there are other family members or individuals who need to be involved. These individuals may not be blood related, but they may function in a highly regarded and critical role within the family. These individuals, referred to as *fictive kin,* may contribute significantly to the daily sustainment and advancement of the family by offering financial support and/or in-kind services (e.g., babysitting, transportation, emotional comfort). Fictive kin is a common practice within communities of color who rely on extended family or non-blood-related individuals (Hall, 2008). For example, a mother's female friend may provide child care and help parents make decisions about the future care of children. These children may refer to her as their aunt and refer to her children as their cousins. The *aunt* and *cousins* may be expected to attend school activities, contribute to family discussions, attend family gatherings during holidays and special occasions, and discipline children. It may be quite beneficial to the outcomes of the youth for the SMH professional to include the parents and the *aunt* in the therapeutic process.

Stage 2: Problem Identification

Upon the closure of the contact stage, SMH professionals should have a preliminary understanding on the psychosocial functioning of the youth and family. During the problem identification stage, African American youth and families may be slow to disclose personal information because of mistrust of authority or shame of experiencing problems in their psychosocial-economic functioning (Thomspon et al., 2004). African American youth may be reticent in expressing depressive symptoms (e.g., feelings of inadequacy, despair, dejection, or hopelessness) because this expression may be viewed as culturally aberrant (Goldston et al., 2008). African American youth and families may engage in a rambling conversation to test the SMH professional reactions and responses. It is important for professionals to recognize this hesitance as a pivotal part of the problem identification, as well as, exercise patience and continue relationship building. One culturally responsive approach during this stage is history taking. It allows the professional to get to know the youth and family by learning cultural factors (e.g., family and life experiences during childhood, family life adjustments, current concerns and expectations for the future, youth and family's present understanding of adjustment difficulties) that promote and deter the youth's psychosocial and academic functioning.

While providing information specific to their history, African American youth and families may describe problems related to oppressive constructs, such as racism, classism, sexism, discrimination, and prejudice. Discussing these constructs and the power and cultural differentials attributed to them may enhance engagement with African American youth and families. Albeit, a discussion about race may be somewhat tricky because not all African Americans are welcoming of engaging in such a discussion, particularly with a professional of a different race (La Roche & Maxie, 2003). This type of discussion may be difficult and even uncomfortable, but it is still needed for understanding the social community and environmental issues that may be affecting them. La Roche and Maxie recommended that professionals whose racial identity differed from that of their client seek knowledge on racial identity development, racial consciousness, racial differences, and oppression and discrimination. Professionals can improve their knowledge by taking diversity classes offered at universities and technical colleges, registering for continuing education trainings on cultural competence, reading race conscious literature (e.g., magazines, books, newspapers), joining sociopolitical grassroots organizations, and conversing with colleagues of different cultural backgrounds about race, class, culture, etc.

Stage 3: Assessment and Diagnoses

The role of assessment is to gather and analyze information, set goals, and plan for interventions (Lum, 2004). During this phase, SMH professionals should focus on the strengths, resources, and healthy functioning of clients as well as on the problems, difficulties in acquiring, accessing, or using resources, and limitations in functioning. African American youth are frequently diagnosed with Attention Deficit/Hyperactivity Disorder (ADHD), Conduct Disorder, and Oppositional Defiant Disorder and SMH professionals describe these youth as exhibiting poor impulse control, externalizing behaviors, conduct problems, acting-out behaviors, noncompliance, antisocial behaviors, behavior disorders, or oppositional behaviors (Rainey & Nowak, 2005; Wu et al., 2001). Furthermore, these youth are labeled with emotional disorders, behavioral disorders, or both (Rainey & Nowak, 2005). Consequently, African American youth, especially males, are consistently overrepresented among youth in special education classes and labeled with emotional and behavioral disorder (EBD; Osher, Woodruff, & Sims, 2002). Regardless of racial/ethnic identity, youth labeled with EBD consistently demonstrate poor academic and social outcomes (Bradley, Doolittle, & Bartolotta, 2008; Frank, Sitlington, & Carson, 1995; Wagner, Newman, & Cameto, 2004), which may be indicative of the school's response and treatment towards them. Approximately 28% of African American youth with EBD graduate from high school and as many as 50% dropout (Blackorby & Wagner, 1996). The negative outcomes of high dropout rates among these youth result in them experiencing difficulties in their adulthood—including difficulties obtaining and sustaining employment, poor personal relationships, substance abuse, incarceration, and early death (e.g., Bullis & Cheney, 1999; Greenbaum, Johnson, & Petrila, 1996).

Clearly there is a critical need for empirically supported and culturally responsive mental health assessment measures and strategies, and interventions that are effective in addressing the needs of African American youth. However, many of the measures being used to address the specific needs of African American families and youth have not been empirically tested with a large or representative African American sample (Rainey & Nowak, 2005). Replication studies may demonstrate that methods and procedures are effective, but when carefully examining the sample population the sample size of African American youth are typically small. Using measures and strategies that were developed for Black populations and subject areas would accurately reflect their psychosocial characteristics and behaviors more than conventional methods (Jones, 1996).

The Diagnostic Statistical Manual of Mental Health Disorders (DSM-IV TR) (American Psychiatric Association, 2000) remains the primary source for diagnosing mental illness. It is based on a multiaxial coding system that allows professionals to rate mental health functioning according to five axes. Most of these diagnostic categories have been derived from White populations, thus, its appropriateness as a tool with other racial/ethnic groups is questionable (Harris & Graham, 2007). The DSM-IV-TR has been criticized for failing to account for the cultural, sociopolitical, and environmental factors contributing to mental health functioning of African Americans, generally and African American children, specifically (Whaley, 2001). Because the expression of mental illness differs among people of color, the patterns of onset, duration, and the clustering of specific symptoms varies. Harris and Graham (2007) caution that mental health professionals should be aware of these cultural differences, which if not attended to increase the chances of inaccurate diagnoses and pejorative labeling. .

Limited knowledge specific to the cultural differences of mental and physical health functioning of African Americans may increase the chances for misdiagnosis. Mental health professionals of different cultural backgrounds should seek understanding of the client with an intentional approach to cultural sensitivity (Constantine, 2007). Engagement with African American youth and family may be improved by actively listening and understanding their definition of the problem, identifying the components that interfere with solving the problem, extracting themes, constructs, and language specific to the problem, and creating an alternative definition (Morris, 2001). For example, SMH professionals should seek clarity from African American youth and families of what they perceive is happening in their lives and ask whether what is happening is common to members of that particular culture. Seeking clarity from youth and families may provide SMH professionals with an opportunity to understand the cultural and environmental context of their problems, which permit them to be flexible in their skills and strategies (Morris, 2001; Rainey & Nowak, 2005).

Stage 4: Intervention

Stigma of mental illness in African American communities, lack of knowledge about mental illness, mistrust of counseling and professionals, impersonal services that are not tailored to the experiences of African American youth and families, and a lack of cultural understanding about the life and cultural experiences of African Americans living in an oppressive society are barriers to mental health treatment among African Americans that SMH professionals should be aware of (Thomspon et al., 2004). To be culturally competent in overcoming these barriers to treatment, SMH professionals should incorporate appropriate evidence-based interventions and culturally responsive perspectives into their practice. The predominant theoretical orientation in mental health training is cognitive-behavioral therapy (CBT) so integrating a culturally responsive perspective, such as Africentrism, into CBT would help enhance understanding of the characteristics and dynamics of African Americans (e.g., emphasis on extended family structure, maturity, here-and-now orientation, speaking with affect, status, and power measured by non-economic possessions, and status in the community; also see Morris, 2001). Africentrism would provide an understanding of "the philosophical premise of African Americans as individuals and as a cultural group" (p. 565). Even being an African American SMH professional does not assure that the individual is culturally competent because of the variety of characteristics and dynamics within this racial/ethnic group.

Stage 5: Service Closure

From the beginning of service delivery, SMH professionals should begin preparing for closure (notice our specific avoidance of the term "termination"). As part of the aftercare plan, African

American families and youth should identify individuals who will continue serving in an active role in their lives. SMH professionals should establish connections with community supports and resources and assist families with making appointments. Assistance in this context means more than simply giving families names and contact information of community resources. It entails giving them this information in addition to exploring whether families have any intention of using the resource(s). Further, professionals should explore with families their positive and negative thoughts about using resources, the barriers to using them, the likelihood of whether contact will actually be made, and hone in on when first contact will be made. For example, if a youth identifies enjoying religious-oriented activities, then SMH professional may give families community resources that are offered by churches of the family's choosing (see Owens et al., 2004). Because African American youth report being more engaged in youth-oriented religious activities than youth of other racial/ethnic groups (Bachman, Johnston, & O'Malley, 2005; Moore-Thomas & Day-Vines, 2008; Warren, Lerner, & Phelps, 2011), SMH professionals may consider including a spiritual leader into the aftercare plans. When professionals close services for students, either the goals have been obtained or additional services within the community that the professional is incapable of providing are needed. Because of stigma of mental health services among African Americans, SMH professionals should discuss the families' attitudes, beliefs, and obstacles about connecting to community resources and troubleshoot overcoming identified obstacles. Additionally, SMH professionals should follow-up with families verifying whether they have followed through with making and keeping appointments with community agencies. Periodically, they could check-in with families postclosure of SMH services as a means of proactively supporting families. Schools provide an opportunity to remain connected to families differently than community-based services because students usually remain enrolled and accessible in the school.

Conclusion

Research Implications

Presently, research on people of color continues to use a comparative methodology. Groups of people from diverse racial ethnic backgrounds are compared and most often education and socioeconomic status are controlled for or partitioned. Partitioning these two variables and determining whether there are differences among racial/ethnic groups does not fully account for the unique nuances that are specific to African Americans and other people of color. This methodological approach is flawed because one group (e.g., White Americans) has sustained an extensive history of obtaining majority rule, privileges, and advancement (Rainey & Nowak, 2005). African Americans have experienced oppression and discrimination—legacy of enslavement, oppression, and unfair treatment while only a small proportion of this population have experienced privilege and advancement (Rainey & Nowak). During data analyses, simply partitioning or separating the population by education, income, and employment and assuming that African Americans are similar to their racial/ethnic counterparts presents a distorted picture of their lived experiences. What is missing from the analysis is a representation of the psychosocial characteristics and dynamics of African Americans specific to their adjustment within overarching systems of oppression (e.g., racism and classism) (Dotterer, McHale, & Crouter, 2009). These systems subject an individual or a group to domination (being controlled), subjugation (made subservient), exclusion (omitted), devaluation (reduced in value), or relegation (assigned to an undistinguished task, place, or category).

Racism is mistreatment based on skin color or other distinctive physical attributes (Hutchison, 2003) and classism is mistreatment based on socioeconomic status, education, and prestige of occupation (Lott, 2002). Bryant (2011) found that African American male youth who experienced frequent racism were likely to internalize racist messages. Internalized racism was then found to be a better predictor in explaining the likelihood of violence among African American male youth than traditional risk factors typically examined in social science research, such as delinquent friends, poverty, drug use, and carrying a weapon. Guthrie and Low (2000) found that institutional, neighborhood, and individual classism limited the living conditions, life chances, material resources, and relative power and privilege of African Americans. These limitations have been found to be reliable markers for measuring their health and health status as suggested by high incidents of chronic illness (asthma, other lung problems, diabetes, heart disease, kidney problems, anemia, and weakened immune system) (CDC, 2011).

Assessment Implications

Additionally, SMH professionals should question and test the validity and reliability of assessment tools developed with normative populations that may not adequately include African American youth. As noted, mental health symptoms are expressed differently in communities of color than they are in White communities. Many of the diagnostic and assessment tools used in mental health treatment have limited reliability and validity with African American populations because of the limited number of African American people used in the studies (Rainey & Nowak, 2005). Thus, it is unknown as to what extent these diagnostic and assessment tools are appropriate for this population. SMH professionals diagnosing and assessing African American families and students should utilize testing methods and tools that have been demonstrated to be reliable and valid with African American populations instead of assuming that what works well for one racial/ethnic group will work well for other groups. SMH professionals should refer to the *Handbook of Tests and Measurements for Black Populations (Vol. 1 & 2)* (Jones, 1996) to use measurement tools that demonstrate reliability and validity with African Americans, while at the same time using more current sources to guide culturally competent efforts (see Clauss-Ehlers, Weist, Gregory, & Hull, 2010).

Culturally specific assessment tools help professionals to delineate differences in the expression of mental illness across racial/ethnic groups (Rainey & Nowak, 2005; Whaley & Hall, 2009). New and specific to the DSM IV TR (American Psychiatric Association, 2000) is an acknowledgement that communities of color express mental illness differently. In the multiaxial system, on Axis 4, culturally specific notations can be made that illustrate a different cultural display of challenges to ones' mental health functioning. Although Axis 4 in the DSM-IV is available, the axis is futile if mental health professionals lack knowledge of the specific indicators attributed to that cultural expression of mental illness. Reading literature about that cultural expression and engaging in discussions with individuals from that culture could enhance professionals understanding.

Practice, Training, and Education Implications

Improving the engagement of African American families and youth for SMH professionals must be done with cultural intentionality and enhanced cultural consciousness. According to the 1999 Surgeon's General Report, African Americans comprise a small percentage of mental health practitioners in the U.S.—2% of psychiatrists, 2% of psychologists, and 4% of social workers (U.S. Department of Health and Human Services, 2001). However, the majority of students disproportionately overrepresented as having social, emotional, or behavioral difficulties are students of color, particularly African American students (U.S. Department of Health and Human Services, 2001). It is likely then that these students will be seeing a professional of a different race, thus, professionals need to include culture-specific perspectives into their practice (e.g., integrating Africentrism perspective into Cognitive Behavioral therapy (Cokley, 2005)). Despite the need for integrating culture-specific interventions into one's practice and the call by most helping professions (American Psychological Association, National Association for Social Workers, etc.), it is difficult to find ones that are evidence based and accessible.

Educational programs could serve as the launching point for enhancing culture-specific discussion within the therapeutic relationship. It has been noted that half of doctoral-level professionals have reported feeling incompetent to work with African Americans despite their level of training and exposure to diverse client populations (Allison, Crawford, Echemendia, Robinson, & Kemp, 1994). The Educational Policies and Accreditation Standards (EPAS) now require undergraduate and graduate social work programs to offer coursework on practice with diverse and oppressed populations. Within such coursework, two main objectives occur: (1) students learn about specific cultural group's cultural characteristics (i.e., family patterns, religiosity, and significant contributions made by members of the group) and (2) students engage in self-reflection and self-analysis on their attitudes, behaviors, and ideas about these groups. These two objectives have been reported to be the most effective way of improving cultural competency within helping professionals (Kelly & Greene, 2010).

In addition to cultural specific educational training, SMH professionals should adopt an attitude of learner, instead of expert within their practice with African American youth and families. SMH professionals are not the experts in their client's lives. Because individual-level differences exist among African Americans, getting to know each client's ideas, beliefs, values, attitudes, customs, and interests would reduce the need to rely on generalizations (Flaskerud, 2007). Cultural diversity training is oftentimes packaged as generalizations of racial/ethnic groups, thus, after "being educated" about these generalizations, professionals may erroneously deem themselves as culturally competent (Kelly & Greene, 2010). Instead of relying on cultural generalizations, SMH professionals should use these generalizations to establish a broad framework and permit families and youth to provide the details. For instance, the racial label "Black" and "African American" are often used interchangeably. However, subtle distinctions exist between the two words because "Black" connotes a family heritage related to African descent. However, individuals of African descent may not identify as African Americans because of their ancestry to other countries (e.g., Haiti, Jamaica, Trinidad, Cuba, etc.). Professionals would exercise a culturally responsive approach by inquiring how a youth self-identifies racially or ethnically, instead of assuming that the youth is African American.

Policy in Action Implications

School policies (both informal and formal) that are not culturally responsive may deter the engagement and involvement of African American families and youth in school settings. Compared to other racial/ethnic groups, African American students do not exhibit higher rates of disruptive behaviors in schools than any other students, but they still account for the highest amount of placements in special education classrooms (Townsend, 2000). Further, African American males tend to receive harsher disciplinary actions (e.g., suspension or expulsion) even when exhibiting lower rates of disruptive behavior (Townsend, 2000). Unjust distribution of punitive actions against African American students (placement in restrictive settings or unwarranted punishments) represents discriminatory and oppressive application of policies by school personnel. Racial/ethnic differences and other differences in cultural background between school personnel and families may influence how school personnel view normality/abnormality, function/dysfunction, and well-being/distress among these families as well as how they create and enforce school policies and practices (Mock, 2003).

To work against these negative influences, SMH professionals could serve in the role of an advocate, helping to assess, analyze, draft, and implement school policies and practices that would improve the engagement of African American youth and their families in SMH services. By helping African American youth and families identify and navigate the school system, the appropriate school personnel would be contacted if behavioral or emotional issues became an issue in the school setting (Koonce & Harper, 2005). School systems can appear intimidating to uninformed families; the lack of support by a school personnel (an insider) may increase levels of intimidation and deter the involvement of some African American families. Ultimately, when SMH professionals discover that school policies or the application of them are oppressive, they should engage in corrective actions to modify or eradicate them altogether.

Wilson (2005) claimed that mental health professionals can help assist African Americans through mental health services by recognizing and addressing historical hostility, acknowledging and validating experiences of external challenges, and integrating spirituality in therapy. Many African Americans experience historical hostility, which may be directed outward through anger, violence, and verbal aggression or inward, for example as depression, alcohol, and substance abuse. Integrating spirituality into therapy may aid them in understanding and attributing spiritual meanings to their experiences, which has been associated with bolstering coping, resilience, and well-being (Owens, 2004). Improving the engagement of African American youth and families to deal with these challenges not only improves youths' psychosocial and academic functioning, but potentially their ability to make positive life choices in general.

References

Allison, K. W., Crawford, I., Echemendia, R., Robinson, L., & Kemp, D. (1994). Human diversity and professional competence: Training in clinical and counseling psychology revisited. *American Psychologist, 49*, 792–796.

Alvidrez, J., Snowden, L. R., & Patel, S. G. (2010). The relationship between stigma and other treatment concerns and subsequent treatment engagement among Black mental health clients. *Issues in Mental Health Nursing, 31*(4), 257–264.

American Psychiatric Association. (2000). *Diagnostic and statistical manual of mental disorders (4th ed. text rev.)*. Washington, DC: American Psychiatric Association.

Anderson, E.L. (1994). The effect of parental involvement on academic achievement. *Doctoral Dissertation, Walled University. Dissertation Abstracts International.* 251.

Austin, A. A., & Wagner, E. F. (2010). Treatment attrition among racial and ethnic minority youth. *Journal of Social Work Practice in the Addictions, 10*(1), 63–80.

Bachman, J. G., Johnston, L. D., & O'Malley, P. M. (2005). *Monitoring the future: A continuing study of American youth (8th, 10th, and 12th-grade surveys), 1976-2003* [Computer files]. Conducted by University of Michigan, Survey Research Center, Ann Arbor.

Baker-Sinclair, M. E., Weist, M. D., & Petroff, H. J. (1996). Language and rapport in cognitive-behavioral therapy with African-American teenagers. *The Behavior Therapist, 19*, 118–119.

Bennett, M. D., Jr. (2007). Racial socialization and ethnic identity: Do they offer protection against problem behaviors for African American youth? *Journal of Human Behavior in the Social Environment, 15*(2–3), 137–161.

Bierman, A. (2006). Does religion buffer the effects of discrimination on mental health? Differing effects by race. *Journal for the Scientific Study of Religion, 45*(4), 551–565. doi:10.1111/j.1468-5906.2006.00327.x.

Bishop, D. (1992). Religious values as cross-cultural issues in counseling. *Counseling & Values, 36*(3), 179.

Blackorby, J., & Wagner, M. (1996). Longitudinal post-school outcomes of youth with disabilities: Findings from the National Longitudinal Transition Study. *Exceptional Children, 62*(5), 399–413.

Boyd-Franklin, N. (2010). Incorporating spirituality and religion into the treatment of African American clients. *The Counseling Psychologist, 38*(7), 976–1000. doi:10.1177/0011000010374881.

Bradford, L., Newkirk, C., & Holden, K. (2009). Stigma and mental health in African Americans. In R. L. Braithwaite, S. E. Taylor, H. M. Treadwell, R. L. Braithwaite, S. E. Taylor, & H. M. Treadwell (Eds.), *Health issues in the Black community* (3rd ed., pp. 119–131). San Francisco, CA: Jossey-Bass.

Bradley, R., Doolittle, J., & Bartolotta, R. (2008). Building on the data and adding to the discussion: The experiences and outcomes of students with emotional disturbance. *Journal of Behavioral Education, 17*(1), 4–23.

Brookover, W. B., & Schneider, J. (1975). Academic environments and elementary school achievement. *Journal of Research and Development in Education, 9*, 83–91.

Bryant, W. W. (2011). Internalized racism's association with African American male youth's propensity for violence. *Journal of Black Studies, 42*(4), 690–707. doi:10.1177/0021934710393243.

Bullis, M., & Cheney, D. (1999). Vocational and transition interventions for adolescents and young adults with emotional or behavioral disorders. *Focus on Exceptional Children, 31*(7), 1–24.

Burkard, A. W., & Knox, S. (2004). Effect of therapist color-blindness on empathy and attributions in cross-cultural counseling. *Journal of Counseling Psychology, 51*(4), 387–397. doi:10.1037/0022-0167.51.4.387.

Carothers, J. L. (1947). A study of mental derangement in Africans and an attempt to explain it's peculiarities, more especially in relation to the African attitude to life. *Journal of Mental Science, 101*, 548–597.

Centers for Disease Control and Prevention. (2011). Rationale for regular reporting on health disparities and inequalities—United States. *MMWR, 60*(Suppl), 3–10. Available at http://www.cdc.gov/mmwr/pdf/other/su6001.pdf

Clauss-Ehlers, C., Weist, M. D., Gregory, W. H., & Hull, R. (2010). Enhancing cultural competence in schools and school mental health programs. In C. Clauss-Ehlers (Ed.), *Encyclopedia of cross-cultural school psychology* (pp. 39–44). New York: Springer.

Coard, S. I., & Sellers, R. M. (2005). African American families as a context for racial socialization. In V. C. McLoyd, N. E. Hill, & K. A. Dodge (Eds.), *African American family life: Ecological and cultural diversity* (pp. 264–284). New York: Guilford Press.

Cohen, J., McCabe, E. M., Michelli, N. M., & Pickeral, T. (2009). School climate: Research, policy, practice, and teacher education. *Teachers College Record, 111*(1), 180–213.

Cokley, K. O. (2005). Racial(ized) identity, ethnic identity, and Afrocentric values: Conceptual and methodological challenges in understanding African American identity. *Journal of Counseling Psychology, 52*(4), 517–526. doi:10.1037/0022-0167.52.4.517.

Coleman, S. (2011). Addressing the puzzle of race. *Journal of Social Work Education, 47*(1), 91–108. doi:10.5175/JSWE.2011.200900086.

Constantine, M. G. (2007). Racial microaggressions against African American clients in cross-racial counseling relationships. *Journal of Counseling Psychology, 54*(1), 1–16. doi:10.1037/0022-0167.54.1.1.

Cuffe, S. P., Waller, J. L., Cuccaro, M. L., Pumariega, A. J., & Garrison, C. Z. (1995). Race and gender differences in the treatment of psychiatric disorders in young adolescents. *Journal of the American Academy of Child and Adolescent Psychiatry, 34*(11), 1536–1543.

Cunningham, P. B., Foster, S. L., & Henggeler, S. W. (2004). The elusive concept of cultural competence. *Children's Services: Social Policy, Research & Practice, 5*(3), 231–243.

Dana, R. H. (2002). Mental health services for African Americans: A cultural/racial perspective. *Cultural Diversity and Ethnic Minority Psychology, 8*(1), 3–18. doi:10.1037/1099-9809.8.1.3.

Dotterer, A. M., McHale, S. M., & Crouter, A. C. (2009). Sociocultural factors and school engagement among African American youth: The roles of racial discrimination, racial socialization, and ethnic identity. *Applied Developmental Science, 13*(2), 61–73.

Fisher, C. B., Wallace, S. A., & Fenton, R. E. (2000). Discrimination distress during adolescence. *Journal of Youth and Adolescence, 29*, 679–695.

Flaskerud, J. H. (2007). Cultural competence: What is it? *Issues in Mental Health Nursing, 28*(1), 121–123. doi:10.1080/01612840600998154.

Frank, A. R., Sitlington, P. L., & Carson, R. R. (1995). Young adults with behavioral disorders: A comparison with peers with mild disabilities. *Journal of Emotional and Behavioral Disorders, 3*, 156–164.

Garretson, D. J. (1993). Psychological misdiagnosis of African Americans. *Journal of Multicultural Counseling and Development, 21*(2), 119–126.

Gibson, P. A., & Denby, R. W. (2007). African-American mental health: A historical perspective. In S. L. Logan, R. W. Denby, P. A. Gibson, S. L. Logan, R. W. Denby, & P. A. Gibson (Eds.), *Mental health care in the African-American community* (pp. 3–14). New York, NY: Haworth Press.

Goldston, D. B., Molock, S. D., Whitbeck, L. B., Murakami, J. L., Zayas, L. H., & Hall, G. C. (2008). Cultural considerations in adolescent suicide prevention and psychosocial treatment. *American Psychologist, 63*(1), 14–31.

Greenbaum, P. E., Johnson, L. F., & Petrila, A. (1996). Co-occurring addictive and mental disorders among adolescents: Prevalence research and future directions. *The American Journal of Orthopsychiatry, 66*(1), 52–60.

Guthrie, B. J., & Low, L. (2000). A substance use prevention framework: Considering the social context for African American girls. *Public Health Nursing, 17*(5), 363–373. doi:10.1046/j.1525-1446.2000.00363.x.

Hall, J. C. (2008). The impact of kin and fictive kin relationships on the mental health of Black adult children of alcoholics. *Health & Social Work, 33*(4), 259.

Harris, Y. R., & Graham, J. A. (2007). *The African American child*. New York: Springer Publishing Co.

Harris-Britt, A., Valrie, C., Kurtz-Costes, B., & Rowley, S. (2007). Perceived racial discrimination and self-esteem in African American youth: Racial socialization as a protective factor. *Journal of Research on Adolescence, 17*, 669–682.

Harry, B. (1992). Restructuring the participating of African-American parents in special education. *Exceptional Children, 59*, 123–131.

Hines-Martin, V., Brown-Piper, A., Kin, S., & Malone, M. (2002). Enabling factors of mental health service use among African Americans. *Archives of Psychiatric Nursing, 17*(5), 197–204.

Hughes, D., Rodriguez, J., Smith, E. P., Johnson, D. J., Stevenson, H. C., & Spicer, P. (2006). Parents' ethnic-racial socialization practices: A review of research and directions for future study. *Developmental Psychology, 42*(5), 747–770.

Hughes, D., Witherspoon, D., Rivas-Drake, D., & West-Bey, N. (2009). Received ethnic-racial socialization messages and youths' academic and behavioral outcomes: Examining the mediating role of ethnic identity and self-esteem. *Cultural Diversity and Ethnic Minority Psychology, 15*(2), 112–124.

Humes, K. R., Jones, N. A., & Ramirez, R. R. (2011). *Overview of race and Hispanic origin: 2010*. U.S. Department of Commerce: U.S. Census Bureau. Washington, DC.

Hunter, C. D., & Lewis, M. E. (2010). Coping with racism: A spirit-based psychological perspective. In J. Chin & J. Chin (Eds.), *The psychology of prejudice and discrimination: A revised and condensed edition* (pp. 209–222). Santa Barbara, CA: Praeger/ABC-CLIO.

Hutchison, E. (2003). *Dimensions of human behavior in the social environment: The changing life course* (2nd ed.). Thousand Oaks, CA: Sage Publications Inc.

Jones, R. L. (1996). Introduction and overview. In R. L. Jones (Ed.), *Handbook of tests and measurements for Black populations* (Vol. 1, pp. 3–15). Hampton, VA: Cobb & Henry Publishers.

Jung, C. (1930). Your negroid and Indian behavior. *Forum, 83*(4), 193–199.

Kelly, J. F., & Greene, B. (2010). Diversity within African American, female therapists: Variability in clients' expectations and assumptions about the therapist. *Psychotherapy: Theory, Research, Practice, Training, 47*(2), 186–197. doi:10.1037/a0019759.

Koonce, D. A., & Harper, W., Jr. (2005). Engaging African American parents in the schools: A community-based consultation model. *Journal of Educational and Psychological Consultation, 12*(1&2), 55–74.

La Roche, M. J., & Maxie, A. (2003). Ten considerations in addressing cultural differences in psychotherapy. *Professional Psychology: Research and Practice, 34*, 180–186.

Logan, S. S. (2007). *Mental health care in the African-American community*. New York, NY: Haworth Press.

Lott, B. (2002). Cognitive and behavioral distancing from the poor. *American Psychologist, 57*, 100–110.

Lum, D. (2004). *Social work practice and people of color: A process-stage approach* (5th ed.). Brooks/Cole: Sacramento.

McMiller, W. P., & Weisz, J. R. (1996). Help-seeking preceding mental health clinic intake among African-American, Latino, and Caucasian youths. *Journal of the American Academy of Child and Adolescent Psychiatry, 35*, 1086–1094.

Mock, M. R. (2003). Cultural sensitivity, relevance, and competence in school mental health. In M. D. Weist, S. W. Evans, N. A. Lever, M. D. Weist, S. W. Evans, & N. A. Lever (Eds.), *Handbook of school mental health: Advancing practice and research* (pp. 349–362). New York, NY: Kluwer Academic/Plenum Publishers.

Moore-Thomas, C., & Day-Vines, N. L. (2008). Culturally competent counseling for religious and spiritual African American adolescents. *Professional School Counseling, 11*(3), 159–165.

Morris, E. F. (2001). Clinical practices with African Americans: Juxtaposition of standard clinical practices and Africentrism. *Professional Psychology: Research and Practice, 32*(6), 563–572.

Nasir, N. I. S., McLaughlin, M. W., & Jones, A. (2009). What does it mean to be African American? Constructions of race and academic identity in an urban public high school. *American Educational Research Journal, 46*(1), 73–114.

National Institute of Mental Health. (2001). *Blueprint for change: Research on child and adolescent mental health*. Rockville, MD: U.S. Department of Health and Human Services Administration, Center for Mental Health Services, National Institutes of Health, National Institutes of Mental Health.

Neblett, E. W., Philip, C. L., Cogburn, C. D., & Sellers, R. M. (2006). African American adolescents' discrimination experiences and academic achievement: Racial socialization as a cultural protective factor. *Journal of Black Psychology, 32*, 199–218.

Neblett, E. W., White, R. L., Ford, K. R., Philip, C. L., Nguyen, H. X., & Sellers, R. M. (2008). Patterns of racial socialization and psychological adjustment: Can parental communications about race temper the detrimental effects of racial discrimination? *Journal of Research on Adolescence, 18*(3), 477–515.

Osher, D., Woodruff, D., & Sims, A. (2002). Schools make a difference: The relationship between education services for African American children and youth and their overrepresentation in the juvenile justice system. In D. Losen (Ed.), *Minority issues in special education* (pp. 93–116). Cambridge, MA: The Civil Rights Project, Harvard University and the Harvard Education Publishing Group.

Owens, C. C., Bryant, T. N., Huntley, S. S., Moore, E., Sloane, T., Hathaway, A., et al. (2004). Enhancing child and adolescent resilience through faith-community connections. In C. Clauss-Ehlers & M. D. Weist (Eds.), *Community planning to foster resilience in children* (pp. 283–296). New York, NY: Springer.

Owens, K.M., Asmundson, G.J., Hadjistavropoulos, T., & Owens, T.J. (2004). Attentional bias toward illness threat in individuals with elevated health anxiety. *Cognitive Therapy and Research, 28*, 57–66. doi:10.1023/B:COTR.0000016930.85884.29.

Purkey, S., & Smith, M. (1985). School reform: The district policy implications of the effective school literature. *The Elementary School Journal, 85*(3), 353–89.

Rainey, J. A., & Nowak, T. A. (2005). Mental health assessment with African American children and adolescents. In D. Harley & J. M. Dillard (Eds.), *Contemporary mental health issues among African Americans*. Alexandria, VA: American Counseling Association.

Roa, S. S. (2000). Perspectives of an African American mother on parent-professional relationships in special education. *Mental Retardation, 38*(6), 475–488.

Roberts, R. E., Phinney, J. S., Masse, L. C., Chen, Y. R., Roberts, C. R., & Romero, A. (1999). The structure of ethnic identity of young adolescents from diverse ethnocultural groups. *The Journal of Early Adolescence, 19*, 301. doi:10.1177/0272431699019003001.

Rodriguez, J., Cavaleri, M. A., Bannon, W. M., & McKay, M. M. (2008). An introduction to parenting and mental health services utilization among African American families: The role of racial socialization. *Social Work in Mental Health, 6*(4), 1–8.

Ryan, D. S. (2011). Ministry solutions for substance abuse. In C. Franklin, R. Fong, C. Franklin, & R. Fong (Eds.), *The church leader's counseling resource book: A guide to mental health and social problems* (pp. 27–39). New York, NY: Oxford University Press.

Sanders, J. L., & Bradley, C. (Eds.). (2002). *Counseling African American families*. Alexandria, VA: American Counseling Association.

Sellars, B., Garza, M. A., Fryer, C. S., & Thomas, S. B. (2010). Utilization of health care services and willingness to participate the future medical research: The role of race and social support. *Journal of the National Medical Association, 102*(9), 776–786.

Sellers, R. M., Copeland-Linder, N., Martin, P. P., & Lewis, R. L. (2006). Racial identity matters: The relationship between racial discrimination and psychological functioning in African American adolescents. *Journal of Research on Adolescence, 16*, 187–216.

Serpell, Z., Hayling, C. C., Stevenson, H., & Kern, L. (2009). Cultural considerations in the development of school-based interventions for African American adolescent boys with emotional and behavioral disorders. *Journal of Negro Education.* http://findarticles.com/p/articles/mi_qa3626/is_200907/ai_n42857095/?tag=content;col1

Smith, L. C., Friedman, S., & Nevid, J. (1999). Clinical and sociocultural differences in African American and European American patients with panic disorder and agoraphobia. *The Journal of Nervous and Mental Disease, 187*(9), 549–560.

Spriggs, J., & Sloter, E. (2005). Counselor-clergy collaboration in a church-based counseling ministry. In M. R. McMinn, A. W. Dominquez, M. R. McMinn, & A. W. Dominquez (Eds.), *Psychology and the church* (pp. 65–70). Hauppauge, NY: Nova.

Stanford, M. S. (2007). Demon or disorder: A survey of attitudes toward mental illness in the Christian church. *Mental Health, Religion and Culture, 10*(5), 445–449. doi:10.1080/13674670600903049.

Stepanikova, I., & Cook, K. S. (2008). Effects of poverty and lack of insurance on perceptions of racial and ethnic bias in health care. *Health Services Research, 43*(3), 915–930. doi:10.1111/j.1475-6773.2007.00816.x.

Stevenson, H. C. (1994). Racial socialization in African American families: The art of balancing intolerance and survival. *The Family Journal: Counseling and Therapy for Couples and Families, 2*(3), 190–198.

Stevenson, H. C., & Arrington, E. G. (2009). Racial/ethnic socialization mediates perceived racism and the racial identity of African American adolescents. *Cultural Diversity and Ethnic Minority Psychology, 15*(2), 125–136. doi:10.1037/a0015500.

Stevenson, H. C., & Renard, G. (1993). Trusting ole' wise owls: Therapeutic use of cultural strengths in African-American families. *Professional Psychology: Research and Practice, 24*(4), 433–442. doi:10.1037/0735-7028.24.4.433.

Terrell, F., Taylor, J., Menzise, J., & Barrett, R. K. (2009). Cultural mistrust: A core component of African American consciousness. In H. A. Neville, B. M. Tynes, S. O. Utsey, H. A. Neville, B. M. Tynes, & S. O. Utsey (Eds.), *Handbook of African American Psychology* (pp. 299–309). Thousand Oaks, CA: Sage Publications, Inc.

Thomas, K. R., & Weinrach, S. G. (2004). Mental health counseling and the AMCD multicultural counseling competencies: A civil debate. *Journal of Mental Health Counseling, 26*(1), 41–43.

Thompson, V., & Alexander, H. (2006). Therapists' race and African American clients' reactions to therapy. *Psychotherapy: Theory, Research, Practice, Training, 43*(1), 99–110. doi:10.1037/0033-3204.43.1.99.

Thomspon, V. L., Bazile, A., & Akbar, M. (2004). African Americans' perceptions of psychotherapy and psychotherapists. *Professional Psychology: Research and Practice, 35*(1), 19–26.

Townsend, B. L. (2000). The disproportionate discipline of African American learners: Reducing school suspensions and expulsions. *Exceptional Children, 66*, 381–391.

Trivedi, P. (2002). Racism, social exclusion and mental health: A Black user's perspective. In K. Bhio (Ed.), *Racism and mental health: Prejudice and suffering* (pp. 71–82). Philadelphia: Jessica Kingsley Publishers.

Trotman, M. F. (2002). Involving the African American parent: Recommendations to increase the level of parent involvement within African American families. *The Journal of Negro Education, 70*, 275–285.

U.S. Department of Health and Human Services. (2001). *Mental health: Culture, race, and ethnicity—A supplement to mental health: A report of the Surgeon General.* Rockville, MD: U.S. Department of Health and Human Services.

Vera, E. M., Buhin, L., Montgomery, G., Shin, R., & Carter, R. T. (2005). Enhancing therapeutic interventions with people of color: Integrating outreach, advocacy, and prevention. In R. T. Carter (Ed.), *Handbook of racial-cultural psychology and counseling, Vol 2: Training and practice.* Hoboken, NJ: Wiley.

Wade, P., & Bernstein, B. L. (1991). Culture sensitivity training and counselor's race: Effects on Black female clients' perceptions and attrition. *Journal of Counseling Psychology, 38*, 9–15.

Wagner, M., Newman, L., & Cameto, R. (2004). *Changes over time in the secondary school experiences of students with disabilities. A report of findings from the National Longitudinal Transition Study (NLTS) and the National Longitudinal Transition Study-2 (NLTS2).* Menlo Park, CA: SRI International. Available at http://www.nlts2.org/reports/changes-time_report.html

Warren, A. E., Lerner, R. M., & Phelps, E. (2011). *Thriving and spirituality among youth: Research perspectives and future.* Hoboken: Wiley.

Weitock, T. (1991). *The development and implementation of a parent outreach program to increase school involvement of fourth grade parents.* Unpublished manuscript, Nova Southeastern University, Ft. Lauderdale, FL.

Whaley, A. L. (2001). Cultural mistrust: An important psychological construct for diagnosis and treatment of African Americans. *Professional Psychology: Research and Practice, 32*(6), 555–562. doi:10.1037/0735-7028.32.6.555.

Whaley, A. L., & Hall, B. N. (2009). Cultural themes in the psychotic symptoms of African American psychiatric patients. *Professional Psychology: Research and Practice, 40*(1), 75–80. doi:10.1037/a0011493.

Wiggan, G. (2008). From opposition to engagement: Lessons from high achieving African American students. *The Urban Review, 40*(4), 317–349. doi:10.1007/s11256-007-0067-5.

Wilson, K. B. (2005). Cultural Characteristics of the African American Community. In D. A. Harley, J. Dillard (Eds.), *Contemporary mental health issues among African Americans* (pp. 149–162). Alexandria, VA US: American Counseling Association.

Wu, P., Hoven, C. W., Cohen, P., Liu, X., Moore, R. E., Tiet, Q., et al. (2001). Factors associated with use of mental health services for depression by children and adolescents. *Psychiatric Services, 52*(2), 189–195.

Zweig, M. (2004). *What's class got to do with it?* New York: Cornell Press.

Black Parents Strengths and Strategies (BPSS) Program: A Cultural Adaptation of the Strong-Willed Child Program

6

Stephanie Irby Coard, Melvin H. Herring, Monica H. Watkins, Shani A. Foy-Watson, and Shuntay Z. McCoy

Introduction

Prevention scientists have become increasingly more aware of the need to include populations of color in their research. Historically, effective universal, selective and indicated prevention models endorsed by major funders, such as the National Institute of Drug Abuse (NIDA), Substance Abuse and Mental Health Services Administration (SAMHSA), Center for Mental Health Services (CMHS), and the Office of Juvenile Justice and Delinquency Prevention (OJJDP), have been based on models targeting non-minority populations, often neglecting the specific needs of individuals and groups of color. While minority populations have long been overrepresented in disparity data in terms of economic conditions, mother-headed households, academic underachievement, and involvement with the criminal justice system, they have remained underrepresented in prevention scholarship (Kumpfer & Alvarado, 2003). Lawmakers and funders began to scrutinize evidence-based programs to consider racial, ethnic and cultural factors in the reduction of these epidemic-level social, health and academic problems (Kellam & Langevin, 2003).

In response to these pressures, many prevention interventionists have begun collaborating with stakeholders, advocates, and local institutions in communities of color to expand outreach efforts in the recruitment of minority groups. This process has generated new questions regarding the challenges of recruiting and retaining minorities, the relevance of research in minority communities, engaging community members in research, assessing minority community needs, and the program fidelity and cultural adaptation of interventions in minority communities.

The Great Adaptation Debate: Program Fidelity Versus Cultural Specificity

As researchers have expanded their prevention efforts to be more inclusive of and receptive to minority populations, the use of program adaptation methods to address contextual issues has become more common. For example, there have been early efforts to develop contextually focused parenting intervention models that target the multiple environments (e.g., adverse effects of poverty and its accompanying stressors) in which economically disadvantaged youth operate (Webster-Stratton, 1995, 1998a, 1998b). Along with such parenting training efforts with low-income and disadvantaged families has come an increased awareness that these programs should be responsive to the social context (that is, the

S.I. Coard (✉) • M.H. Herring • M.H. Watkins
S.A. Foy-Watson • S.Z. McCoy
The University of North Carolina at Greensboro,
Greensboro, NC, USA
e-mail: sicoard@uncg.edu

needs and characteristics) of the community it serves. While such efforts have been key in emphasizing the importance of the social context and needs of economically disadvantaged parents and children, specific cultural/ethnic factors have not traditionally been addressed.

The prevention field remains divided on the cultural relevancy issue, as the theoretical and empirical evidence is equivocal (Dent, Sussman, Ellickson, Brown, & Richardson, 1996). The research community's debate over program fidelity vs. cultural "fit" continues to gain momentum. Many have acknowledged the challenge of culturally-modified versions maintaining the fidelity and effectiveness of their original format (Castro, Barrera, & Martinez, 2004). Proponents of program fidelity argue the criticality of maintaining the integrity of established preventive interventions and that any modifications to the established protocol may reduce the effectiveness of the program.

Contrary to this perspective, prevention interventionists targeting communities of color assert that because established protocols fail to adequately address racial, ethnic and cultural issues relevant to these communities of color, they have limited effectiveness with them. Some researchers believe that culturally modified programs are essential for the success of prevention (Kumpfer & Alvarado, 1995; Turner, 2000) and contend that adaptations to content and delivery may be necessary to engage families of color from urban neighborhoods to promote interest, participation and satisfaction with the intervention (Coard, Wallace, Stevenson, & Miller Brotman, 2004; Dumka, Roosa, Michaels, & Suh, 1995; Roosa, Dumka, Gonzales, & Knight, 2002). Researchers acknowledge that program infidelity will reduce positive outcomes and overall effectiveness of generic prevention intervention programs, even when cultural adaptations are successful (Kumpfer, Alvarado, Smith, & Bellamy, 2002). This debate suggests that the resolution is a "both/and" approach rather than an "either/or" approach to fidelity and cultural "fit." The authors contend that a "both/and" approach to culturally-specific adaptation and fidelity is an optimally effective strategy when working with minority populations and implemented with the proper balance.

This chapter outlines the process by which the authors' balanced the need for fidelity and cultural specificity in the development of the Black Parenting Strengths and Strategies (BPSS) program, a culturally- and strengths-based parenting preventive intervention designed to improve aspects of parenting associated with the early development of conduct problems and the promotion of social and cultural competence (Coard, Foy-Watson, Zimmer, & Wallace, 2007). The authors illustrate the challenges, added value and lessons learned in addressing racial, ethnic, and cultural factors, nuances, and competencies in both content and delivery adaptations.

Black Parents Strengths and Strategies: The Development Process

Goals

Program developers set out to develop a program that could address conceptual and practical issues in the field of prevention in a manner that was not only sensitive but directly relevant to the targeted families. The aim was for a program that: (a) was evidence-based; (b) was culturally- and strengths-based; (c) was tailored to economically disadvantaged African American families; (d) was easy to deliver; (e) did not require specialized professional staff; and (f) intervened prior to the development of conduct problems and impaired social and cultural functioning. A major goal of the intervention was to instill optimal parenting practices along with fostering African American parents' use of proactive racial socialization with their children in order to prevent the development of conduct problems and to enhance children's social and cultural competence. With this in mind, the program was specifically designed to be acceptable to and appropriate with African American families.

Standard Intervention

One of the most established and carefully evaluated parent training programs, (PSWC) *Parenting the Strong-Willed Child* (Long & Forehand,

2002), is a six-session evidence-based behavioral parent training program, recognized nationally and internationally for its general effectiveness. Weekly 2-h classes cover the material in 6 weeks. The original version of this parenting program, *Helping the Noncompliant Child*, was developed by Forehand and McMahon (1981) for use in the secondary prevention of serious conduct disorder problems in preschool and early elementary school-aged children, and for use as a primary tool for prevention of subsequent juvenile delinquency. The (PSWC) *Parenting the Strong-Willed Child* version of *Helping the Noncompliant Child* was developed to address significant restrictions caused by managed care and access to traditional mental health services where the original program was developed and utilized. The program and approach are outlined in the book (PSWC) *Parenting the Strong-Willed Child: The Clinically Proven Five-week Program for Parents of Two- to Six-Year Olds* (Forehand & Long, 2002). The program teaches skills (attending, rewards, ignoring, effective directions, time out) that assist parents in dealing with and preventing noncompliance and other problematic behavior. While the effectiveness of PSWC is established, and it has increasingly been used with ethnically diverse populations, it does not consider the "deeper" structural cultural adaptations (specific values, traditions, conditions) that may prove critical to optimal effectiveness.

To effectively make the adaptations, BPSS developers remained cognizant of the importance of maintaining the balance between fidelity and adaptation. Backer (2001) encouraged program developers to utilize a 12-step process when making adaptations to a universal program. BPSS developers used a modified version of Backer's 12-step process to incorporate the adaptations to the original program. The modified process consisted of the following steps: (a) identifying and understanding the theory and logic behind the program, (b) consulting with original program developers, (c) identifying and assessing the core components of the program, (d) assessing the adaptation and fidelity concerns of the African American community, (e) engaging the African American community in the program development process, (f) developing strategies for the implementation phase, and (g) evaluating the on-going fidelity and adaptation analysis.

Theory and Logic

Perhaps the most critical aspect of establishing a balance between program fidelity and adaptation is identifying an original program with a theoretical framework that effectively describes the targeted population once ethnic, demographic and/or cultural differences are considered. For BPSS developers, validating the transferability of PWSC theoretical underpinnings to the African American community was a vital step.

The PSWC program approach is a three-dimensional strategy that addresses strong-willed behavior by:

> First, helping parents understand their child's strong-willed behavior and how various factors influence such behavior. Second, involves teaching-specific parenting techniques for addressing the behavior problems most commonly exhibited by strong-willed children who are two to six years old. Third, involves helping to foster a climate within the family and home that will make these parenting techniques most effective (Forehand & Long, 2002, p. 2).

Consistent with the beliefs of the BPSS developers, the developers of the PSWC program ascribed to the notion that strong-willed children are born with a certain temperament-type that is predisposed to negative behavioral outcomes when appropriate interventions are absent during early childhood. Furthermore, neglectful parenting or an inadequate parenting style may exacerbate the situation and reinforce the negative developmental trajectory of the child and, in some cases, even expedite the process. Once confirmation of the alignment between the PSWC program and BPSS program objectives were established, the program developers were prepared to advance to the next phase; a consultation with the original program developers.

Consultation with Program Developers

Throughout the adaptation process, it was essential that the key elements of the standard parenting program were maintained and not diluted by the addition of new content or the omission of existing content. The BPSS developers received training on the standard program and received consultation from the original program developers throughout the adaptation process to ensure fidelity to the standard program. For example, one important aspect of the standard program that could not be altered was the order in which specific parenting skills were taught; only the companion parenting issues could be shifted and altered (e.g., inclusion of more culturally relevant examples when teaching the standard skills).

Drs. Long and Forehand provided consultation during the duration of this phase and reviewed the adaptations to ensure fidelity to the standard program. Additionally, they agreed to continue consultation through the latter stages of the process, including the pilot study.

Another critical fidelity issue that had to be addressed was dosage equivalency. The PSWC program was designed to be administered in six 2-h sessions over 6 weeks, while the culturally-modified version (BPSS) resulted in a program administered in twelve 2-h sessions over 12 weeks. In order to test equivalent dosage versions (interventions of equal length) in future evaluations, additional consultation from Drs. Long and Forehand was sought. How would the differences in program length and dosage of the intervention be addressed? It was decided that in order to address the imbalance in program length, each session of PSWC would be taught separately. For example, PSWC Session 2 topics *Rewards* and *Creating a More Positive Home* would be held in two separate sessions. Doing so throughout the entire program would result in the *PSWC* format being converted from a 6-week format to a 12-week format.

Core Components

Identifying components that were essential to the success of the original program was a necessity. Backer (2001) referred to these core components as "the main program ingredients." Conducting an analysis helped to determine the core of the program that was crucial to yielding the desired outcomes intended by the developers. For the purposes of this adaptation, the "analysis" refers to what the original program developers identified as core components (based on replicated evaluation data and the extant literature). The core components served as the foundation from which the modified program was created, as well as represented the section of the program that is more amenable to modifications. Furthermore, the extraction of these components establishes the bridge between the original and modified programs. BPSS developers were fortunate in that the original developers provided this information in consultation. Component analysis (based on earlier evaluation by and experience of original developers) concluded that all parenting skills taught in the original program must remain in their precise order and as designed for maximum effectiveness. The PSWC core components were the original five skills: *Attending, Rewarding, Ignoring, Giving Directions, and Using Time-Outs*. Therefore, the BPSS developers were challenged with determining the necessary adaptations to be made.

Adaptation Assessment

When considering adaptations for a particular population or group, the developers must assess a number of influential factors relevant to the feasibility of the modifications. For example, prior to implementing adaptations to the original program, BPSS developers conducted an assessment to identify specific issues or concerns when addressing the African American community such as available resources, demographic characteristics, and cultural nuances. More specifically, the developers had to determine which dimensions of adaptation were necessary for the African American community.

Castro et al. (2004) identified three dimensions of adaptations that developers should consider when addressing program-consumer fit. The *cognitive-information processing dimension* refers to adaptations made to program characteristics such as the language used and age appropriateness of content. Adaptations related to characteristics such as gender, ethnic background, religious background, and socioeconomic status describe the *affective-motivational dimension*. The third dimension assesses the *environmental* characteristics, such as the local community, that may be modified to increase the program's effectiveness with the targeted population.

Although BPSS developers incorporated adaptations on all three dimensions, the most defining adaptations occurred in the *affective-motivational dimension*. This dimension was critical in the adaptation process because it adequately addressed contextual (e.g., racial, ethnic, and cultural) issues relevant to Black communities. While maintaining program fidelity, BPSS developers made both surface (e.g., changing ethnicity of visible models and program representatives) and deep (e.g., core values, beliefs, norms, and cultural worldviews) structure changes (Castro et al., 2004). This was done to attend to the unique challenges that Black parents face in instilling common childrearing competencies and the racial realities in which Black children live that cannot be ignored: improve understanding of Black children's social and emotional development; increase children's confidence in school environments; develop positive self-image in Black children; promote positive discussion about race; and enhance children's problem solving skills (Coard et al., 2007). Studies of African American families suggest that the parenting of African American children involves specific parenting strategies (*racial socialization*) that are not accounted for in the general parenting or prevention literature. Racial socialization is important because: (1) It influences children's beliefs about the way the world works; (2) It informs children's beliefs and attitudes regarding "the self"; (3) It helps shape children's repertoire of strategies and skills for coping with and navigating racism; and (4) It impacts the nature of the children's inter- and intra-racial relationships and interactions. For a review of racial socialization in African American families see Coard and Sellers (2005).

The primary objective of the adapted components of the program was to assist African American parents in fostering cultural, social, and emotional health in their children. The program aimed to *strengthen* parenting skills; *improve* parental involvement; *empower* parents to advocate for their children and access community resources; and *guide* parents in preparing African American children for success.

Community Engagement

Involving the community or targeted population in the developmental process is vital to the overall success of the program. This step of the process serves three main functions: it allows the developer to identify specific issues challenging the local community or the community at large; it allows the end-user (program participant) to interject valuable information that may have been undetected by the developer; and it allows the developer and community an opportunity to foster a working relationship. Two major areas of concern consistently identified in the African American community by numerous researchers are low participant recruitment and retention rates.

To address the issue of recruiting African American parents, the BPSS developers employed culturally specific strategies to identify, market, and educate African American parents on the program's philosophy, opportunities, and community relevance. Additionally, the program developers utilized local economic (e.g., low income) and environmental factors (e.g., neighborhood violence and crime) to further distinguish among the communities in which BPSS would be most beneficial. Culturally familiar marketing materials, such as brochures displaying pictures and biographical narratives of Black staff and uplifting language, were also developed and distributed in targeted locations (e.g., barber shops, salons, street vendors, churches, block parties, the Department of Motor Vehicles). Once interest was expressed, BPSS staff continued to frequent sites targeted for recruitment and spent many hours developing rapport with parents and caregivers through telephone contacts and face-to-face home visits explaining, in further detail, the study's logistics (i.e., program purpose, intervention strategies, and participation requirements). The purpose of this rapport building was to be identified and perceived as committed "faces" of the community and not mere outsiders, recruiters or University personnel. This formal (yet informal) interactive style with the community members informed to a great extend what the community members were in need of, receptive to and most importantly, not going to support.

Another focus of the BPSS developers was to identify ways to maintain high retention and improve parental engagement among the program participants. BPSS achieved retention primarily through two methods: *consistent non-program communication/follow up* and *monetary and service incentives*. Communication and correspondence methods (e.g., frequent phone calls and mailing birthday or holiday cards) were employed to gently remind parents and caregivers of the researchers' interest in their participation and to foster trusting relationships with the families. In addition to communication and correspondence, the program developers provided monetary incentives and service incentives (i.e., participant service and support) to families who participated in the program. More specifically, given the financial constraints of many of the potential participants (i.e., low-income or poor), BPSS provided parents and caregivers a thirty-dollar gift for completing assessments and offered meals and childcare to families during program sessions. BPSS parents and caregivers were also provided with unsolicited periodic "check-ins" to simply let families know that their well-being is our priority.

Implementation

Engaging with the community (parents and caregivers who are potential and current program participants) in a proactive and genuine manner is critical to program implementation. It can provide invaluable information that may be useful in the implementation process. BPSS developers maximized on their interactions with the community by identifying critical resources needed for the implementation process with regard to feasibility testing and subsequent randomization of a control trial.

The first step in the BPSS developers' implementation strategy was to determine if their modified program was viable for the targeted community. In other words, would the program content meet the needs of the intended population? To answer this question, the developers conducted a feasibility test in the local African American community. Effective collaboration with local agencies allowed the developers to recruit parents and professionals (e.g., teachers, counselors, social workers, etc.) to evaluate and validate the relevance of the adapted materials. During this two hour process, the participants were encouraged to make recommendations for improvements to content and esthetic components of the modified materials, as well as instructed to interject their personal views regarding the sessions' content and to evaluate whether or not the skills taught would benefit their parenting processes and ultimately their children. Similarly, the professionals were invited to scrutinize the merit of the program objectives and to provide feedback regarding the relevance to African American parents in the area. This information was used to make modifications to the materials to maximize the program's effectiveness.

BPSS developers also conducted a randomized controlled trial to evaluate the feasibility of the adapted program. Due to the scarcity of culturally relevant, evidenced-based programs targeting African American parenting, it was critical for the developers to validate the relevance of the program through empirical methodology. The sample used in the trial consisted of 30 families (30 caregivers and 30 children) who self-identified as African American. The participants were from low socio-economic communities (unemployed and/or received public assistance) and had children between the ages of 5 and 6 years old. Prior to the initial assessment, the participants were provided with written materials describing the study. In an effort to alleviate any further concerns and strengthen the rapport with participants, developers conducted face-to-face interviews to address topics such as study rationale, randomization process, study conditions, length and extent of involvement, confidentiality, and other human subject issues (Coard et al., 2007). After the completion of a 2-h baseline assessment, the participants were randomized to the BPSS prevention program or the "wait list" control group. The BPSS group was administered the 12-week curriculum (twelve 2-h sessions/once per week) by two group leaders. Families assigned to the "wait list" group were subjected to group discussions covering various parenting topics, but were not provided with any supplemental educational materials. Both groups completed postintervention assessment at the end of the program. As a result, caregivers that were a part of the intervention program used significantly more racial socialization strategies, positive parenting practices, and less harsh discipline than those caregivers who were in the control group. Additionally, high rates of satisfaction and attendance were achieved, despite the multiple risk factors associated with caregivers. Results of pilot evaluation support the feasibility, acceptability, and potential efficacy of a culturally relevant intervention program. For a detailed report of randomized controlled trial evaluation findings please see Coard et al. (2007)

Content Adaptation

Content adaptation involves the modification of the original program curriculum (e.g., incorporation of culturally relevant historical models) to address the specific needs of the minority population. Based on extant literature on Black child development and Black family process, BPSS developers focused on four main areas of content adaptation related to parenting strategies for Blacks: *social exclusion*, *academic achievement*, *racism, and prejudices*. These areas of foci are also consistent with earlier qualitative work conducted by Coard et al. (2004). Similarly, when adapting universal programs for Blacks, it has been noted that researchers should consider extended family supports, strict disciplining practices, spirituality and religion, education, adaptability in family roles (Kumpfer et al., 2002), resiliency through financial and economic hardships, and discrimination; hence the selection of the four main areas of content adaption for BPSS.

Social Exclusion

The first dimension of the PSWC model focuses on helping parents understand and negotiate factors influencing the child's behavior, such as peer acceptance. Although the original model has been successful in achieving this goal with white participants, it fails to address the unique challenges experienced by Black families, such as social exclusion. Social exclusion refers to situations in which the child or parent is alienated from social opportunities because of racial biases.

The BPSS model addresses these issues in week 3 of the program by teaching parents how to discuss and problem solve sensitive social isolation or racial discriminatory situations with their children. One of the session goals is to increase parents' understanding of children's racial awareness. During the racial awareness, exercise parents are taught how to identify their child's level of racial awareness at various developmental stages. Understanding the child's racial awareness helps to prepare parents to address discriminatory situations, such as their child's experiences of racial slurs in school or being excluded from activities because of the color of their skin.

In addition to racial awareness, the BPSS incorporated culturally relevant problem solving techniques to address social exclusion issues. In session 10, parents are encouraged to revisit the basic strategies to problem solving, while simultaneously being introduced to strategies relevant to specific race-related incidences. For example, parents learn to teach their children basic skills for handling racism, such as identifying problems or situations as racial or prejudice, expressing their feelings about the experienced racism, expressing action regarding the experienced racism; involving proper authorities when indicated, and engaging parents in the racial experience by talking about what happened and how it made them feel.

Academic Achievement
Another critically important adaptation to the PSWC model was the consideration of the true

legacy for education and deep-seated cultural quest for academic advancement in the Black community. That is, the black community has long held the education of its children in the highest regard. Education is not only the most important measure of the ability to succeed but also the most powerful tool for challenging stereotypes and overcoming racial barriers. Education disparities exist across racial lines, despite the high regard that the Black community has held about education and long-standing belief that education is critical for a better life (Kantor & Lowe, 2006). Black children are exposed to instructional biases, lowered teacher expectations, discriminatory school climates, while parents are often excluded from decision-making processes and oblivious of their parental rights and school policies (Ladner & DiGeronimo, 2003). The BPSS model acknowledges and directly addresses the specific challenges that self-image plays in their academic achievement; institutional racism in schools; and the importance of parental involvement and advocacy in the educational process.

In week 9, parents are made aware of the impact their children's self-images have on their academic performance. The program acknowledges how racism and discriminatory experiences in school can deteriorate Black students' beliefs in the benefits of academic achievement by adolescence. For example, 80 % of Black children enter school with positive self-images, yet only 5 % maintain that positive self-image through their senior year in high school (Children's Resources for Community Day School Network, 2008). The BPSS model illustrates this influence by examining the harsh realities of institutional racism, including negative stereotyping and low teacher expectations, under-appreciation of non-academic strengths, absence of culturally relevant instructional materials, academic tracking, failure to foster higher-order thinking skills, and test biases for Black children. Parents are taught self-empowerment strategies (e.g., self-motivation, self control, self-reinforcement, communication skills) to provide their children so they have the tools for succeeding under whatever learning conditions exist, including conditions where they will receive very little academic support and encouragement.

Finally, BPSS modified the promotion of Black children's academic achievement by focusing on the parents' involvement and advocacy for their children in the educational process. Often Black parents are excluded from educational decisions regarding their children due to a lack of involvement in the educational process. However, in many cases Black parents have cited a lack of knowledge of rights, intimidation, and feelings of "unwelcomeness" by the school system as reasons for their lack of involvement. Coard et al. (2007) found that in many situations Black parents did not advocate for their children's academic track because of their lack of knowledge of rights and not due to their lack of willingness to be involved. BPSS engaged the parents in exercises that encouraged them to know their rights and school policies as well as to develop healthy communications with teachers and other parents in their children's school.

Racism, Prejudice, and Discrimination

The most significant adaptation made to the PSWC model by the BPSS developers is the incorporation of materials addressing situations of racism, prejudice, and discrimination. The original program based its concepts on white participants' encounters and experiences and neglected to consider those situations common to minority populations. BPSS emphasized a number of strategies to combat racism, prejudice and discrimination such as parental racial socialization practices (see discussion below); engagement in developmentally appropriate race-related discussions with their children; and understanding the influence of racism on family functioning.

Racial socialization is, perhaps, the most important factor in which a Black parent can contribute to the social success and mental well-being of their child. Racial socialization refers to "the process by which messages are transmitted or communicated inter- and intra-generationally regarding the significance and meaning of race and ethnicity" (Coard & Sellers, 2005, p. 266). BPSS addressed racial socialization in week 3 by defining the concept, assisting parents in identifying their own practices and strengthening and reinforcing their parenting skills with a better understanding of the process and its effects on their children. In this session, parents learned that the racial socialization process promotes *racism preparation* by emphasizing racial barriers, strategic racial protocol, and adaptive racial orientation, *racial pride* by emphasizing racial and ethnic pride and commitment in cultural history and heritage, *racial equality* by emphasizing humanitarianism and multi-ethnic co-existence, and *achievement* by emphasizing individual and academic achievement and good work ethic. Additionally, the session emphasized the positive impact racial socialization can have on a child's racial competence, academic achievement, self-efficacy, and self-esteem.

Finally, the BPSS model encouraged healthy and productive communications regarding race-related issues between Black parents and their children. For example, the parents are facilitated in an open group discussion of various race-related topics in order to foster collaborative efforts in developing relevant solutions and a sharing of ideas. Several of the topics of discussion included specific challenges faced by Black boys in society, how to debunk negative stereotypes, how to handle racial incidences, and understanding how race influences behavior. In session 6, BPSS incorporated its model of ineffective communication to illustrate how racism, prejudice, and discrimination cause increased distress for the Black family in addition to the normal daily life stressors. According to the model, this increase in distress perpetuates ineffective communications that often lead to a breakdown of family relationships. Black families' relationships and individual member success may be extremely vulnerable to racism, prejudice, and discrimination, particularly when they lack racial identity. Racial identity refers to one's acceptance and internalization of the race in which they belong. This includes embracing the strengths and weaknesses of the group. Racism, prejudice, and discrimination can exploit a minority member's uncertainty and lack of commitment to their race.

One of the many ways in which the BPSS model addresses the issue of racial identity with Black families is through the illustration of Black culture and success outside of the immediate family structure. The objective of the program was to provide parents with examples of ways in which Blacks have contributed to America and abroad. For example in session 3, BPSS developers exposed parents to a chronological evolution of Blacks plight from the slave trades of the 1500s to current events of the 2000s. An essential purpose of this session was to equip parents with a knowledge base from which to educate their children on the many struggles and accomplishments of Blacks.

Delivery Adaptations

Delivery adaptations involve modifications to how the program content is presented to the target population. Castro et al. (2004) suggest three forms of delivery adaptations that are necessary when modifying a universal program to meet the needs of a minority population: *characteristics of delivery person*, *channel of delivery*, and *location of delivery*. The channel of delivery refers to the median in which the program is delivered such as physical presentation, telephone, or the internet. The delivery adaptations made to this program did not include modifications to the *channel of delivery* and therefore, will not be discussed in the following sections. However, BPSS developers introduced a fourth form of delivery necessary when adapting universal programs to African American needs: *method of delivery*.

Characteristics of Delivery Person(s)

Modifying the characteristics of the delivery person (s) reinforces the rapport and relatedness between the program facilitators and participants. Shared characteristics, such as ethnicity, gender, and dialect/language may provide participants with a sense of familiarity that makes the program process somewhat more intimate. For example, BPSS utilized African American female facilitators, to reflect the demographic characteristics of participants. Research has found that matching ethnicity between facilitator and participant can have positive effects on program outcomes (Griner & Smith, 2006).

Perhaps the most important adaptation made to the characteristics of the delivery person(s) was the selected use of a culturally sensitive dialect or language. Some of the subtle nuances of this strategy were evident by the inclusive language used by BPSS facilitators. For example, facilitators consistently referred to the group as "we," "us," and "our" when discussing various issues. This language expression served a dual purpose with the participants in that it identified the facilitators as a part of the group, as well as maximized on the collectivistic orientation of the African American community.

A more demonstrative example of the use of culturally sensitive language by the BPSS facilitators was the incorporation of pledges, quotes, and poems into the program sessions. For example, at the end of each session the parents were encouraged to recite the pledge "I will show pride by liking myself, the way I look, the way I behave. By feeling good about where I come from, my history." This pledge was used to promote unity within the family while reminding the parents and children to embrace their cultural heritage. Additionally, a number of African Americans' quotes and African proverbs were incorporated into the sessions to articulate the practical messages in the sessions' topic. For instance, session 9s topic of "promoting good study habits" was illustrated in the African Proverb "If you don't know where you are going, then any road will take you there." Finally, the BPSS facilitators used culturally relevant poetry to communicate the uniqueness of African American people through their own words. A good example of this was in session 7 when the facilitators read and analyzed the poem "Lord Why Did You Make Me Black" by Runell Ni Ebo. The poem presented the opportunity to engage participants in discussions regarding ethnically sensitive issues such as skin color, racism, ethnic features, ethnic pride, and spirituality.

Location and Method of Delivery

The BPSS program was delivered at various locations including schools and community agencies. It is a manualized program that consists of explicit guidelines, techniques, and strategies. The manual is used to (1) discuss theory, program philosophy, general characteristics of the intervention process, sequencing of techniques, examples of intervention operations, guidelines for handling deviations, and the external boundaries of the Parent Training Program (e.g., activities not included in the intervention); (2) guide and standardize implementation; and (3) train future trainers and group leaders. The program is delivered to accommodate content designed to address the unique challenges that African American families experience. By taking a collaborative approach to working with parents, the program is sensitive to individual cultural differences and personal values. Furthermore, the program is tailored to each family's individual needs and goals, as well as to each child's strengths and weaknesses

Conclusion

Over the years, many have acknowledged the importance of including minority populations in research and understanding the importance of incorporating culture into intervention programming (Roosa et al., 2002). The BPSS program is an example of how researchers can extend their prevention outreach efforts to Black communities by adapting effective universal prevention programs to meet the culturally specific needs of Blacks (Coard, 2003). These adaptations included important issues that should be considered when making cultural adaptations to the content components of universal prevention programs targeting Black communities and the exploration of culturally adapted delivery strategies aimed at increasing the recruitment, retention, and overall program effectiveness with Blacks. In essence, BPSS serves as a model for incorporating culturally relevant content and processes into established evidence-based interventions that results in positive changes in parenting, including increase in positive parenting practices, increase in use of proactive racial socialization strategies, and positive changes in social and racial competence in African American children.

References

Backer, T. E. (2001). *Finding the balance—program fidelity and adaptation in substance abuse prevention: A state-of-the art review*. Rockville, MD: Center for Substance Abuse Prevention.

Castro, F., Barrera, M., & Martinez, C. (2004). The cultural adaptation of prevention interventions: Resolving tensions between fidelity and fit. *Prevention Science, 5*(1), 41–45.

Children's Resources for Community Day School Network Conference. (2008). *Improving Student Self-Image for Better Academic Achievement.* Community Day School Network 2008 Annual Conference. Sacramento, CA.

Coard, S. (2003). *Black parenting strengths and strategies program (BPSS): Trainer's manual.* Unpublished Manual. Duke University.

Coard, S., Foy-Watson, S., Zimmer, C., & Wallace, A. (2007). Considering culturally relevant parenting practices in intervention development and adaptation: A randomized control trial of the black parenting strengths and strategies (BPSS) program. *The Counseling Psychologist, 35*(6), 797–820.

Coard, S., & Sellers, R. (2005). African American families as a context for racial socialization. In V. C. McLoyd, N. E. Hill, K. A. Dodge, V. C. McLoyd, N. E. Hill, & K. A. Dodge (Eds.), *African American family life: Ecological and cultural diversity* (pp. 264–284). New York, NY US: Guilford Press.

Coard, S., Wallace, S., Stevenson, H., & Miller Brotman, L. (2004). Towards culturally competent preventive interventions: The consideration of racial socialization in parent training with African American families. *Journal of Child and Family Studies, 13*(3), 277–293.

Dent, C., Sussman, S., Ellickson, P., Brown, P., & Richardson, J. (1996). Is current drug use prevention programming generalizable across ethnic groups? *American Behavioral Scientist, 39*(7), 911–918.

Dumka, L., Roosa, M., Michaels, M., & Suh, K. (1995). Using research and theory to develop prevention programs for high-risk families. *Family Relations, 44,* 78–86.

Forehand, R., & Long, N. (2002). *Parenting the strong willed child: The clinically proven five-week program for parents of two- to six-year-olds.* Chicago: Contemporary Books.

Forehand, R., & McMahon, R. (1981). *Helping the non-compliant child: A clinician's guide to parent training.* New York: Guilford.

Griner, D., & Smith, T. (2006). Culturally adapted mental health interventions: A meta-analytic review. *Psychotherapy River Edge, 43*(4), 531–548.

Kantor, H., & Lowe, R. (2006). From new deal to no deal: No Child Left Behind and the devolution of responsibility for equal opportunity. *Harvard Educational Review, 76,* 474–502.

Kellam, S., & Langevin, D. (2003). A framework for understanding 'evidence' in prevention research and programs. *Prevention Science, 4*(3), 137–153.

Kumpfer, K., & Alvarado, R. (1995). Strengthening families to prevent drug use in multi-ethnic youth. In G. Botvin, S. Schinke, & M. Orlandi (Eds.), *Drug abuse prevention with multi-ethnic youth* (pp. 253–294). Newbury Park, CA: Sage Publications.

Kumpfer, K., & Alvarado, R. (2003). Family-strengthening approaches for the prevention of youth problem behaviors. *American Psychologist, 58*(6), 457–465.

Kumpfer, K., Alvarado, R., Smith, P., & Bellamy, N. (2002). Cultural sensitivity and adaptation in family-based prevention interventions. *Prevention Science, 3*(3), 241–246.

Ladner, J., & DiGeronimo, T. (2003). *Launching Black children for success: A guide for parents of kids from three to eighteen.* San Francisco: Jossey-Bass.

Long, N., & Forehand, R. (2002). *Parenting the strong-willed child leader's guide for the 6-week parenting class.* Unpublished manual. University of Arkansas for Medical Sciences.

Roosa, M. W., Dumka, L., Gonzales, N. A., & Knight, G. P. (2002). Cultural/ethnic issues and the prevention scientist in the 21st century. *Prevention and Treatment, 5,* Article 5. Posted January 15, 2002 on http://journals.apa.org/prvention/volume5/pre0050005a.html.

Turner, W. (2000). Cultural considerations in family-based primary prevention programs I drug abuse. *Journal of Primary Prevention, 21*(3), 285–303.

Webster-Stratton, C. (1995). *Preventing conduct problems in Head Start Children: Short term results of intervention.* Paper presented at the meeting of the Society for Research and Child Development. Indianapolis, Indiana.

Webster-Stratton, C. (1998a). Preventing Problems in Head Start children: Strengthening parenting competencies. *Journal of Consulting and Clinical Psychology, 66*(5), 715–730.

Webster-Stratton, C. (1998b). Parent training with low-income clients: promoting parental engagement through a collaborative approach. In J. R. Lutzker (Ed.), *Handbook of Child Abuse Research and Treatment* (pp. 183–210). New York: Plenum Press.

Working with Lesbian, Gay, Bisexual, and Transgender Youth in Schools

Nancy Bearss

The Experience of Lesbian, Gay, Bisexual, and Transgender Youth in US Schools

In 2010, the Gay, Lesbian and Straight Education Network (GLSEN) published the experiences of lesbian, gay, bisexual and transgender (LGBT) youth in our nation's schools. This survey used two methods of accessing this information: the surveys of randomly selected community organizations working with LGBT youth and surveys conducted through Internet sites. The sample consisted of 7,261 students between the ages of 13 and 21. The young people surveyed represented 50 states and the District of Columbia and 2,783 unique school districts. Seventy-four percent were White, 57.1% were female, and 61% of those surveyed were identified as gay or lesbian. The largest numbers of students were in grades 11–12.

The following findings reported by LGBT youth create a concern for all young people in our schools:

- 89% of students reported hearing the word "gay" being used in a negative manner.
- 61.1% of these young people reported feeling unsafe in school.
- 84.6% reported being verbally harassed and 40.1% reported being physically harassed because of their sexual orientation. 18.8% reported being physically assaulted.
- 52.9% of LGBT youth reported harassment by information or communication technologies: cyberbullying.
- 62.4% of youth reported that they did not report these events to school authorities and 33.8% of youth who did report it stated that nothing was done in response to the reports.

These conditions for GLBT youth result in increased days missed from school, decreased performance at school and increased psychological stress among LGBT youth (Kosciw, Greytak, Diaz, & Bartkiewicz, 2010).

Lower academic achievement was documented by the GLSEN study with the following results:

- LGBT students who reported being more frequently harassed because of sexual orientation or gender expression had average grade point averages (GPAs) of 2.7 compared to a 3.1 GPA among students who were less often harassed.
- LGBT students were more likely to report that they did not plan to pursue post-secondary education, including finishing high school or going to college, when compared to a national sample of students.

The GLSEN study revealed that the school environment for LGBT youth may be different based on race/ethnicity.

- African American LGBT youth were less likely to report feeling unsafe at school due to sexual orientation or gender expression than

N. Bearss (✉)
La Red Health Center, Georgetown, DE, USA
e-mail: nbearss@towson.edu

Hispanic/Latino, White/European American and multiracial students.
- African American LGBT youth were less likely to report being harassed or assaulted than Hispanic/Latino, White/European American and multiracial students.
- Asian/Pacific Islander LGBT students were less likely to feel unsafe at school because of sexual orientation or gender expression than Hispanic/Latino, White/European American or multiracial students.
- Asian/Pacific Islander LGBT youth were less likely to report experiencing harassment or assault based on sexual orientation than Hispanic/Latino, White/European American or multiracial students.
- Asian/Pacific Islander LGBT youth were less likely to be harassed or assaulted based on gender expression than multiracial students.

Despite these differences, students of color who are LGBT have consistently reported school environments as hostile. The authors reported that they were unable, from their data, to understand the differences found among different ethnic groups. To date, there is inadequate research available that allows us to understand the specific factors leading to these reported differences.

Conditions in schools for LGBT youth have improved since the first report of the GLSEN network in 1999, but only in schools who have developed inclusive curriculum, identified supportive educators, developed Gay and Straight Alliances and developed comprehensive bullying/harassment policies and laws. In addition to this comprehensive report, the National Education Association (NEA) held a summit in 2009 to look at the issues facing LGBT youth in schools. The purpose of this summit as stated by the NEA was "to elicit the best available research regarding the impact of LGBT issues on students and education and to examine what is working and what is not" (Kim, 2009, p. vi). As is reflected by the research done by GLSEN, the NEA report found similar findings supported by those of GLSEN. According to summit participant Professor Dr. Catherine Lug, who spoke on the role of GLBT youth in society and education, schools are indeed a microcosm of society and American society has a history of viewing LGBT individuals as "criminal, sinful or sick" (Kim, 2009, p. 3).

In 1973, the American Psychiatric Association (APA) declassified homosexuality as a mental disorder. The Diagnostic and Statistical Manual of Mental Disorders (DSM IV, 2000) that is published by the American Psychiatric Association and defines the standards in the field of psychiatry, does not include homosexuality.

There has since been support from all other major health professional organizations in declassifying homosexuality as a mental disorder. In spite of these professional changes and sustained positions by the American Academy of Pediatrics, the American Counseling Association, the American Psychiatric Association, the American Psychological Association, and the American School Counselor Association, there continue to be efforts to change sexual orientation through therapy by some political and religious organizations (Just the Facts Coalition, 2008). Such efforts have serious potential for harm, especially to young people. In addition, it may be difficult for LGBT individuals to find counseling support, especially in rural or economically disadvantaged areas.

Risk Factors among Lesbian, Gay, Bisexual, and Transgender Youth

A recent review of adolescent health services commissioned by the National Research Council/Institute of Medicine Board on Children, Youth and Families (Lawrence, Appleton Gootman, & Sims, 2009) found that the frequent practice in mental health domains is to simply ask young people whether there are any areas of concern. Health personnel, including mental health providers, often rely upon clients to initiate discussions related to high-risk behaviors. The common practice is to use open-ended questions about health or mental health concerns or to use trigger questions around a specific topic. This results in a general lack of communication about high-risk issues for LGBT youth who may perceive themselves as socially distant from mental health providers or primary care providers (Lawrence et al., 2009).

A recent surveillance summary published by the Centers for Disease Control and Prevention (2011) reflects the increased stress felt by GLBT youth. The Youth Risk Behavior Surveillance System monitors priority health-risk behaviors among youth attending schools. These include behaviors that contribute to unintentional injury, violence, attempted suicide, tobacco use, alcohol use, other drug use, sexual behaviors, dietary behaviors, physical activity and sedentary behaviors and weight management. The survey is conducted by state and local health and education agencies. Seven states and six large urban school districts from years 2001–2009 included questions on sexual identity or sex of sexual contacts among students in grades 9–12. Across the nine states the prevalence of high-risk behavior was on an average 63.8% higher among gay and lesbian youth and on the average 76% higher among bisexual youth than heterosexual youth. Behaviors that contribute to violence, attempted suicide, tobacco use, alcohol use, other drug use, sexual behaviors, and weight management were more prevalent among gay or lesbian students than heterosexual students.

National surveys report sexual orientation as an independent predictor of suicide attempts with gay, bisexual and transgender adolescents twice as likely to attempt suicide as heterosexual youth. Smaller studies report young men who are bisexual or gay having suicide attempts as high as seven times those of heterosexual males (Lawrence et al., 2009). Bisexual youth have a greater risk of substance and tobacco use than heterosexual youth, with reported higher rates of marijuana use, binge drinking, getting drunk, drinking alone, and using illicit drugs. These higher rates do not hold for youth reporting same-sex attraction only (Lawrence, et al., 2009).

Risk behaviors relating to eating and body image disorders reveal that young lesbians are at less risk of developing a problem with eating or body image than their heterosexual counterparts but that the opposite is true of young gay or bisexual males. Lesbian and bisexual females report being happier with their bodies than heterosexual females. They are less likely to report trying to look like women in the media. Gay and bisexual males, on the other hand, are more concerned with trying to look like images of men in the media and are more likely to binge eat (Lawrence, et al., 2009).

High-risk sexual behavior is well documented among lesbian, gay, and bisexual youth. Lesbian, gay, and bisexual youth report more unprotected sex and they initiate sexual contact earlier than heterosexual youth. Young gay and bisexual men have a higher incidence of unprotected anal intercourse and young lesbian and bisexual women report having unprotected intercourse with men, putting them at higher risk of unwanted pregnancy. Young lesbians are also less likely to engage in health promotion activities, such as annual pelvic examinations (Lawrence, et al., 2009). Lesbian, gay, and bisexual youth have higher rates of exposure to violence, including being threatened with a weapon, being in a physical fight and being raped (Lawrence, et al., 2009).

The mental health needs of transgender youth are not well understood, with the *Diagnostic and Statistical Manual of Mental Disorders, Fourth Edition* (DSM-IV, 2000) categorizing these youth as having gender identity disorder. *The Diagnostic and Statistical Manual of Mental Disorders, Fourth Edition* (DSM-IV, 2000) requires two components of "Gender Identity Disorder" both which must be present to make the diagnosis. Individuals who self-identity as transgender with no hormonal explanation (such as any individual who has a concurrent physical intersex condition such as androgen insensitivity or congenital adrenal hyperplasia) may or may not be diagnosed with Gender Identity Disorder, dependent upon the discomfort they feel with identifying as the opposite sex. There must also be evidence of a strong and persistent cross-gender identification and there must be persistent discomfort about one's assigned sex or a sense of inappropriateness in the gender role of that sex. This discomfort can manifest in depression, anxiety, relationship difficulties, and personality disorders. Treatment goals include acceptance of the assigned gender and resolution of the depression or anxiety. There is continual discussion of the use of this categorization of transgender youth. There is currently no United States (U.S.) or state-based representative data on transgenderism in adolescence. Smaller studies reveal that transgender youth also suffer higher rates of depression, suicide attempts, risky sexual behavior, violence, HIV infection, and homelessness (Lawrence et al., 2009).

The criminal justice system has not protected LGBT individuals who are incarcerated. In male facilities, gay men, and male to female transgender prisoners have been shown to be especially vulnerable to sexual abuse, sexual exploitation, and rape (Ray, 2006). There is little research available on the treatment of LGBT youth and the criminal justice system although it is clear that these youth are more likely to encounter this system than heterosexual youth, in large part because of the above-mentioned risk factors and the increased risk of homelessness. In February, 2006, an 18-year-old lesbian, a 17-year-old transgender female, and an 18-year-old male who was perceived to be gay filed a lawsuit against the state of Hawaii for abuse in their juvenile justice system. Hawaii will now be accountable for more than a dozen requests of protection from violence related to sexual orientation or sex (Ray, 2006).

Athletics: LGBT athletes face a special set of circumstances in schools. Virtually, no major athletic organization in this country addresses discrimination against lesbian, gay, bisexual, or transgender individuals. The Gay Olympics is a separate event that allows expression of incredible athletic ability among LGBT individuals, but again, it is a separate event in response to this overt prejudice that is present in U.S. national sports. Athletic participation necessarily reinforces gender stereotypes and gender roles, initially on the basis of physiologic differences between young boys and girls. The history of athletics in the United States has been male-dominated. Although Title IX has given support to women in sports, women athletes tend to not share the same rewards as male athletes in the United States. This prejudice lends itself to same sex environments, putting LGBT youth in especially vulnerable areas for victimization. There is little research on the continual impact of this vulnerability, especially in middle and high school sports settings. Special training for coaches is recommended to protect LGBT youth from the increased harassment that may occur during athletic functions in schools.

Religion: The impact of religion on LGBT youth has been profound in the United States. LGBT youth have had severe inhibitions on their ability to develop spiritually. Professor Stacey Horn, a summit participant in the NEA study, stated that "belonging to a particular religious denomination appears to correlate more to higher levels of sexual prejudice than belonging to a particular race or ethnicity" (Kim, 2009).

Since the passage of the executive order in 2002 by President George W. Bush permitting federal funding for faith-based organizations to provide social services, funding for youth services that are not faith-based have decreased. These nonfaith-based organizations often serve LGBT youth, especially those youth who have experienced rejection by their families, and have suddenly found themselves without a safe haven. As a report on homeless youth from the LGBT Task Force states: "If an organization's core belief is that homosexuality is wrong, that organization (and its committed leaders and volunteers) may not respect a client's sexual orientation or gender identity and may expose LGBT youth to discriminatory treatment" (Ray, 2006, p. 5).

As LGBT youth find themselves transitioning into adult American society under hostile circumstances, they face an increased risk of both mental and physical instability. Homelessness, according to the National Gay and Lesbian Task Force, is high among LGBT youth (Ray, 2006). The study conducted by the Task Force in 2006 reports between 20 and 40% of all homeless youth identifying as LGBT. According to this study, "Family conflict is the primary cause of homelessness for all youth, LGBT or straight. Specifically, familial conflict over a youth's sexual orientation or gender identity is a significant factor that leads to homelessness or the need for out-of-home care. According to one study, 50%

of gay teens experienced a negative reaction from their parents when they came out and 26% were kicked out of their homes. Another study found that more than one-third of youth who are homeless or in the care of social services experienced a violent physical assault when they came out, which can lead to youth leaving a shelter or foster home because they actually feel safer on the streets" (Ray, 2006, p. 2).

The increased incidence of mental illness, substance abuse, risky sexual behavior, and exposure to the criminal justice system make LGBT youth particularly vulnerable. The ability of schools to accommodate them is particularly poor. According to the NEA study, "First, we know from community-based surveys and research studies that many students miss or drop-out of school at least in part because of difficulties related to their LGBT identity" (Kim, 2009, p 29). Student victimization appears to be the factor that separates LGBT youth from heterosexual youth as the major reason for missed school or school dropout. LGBT identified youth are 1.75 times as likely to consider dropping out of school when compared to their heterosexual peers (Kim, 2009). Questioning youth, or young people who are in the process of questioning their sexual orientation, are an even more vulnerable population. They are seven times as likely to consider dropping out of school as heterosexual youth, and four times as likely as LGBT youth. This statistic speaks to the continuum of sexual development we all experience and the necessity of understanding and integrating a healthy, supportive model in schools that supports this development.

The experience of LGBT youth in schools is fraught with danger and uncertainty, reflective of society at large. According to the NEA study, the ability of schools to address this danger has been inadequate. Perpetrators of homophobic behavior are not concerned about the actual sexual orientation of their targets, just the perception of gender nonconformity (Kim, 2009). According to the authors, "Students who commit homophobic acts need not rely on actual knowledge that their target is LGBT; heterosexual students, particularly those who are gender-nonconforming, may be targeted as LGBT just as often as LGBT students. Many students, particularly elementary and middle school children both commit and are victimized by homophobic acts even before they have any awareness of their own or others' sexual orientation. Thus, schools can identify youth who are likely targets of homophobia without knowing or inquiring into their actual sexual orientation (which would be legally problematic in any event) and can also foster a climate that is safe for all youth—even those who are not visibly gender-nonconforming" (Kim, p. 31).

In addition, school personnel and parents have reported feeling unsupported when they bring up issues confronting LGBT youth. LGBT school personnel face significant, dangerous obstacles when addressing youth in the context of their professional role. This leaves many LGBT youth without obvious, necessary role models. School administrators have not been successful in eliminating fear among teaching staff for many issues facing at-risk youth. Clear guidelines for teachers are not readily available on how to handle LGBT issues when they arise and there are no guidelines for LGBT teachers or parents when they are feeling marginalized or victimized in the school environment.

In summary, the current status of LGBT youth in schools is wholly inadequate to meet their educational needs. Although there have been improvements since Stonewall in 1969, young people who are gay, lesbian, bisexual, transgender or questioning are still bullied, harassed, violated, isolated and ignored in their attempts to navigate their transition to adulthood. The raid by police on Stonewall Inn, a popular gay bar in New York City in June of 1969 sparked a large resistance estimated to reach 2,000 people with over 400 police officers. This raid on Stonewall mobilized LGBT communities and started the conversation around the civil liberties of gays and lesbians around the globe. It is imperative that as an open society we work to continue to address these inadequacies in a manner that reflects a tolerant, compassionate community.

Strengths and Coping Mechanisms among Gay, Lesbian, Bisexual, and Transgender Youth in Schools

Developmental and Contextual Considerations

The ability of the gay, lesbian, bisexual, or transgender young person to adapt to the dominant culture in the United States is fraught with danger and confusion. The acceptance of homosexuality in the mental health field and in mainstream culture is still evolving, and although there has been progress, young people receive constant mixed messages regarding healthy sexual behavior, including same sex relationships. Human sexuality is a dynamic characteristic, influenced by both socio-cultural and biological factors. Gender identity is formed as early as age 3 with gender constancy established by ages 5–6. A young person who is transgender will identify as the opposite of their phenotypic gender and may be attracted to either male or female independent of their gender constancy (Haffner, 1999).

Sexual attraction, on the other hand, does not develop until pre-adolescence, at the onset of puberty (Haffner, 1999). Dating and the development of intimate relationships in middle and high school begins the realization of same sex attraction in LGBT youth as different than that of heterosexual adolescents. By middle childhood, a young child is able to make social comparisons and form an abstract concept of him or herself. As girls and boys approach adolescence, the gender roles they adapt are heavily influenced by the intense socialization they have received in early development.

The nonacceptance of same sex relationships or of nonconforming gender roles may create shame among LGBT youth during this phase and reinforce conforming sexual roles. Negative peer reactions to nonconforming roles will further this shame and socially isolate LGBT youth, thus leading to the many deleterious outcomes described in the above section. As adolescence approaches, it is important to allow a young person only as much help as they want at the time.

Primary family dynamics, especially if these dynamics are of rejection and nonacceptance, can affect the sexual behavior of a questioning adolescent or result in acting out, unsafe heterosexual behavior.

Coping mechanisms are varied and evolving in adolescents and behavior in school can be a reflection of difficulties coping with the mistreatment and unfairness that gay, lesbian, bisexual and transgender individuals continue to encounter in American society. As with any civil rights dynamic, protective legislation occurs decades before full cultural integration and acceptance. There is a large body of literature that documents that LGBT youth or young people who do not conform to heterosexual norms are at risk for victimization and the psychological harm that comes from such victimization (Toomey, Ryan, Diaz, Card, & Russell, 2010).

This victimization occurs among LGBT youth, with transgender and questioning youth at most risk. Boys experience greater levels of victimization than girls. Consistent with minority stress models hypothesized by Meyer (2003) victimization due to LGBT status is significantly associated with psychosocial adjustment, when measured by life satisfaction and depression.

Furthermore, the development of school policies and practices that affect all students regardless of gender, that prohibit victimization due to LGBT status can help reduce negative psychosocial outcomes in LGBT and gender nonconforming youth. This evidence reinforces the need for clearly articulated and implemented anti-bullying policies in school.

In 1977, Brofenbrenner published an article in *The American Psychologist* that proposed an ecological perspective on human development that puts the child at the center of multiple levels of influence along a proximal-distal dimension based on the immediacy of direct influence (Bronfenbrenner, 1977). LGBT youth bring an array of personal characteristics to school and the application of those characteristics to a school environment shapes their individual experience and future health and well-being. It is in this context that an approach to LGBT youth in schools is offered. It is important for all school personnel to have access to mental health providers who are competent working with LGBT youth and their families.

Horn, Kosciw, and Russell (2009) have suggested a shift in the context in which we frame the experiences of LGBT youth. They suggest that we move beyond studying LGBT youth in the context of at-risk youth and try to focus on understanding ways that LGBT youth can cope and negotiate their development within various social contexts. This allows us to individualize the experience of young people who are LGBT and integrate their unique characteristics such as temperament and gender identity into their social experience.

School Environments

There is an increase in the number of LGBT students who report being in school environments with inclusive policies and programs. Yet there is little evidence that the presence of such programs is protective for LGBT youth. Students who are in school environments where anti-LGBT harassment is frequent or perceived to be frequent are more likely to be victimized than students where such harassment is rare or not tolerated. Chesir-Teran and Hughes (2009) found in their study of heterosexism and victimization of LGBT youth that manifestations of heterosexism in policies, programs, and social features of schools have a moderate correlation with each other. Perceptions of nondiscrimination and harassment policies and the presence of inclusive programs were both predictive of student's perception of the prevalence and tolerance of anti-lesbian, gay and bisexual harassment in schools. They found that effects of perceived programs were stronger than those of policies. They hypothesize that the presence of such programs, such as Gay and Straight Alliances, may be more likely to form in schools who have adapted anti-bullying, anti-harassment policies. Their study further found that personal experiences of victimization were related to the perceived prevalence and tolerance of anti-lesbian, gay, bisexual and questioning harassment in schools. There is sufficient evidence that schools can improve LGBT student capacity and performance by adapting policies and programs that prohibit bullying and harassment.

School climate has long been associated with outcome measures in students. In their study of high-risk behavior among LGBT youth, Birkett and Espelage (2009) found that all children, regardless of sexual orientation, reported the lowest levels of depression, illicit drug and alcohol use and truancy, when in a positive school environment free of homophobic teasing. The most important lesson learned from their study is that schools have a direct responsibility to consider the needs of their sexual minority students. Again, this study suggests that preventing bullying is not enough for a school to improve the lives of LGBT youth, that a general attitude and climate of tolerance will improve outcomes in all school children.

Espelage, Aragon, Birkett, and Koenig (2008) also examined protective measures for LGBT youth in schools. Their study found that a supportive school and parental environment provided protection for gay, lesbian and bisexual and questioning youth from depression and illicit drug use. Of particular interest in this study was the impact of a hostile school and home environment on questioning youth, making this population more vulnerable, perhaps because they do not perceive themselves as having the support of other gay, lesbian and bisexual youth. Anti-bullying policies and anti-harassment policies have been developed across the country to assist schools in dealing with this victimization. These are described in the next section.

Sex education has a rich, tumultuous history in the United States, with sound evidence-based curriculum and training available to every educator in the country (National Guidelines Task Force, 2004). This curriculum embraces an open, respectful approach to sexual development, enhancing respectful and mutual relationships regardless of gender preference.

In spite of this availability, U.S. health educators are bound by local school boards to teach a limited curriculum. Abstinence only or curricula that excludes open acceptance of same sex relationships occurs throughout the country with little or no effective resistance. Other areas of the school curriculum such as social studies and literature have yet to embrace LGBT culture as an open part of the curriculum. To date, there is very little literature on the ability of public schools to fully integrate LGBT issues into schoolwide curriculum (Bearss, 2010).

Media Presentation of Role Models

While risk factors associated with athletics were discussed above, LGBT role models in sports also present a protective factor. In fact LGBT role models in entertainment and society at large have increased dramatically over the past two decades. The normalization of gay culture for many Americans who have been able to find supportive, open environments has transferred to young LGBT individuals. As young people find accepting environments in the larger society, LGBT youth find it less necessary to focus on their sexuality and instead focus on other characteristics that will make them successful adults. In his book, *The New Gay Teenager (Adolescent Lives)*, Savin-Williams (2005) explains this generational shift. He presents the argument and supportive evidence through interviews with young developing adolescents, that young people have same sex attractions and desires but, unlike earlier generations, are not labeling themselves as gay. He argues that "teenagers are increasingly redefining, reinterpreting, and renegotiating their sexuality such that possessing a gay, lesbian, or bisexual identity is practically meaningless" (Savin-Williams, 2005, p. 1). He states that "rather than obsessing over their sexuality, young adults are occupied with typical college pursuits, including sports, fraternities and careers. The sex scene is similar to that of straights, with lots of hook ups and few long term relationships. Few assert a gay identity or define themselves in relation to straight culture" (Savin-Williams, 2005, pp. 200–201). Savin-Williams asserts that this mainstreaming of sexual identity has not yet made its way into the school system. Young people interviewed by him reported being hesitant to be open about their same-sex relationships in school settings.

Cultural Considerations among LGBT Youth in Schools

There is no evidence that the formation of sexual identity is significantly influenced by cultural factors. In addition, Black and Latino youth do not differ from White youth in their acceptance of their own sexuality (Bridges, 2007). There are many dimensions of disparity that exist in the United States and contribute to poorer health outcomes. These include race or ethnicity, sex, sexual identity, age, disability, socioeconomic status, and geographic location. For the past two decades, *Healthy People* has focused on disparities and the reduction of health disparities as one of its overarching goals (www.healthypeople.gov). These disparities contribute to an individual's ability to achieve good health. The double burden of discrimination due to race/ethnicity and sexual identity falls on young people and increases their risk of social stress and poor health outcomes. The following disparities have been found in young people of color who are LGBT or questioning:

- LGBT youth of color are significantly less likely to have told their parents about their sexuality.
- African-American same-sex attracted youth are more likely to have low self-esteem and experience suicidal thoughts than young people of other racial/ethnic backgrounds. Young LGBT African American men are more likely to be depressed.
- Latino communities report that homophonic attitudes reinforced by machismo and Catholicism prevent young LGBT youth from accessing information about safe sex practices.
- LGBT youth of color feel pressure to choose between their racial/ethnic and their sexual identities and often miss gay-centered activities that may help combat homophobia when compared to their White counterparts.

In addition, the following disparities have been found with regard to LGBT youth of color and sexual activity:

- HIV rates for African American men ages 15–22 is 16% when compared to 7% for Latino male youth and 3% for White male youth.

- Transgender youth of color have experienced forced sex with one study stating that almost 60% of transgender minority youth had traded sex for money or resources.
- The majority of LGBTQ youth of color have experienced victimization in school because of either race or sexual identity, while half report being victimized because of both race and sexual identity.
- More than a third of LGBTQ youth of color have experienced physical violence because of their orientation.

The combined exposure to racism and homophobia make minority LGBT youth especially vulnerable in schools. Programs and policies should be evaluated in their ability to capture and access minority youth in an equitable, open manner. There is a strong need for more evidence-based approaches to reaching minority students in schools.

Successful Interventions in Schools

The final section of this chapter deals with recommended school interventions to promote well-being for LGBT youth. Many of these interventions have been shown to improve school climate for all youth. The approach taken is one of a coordinated school health (CSH) model. It will be presented in a manner where individual student needs are addressed, and school policies as well as the development of model programs are described. This section attempts to provide the resources needed for all educators and individuals working with LGBT youth.

It is well established that when student mental health needs are met, the likelihood of school success increases (Hurwitz and Weston, 2010). This allows researchers to focus on broad school achievement as an outcome measure when looking at CSH and mental health. In addition, school mental health promotion activities have been shown to create an environment where students can learn. School climate is indirectly related to school achievement but as we have seen, for LGBT youth, a safe school climate is essential to prevent bullying and victimization. The presence of school mental health services allows teachers and school staff to enhance their ability to teach and serve students. Finally, schools are where children are located, allowing an increased impact of prevention, early intervention and treatment. The provision of these services on site at school reduces the cost of overall mental health services.

There are five overarching tenets or "pillars" that can and should be addressed when focusing on diversity in education and LGBT populations (Kim, 2009). These include:

1. *Cultural competency*: Awareness of LGBT youth in language, diversity, celebrations, events, and publications.
2. *School leadership*: Implementing policies, procedures, professional development, and programs on LGBT issues.
3. *Environmental and behavioral monitoring*: Vigorously promoting safety and protecting all members of the school community.
4. *Mental and physical needs*: Helping students and staff cope with physical needs, stress and marginalization.
5. *Engagement and socialization*: Linking with community activities and outside organizations.

The public health and school health community have adapted the CSH model first described by Allensworth and Kolbe (1987). This approach has eight interrelated components:

1. Comprehensive health education
2. Physical education
3. Health services
4. Nutrition services
5. Counseling, psychological and social services
6. Healthy school environment
7. Health promotion for staff and
8. Family/Community involvement

The Centers for Disease Control and Prevention (CDC) have used the same CSH model to prevent injury and harm to young people in schools (CDC, 2001). These guidelines were developed by the CDC in collaboration with specialists from universities, national, federal, state, and local organizations. They are based on an in-depth review of the research, theory and current practice in preventing injury to young people using the public health model. The following describes the CDC recommendations:

- *Recommendation 1: Social environment*: Establish a social environment that promotes safety and prevents unintentional injuries, violence, and suicide.
- *Recommendation 2: Physical environment*: Provide a physical environment, inside and outside school buildings, that promotes safety and prevents unintentional injuries and violence.
- *Recommendation 3: Health education*: Implement health and safety education curricula and instruction that help students develop the knowledge, attitudes, behavioral skills, and confidence needed to adopt and maintain safe lifestyles and to advocate for health and safety.
- *Recommendation 4: Physical education and physical activity programs*: Provide safe physical education and extracurricular physical activity programs.
- *Recommendation 5: Health services*: Provide health, counseling, psychological, and social services to meet the physical, mental, emotional, and social health needs of students.
- *Recommendation 6: Crisis response*: Establish mechanisms for short- and long-term responses to crises, disasters, and injuries that affect the school community.
- *Recommendation 7: Family and community*: Integrate school, family, and community efforts to prevent unintentional injuries, violence, and suicide.
- *Recommendation 8: Staff members*: For all school personnel, provide staff development services that impart the knowledge, skills, and confidence to effectively promote safety and prevent unintentional injuries, violence, and suicide, and support students in their efforts to do the same.

A stepwide approach is not feasible when adapting these models to school environments. All of these approaches must take place concurrently and in conjunction with each other. Regular meetings should occur that ensure that individual, schoolwide, and community services are well coordinated. Support for these approaches should be mandated at the very top, and not marginalized to a "special service."

The first approach discussed that uses this public health model is the provision of individual support to LGBT youth and LGBT faculty. On an individual level, school staff and students should be alert to signs of distress from harassment or victimization and be able to refer individuals for support to address these cases. Addressing health services by providing counseling, psychological and social services, treatment, referral and follow-up services should be implemented either through student support services, the school nurse or ideally, a school-based wellness program. These services should be offered to all students or faculty who present with mental health or behavioral problems that interfere with their functioning at home, in school, with peers, or in the classroom. The APA Healthy Lesbian, Gay and Bisexual Students Project is an example of this approach. It was designed to help schools improve mental health outcomes for sexual minority youth. With the help of the CDC, this program provided science-based workshops for school personnel on how to reach LGBT youth with prevention messages. Education societies in Connecticut, Massachusetts, Delaware and San Diego have since formed their own training staff to continue the trainings locally (CDC, 2011).

For LGBT youth who present with mental health issues or who need support, it is essential that services are provided by providers who are developmentally appropriate, research-based, family centered and culturally competent. Efforts should be made to identify supportive counseling centers in the community and to regularly evaluate that LGBT youth benefit from the services provided. Support for parents should be sought out in cases where LGBT youth express discrimination or problems at home.

Advocates for Youth established a Health Care Bill of Rights for LGBTQ youth that includes the tenets listed below. LGBT youth can be asked if these rights are being met when they encounter individual providers in the school or community (Gilliam, 2002). This states:

- You have a right to receive treatment without discrimination on the basis of race/ethnicity,

religion, gender, gender identity, disability, or sexual orientation.
- You have a right to receive respect and positive, caring treatment.
- You have a right to ask questions. You have a right to ask for clarification and to receive explanations of tests, treatments, treatment options, and all aspects of your care.
- You have a right to receive confidential and affordable care. Your provider should assure you that the information you share is confidential and will not be disclosed to a parent or guardian unless you provide permission.
- If the provider will not guarantee your confidentiality, you have a right to find a provider who will. You should not be denied care based on your ability to pay.
- You have a right to accurate, uncensored information.
- You have a right to demand youth-friendly services that are flexible and culturally appropriate.
- You have a right to nonjudgmental health care. Your provider should not make assumptions about your behavior.
- You have a right to disclose your sexual identity, gender identity, and sexual activities. This information may help providers understand what types of tests, referral, and health information you need.
- You have a right to say "no" to care and to learn about the effect this may have on your health.
- You have a right to change providers at any time and for any reason. You also have a right to a second opinion.

Schools are encouraged to be proactive about providing this level of support. School counselors should identify the counselors in their area that are competent in dealing with LGBT youth and issues of sexual development. National mental health organizations that can help identify individual counselors throughout the country are provided in the resource list included in the chapter. The APA also publishes a primer of sexual orientation and youth that should be available to all school personnel (Just the Facts Coalition, 2008).

The next concurrent approach in this comprehensive school health/public health model is to enhance school policies. School policies should be evaluated with their respect to LGBT youth and faculty. All of the evidence reviewed supports a specific anti-bullying policy. Schools who adapt anti-bullying policies must clarify that any teasing and exclusion based on sexual orientation is fully prohibited. The National School Climate Study recommends that schools "adopt and implement comprehensive harassment/assault policies that specifically enumerate sexual orientation, gender identity, and gender expression in individual schools and districts, with clear and effective systems for reporting and addressing incidents that students experience" (Kosciw et al., 2010 p.127).

The first major anti-bullying intervention program in schools was conducted in Bergen, Norway in 1983 by Dan Olweus. Since 1983, bullying prevention programs have been implemented in 11 countries and on three continents. The on-line website www.teachsafeschools.org, a product of The Melissa Institute for Violence Prevention and Treatment, gives a step-by-step approach to implementing anti-bullying policies in schools with a full component of resources. As mentioned above, the approach suggested is one of comprehensive school health, with the recommendation of an initial needs assessment and participation at all levels of the school. The NEA recommends using the language utilized in the Massachusetts anti-bullying policy for programming (Kim, 2009).

The Massachusetts Department of Elementary and Secondary Education states:

> Schools are encouraged to develop policies protecting gay and lesbian students from harassment, violence, and discrimination. In order to guarantee the rights of all students to an education and to prevent dropping out, school policies should include sexual orientation within anti-discrimination policies, as well as within policies which guarantee students' rights to an education and to equal access to school courses and activities. In order to make schools safe for all students and to prevent violence and harassment, schools should amend existing anti-harassment policies to include prohibiting violence, harassment, and verbal abuse directed against gay and lesbian students and those perceived to be gay or lesbian. Incidents of anti-gay abuse should be treated with the same discipline procedures as other incidents involving bias and hatred (Kim, 2009, p. 47).

Recommendations from the US Department of Health and Human Resources to stop bullying include the following (www.stopbullyingnow.hrsa.gov):

- Add sexual orientation and gender identity to school polices on discrimination and harassment if these do not already exist.
- School clubs, camps, after school and summer programs, and every youth-serving organization should train staff and volunteers on effective anti-bullying prevention methods and interventions.
- Safe havens must be created for LGBT youth. These havens should promote non-biased supportive environments that have been evaluated to reduce the hazards and stresses experienced by LGBT youth.
- Age-appropriate instruction on sexuality, including sexual orientation, should be implemented into the school curriculum. Inclusiveness should be promoted in social, recreational, and sports programming in the community.
- Open discussion about harassment and bullying should occur with concerned youth and direct intervention to prevent this should occur immediately.
- Access to qualified mental health providers and health care providers who have experience working with LGBT youth should be provided.
- Local pediatricians and health care providers should be engaged to help raise awareness among community leaders on issues of adolescent sexuality and those issues specifically related to LGBT youth. Efforts should be made, if deemed necessary to provide support groups for LGBT youth and their families.

Evidence-Based Programs

As is true with many issues of school services, model programs are instrumental to provide guidance to enhance school climate. There are two evidence-based programs that address issues of LGBT youth (Stiegler and Lever, 2008). These are described below.

The *Olweus Bullying Prevention Program* is a comprehensive schoolwide program designed for use in grades kindergarten through ninth grade. School staff are trained and a Bullying Prevention Coordinating Committee is formed. Outcome measures include reduction of bullying problems among school children and improvement of peer relations at school. Evaluations of this program have shown a reduction in bullying among children, improvement of the school climate of classrooms, and a reduction in related antisocial behaviors such as vandalism and truancy. Classroom-level competencies and individual support of children who bully and are bullied comprise the structure of the curriculum. The curriculum includes a targeted approach for LGBT youth who are at risk for bullying. It encourages a no tolerance approach to anti-homosexual slurs, working with student government and other student organizations to promote respect and anti-bullying, reporting bullying behavior and providing confidential support to students. Finally, this program promotes education and training for staff (www.olweus.org).

The *Steps to Respect* program is operated by the Committee for Children and designed for grades 3–6. This program focuses on providing support to all students who are concerned about harassment. It promotes the message that concerns will be addressed when brought to administrators and school personnel. A comprehensive program guide is available with step-by-step tools for developing policies and implementing the program. Training occurs for all staff who have contact with students. The curriculum is divided into different levels. Level 3 specifically addresses issues of sexual harassment among students with a global focus on a no tolerance approach to sexual harassment for all youth (www.cfchildren.org/steps-to-respect.aspx).

There have also been local attempts to offer training programs for safe schools for LGBT youth. The HIV/AIDS Prevention Unit of the Los Angeles Unified School District has developed a chapter about sexual orientation in their required health education courses. The Michigan Department of Education, in response to requests for creating safe school environments, created its own training guide. *A Silent Crisis: Creating Safe Schools for Sexual Minority Youth*, a training guide for schools has been widely distributed among Michigan and 20 other states. Rhode Island established a statewide task force on LGBT youth. It has released a plan that makes comprehensive recommendations about education, policy, child welfare, mental health, and data collection including training programs (CDC, 2011).

School Climate

The recent survey by GLSEN examined principal's perspectives on bullying and anti-harassment and reported that "all schools report that their school or school district has a 'safer school' or anti-bullying/harassment policy" (GLSEN & Harris Interactive, 2008, p. 16). These policies are most often characterized by procedures for students to report incidents of bullying or harassment and a description of consequences to students for engaging in bullying or harassing behavior. Interestingly, only seven in ten schools whose district has a policy are required to notify school personnel, students, and families of the policy. Relatively few of schools' anti-bullying or anti-harassment efforts are focused on increasing the safety of LGBT students or families, although principals indicate that LGBT students are among the least likely to feel very safe at their schools.

A majority of school/district policies do not specifically mention sexual orientation or gender identity or expression, compared to the two-thirds that mention other characteristics such as religion or race/ethnicity. Furthermore, only four in ten secondary schools and one in nine elementary schools have engaged in efforts specifically designed to create a safe environment for "LGBT students" (GLSEN & Harris Interactive, 2008, pp. 11–12). This reinforces the need for schools to make sure they have successfully implemented anti-bullying policies and programs.

Another component of a comprehensive school approach is the provision of an onsite peer support program such as a Gay-Straight Alliance (GSA). The GSA is a school group designed to promote a safe school environment for LGBT youth in schools. GSAs meet regularly and members include both gay and straight students along with faculty advisors. GSAs are an important contemporary example of a site where LGBT youth can feel safe and empowered. They were developed by adults committed to forming alliances among youth of different sexual orientation. They also reflect the need for youth organizations to be organized and led by youth (Russell, Muraco, Subramaniam, & Laub, 2009). The presence of GSAs can assist in the actual implementation of safer school policies such as those described above. They can be the source of new information and perspectives for students and all school staff. They also have the ability to increase awareness for all students about issues of diversity and culture in addition to those issues related to sexual orientation.

Although GSAs can function as any other school club, their ability to have an impact on the school environment can be very powerful (Griffin & Ouellett, 2002). Students who participate in GSAs have found support and been able to voice their concerns freely on a regular basis. In addition, they have been able to influence the school environment as issues of harassment become evident and the manner in which they are handled is addressed (Unks, 1995). They are a necessary component of changing school environment to create a safe haven for nonconforming adolescents in schools. One of the recommendations of the Rhode Island task force was that GSAs be established when requested by students (CDC, 2011). The Los Angelos Unified School District also has many active GSAs.

Schools can create forums to support LGBT parents, who often feel the isolation of their children and find schools unsupportive of their concerns (Kosciw & Diaz, 2008). As stated in their study, GLSEN revealed that "LGBT parents are highly engaged in their children's school experiences, qualities which can be of great benefit to teachers, school administrators and parent–teacher associations in America's schools. When LGBT parents are made to feel invisible in their children's school, schools risk alienating these parents and risk losing the rewards of actively engaged school community members. And when children from LGBT families are subjected to harassment and other mistreatment at school, schools are not providing a safe learning environment and are failing an entire community of students" (Kosciw & Diaz, 2008, p. viii).

School climate is a final component of school environments where LGBT youth can excel. The quality of this component will depend heavily on the ability of schools to implement the previous three components. For example, if there is resistance to anti-bullying policies and schools are unable to police and reverse harassment, then school climate interventions are going to need to be very specific and targeted to identify what factors are responsible for this resistance. Schools may need to look at internal factors of prejudice and rely on outside evaluators should the culture of abuse be widespread in a school district. In these cases, youth should be encouraged to form strong GSAs for safe havens. Administrators and faculty should undergo training and supervision around identifying victims, perpetrators, and school climate issues that lead to bullying.

For districts that have implemented successful policies, and thus have strong active support for GSAs, there are several programs that can further enhance school climate. *Welcoming Schools* is an innovative comprehensive education program for administrators, educators, and parents/guardians who want to provide a comprehensive schoolwide approach to family diversity, gender stereotyping, and bullying. Developed by the Human Rights Campaign, *Welcoming Schools* starts in elementary schools and addresses the issues of policy and bullying mentioned above in addition to global climate issues such as teacher language and curriculum. The program attempts to integrate all components of education to include diversity at all levels of education. It is one of the few resources available to elementary schools that is inclusive of LGBT families and individuals (www.welcomingschools.org).

Schoolwide efforts to improve school climate should include teacher support. The NEA has published a guide for teachers to address schoolwide language and curricular changes (Griffin & Ouellett, 2002). Evaluation of these efforts can occur through reports from the GSAs in the school and CSH coordinators. Curricular changes can include LGBT role models. Studies have shown that inclusion of LGBT issues in the school curriculum improves students' health, safety, and performance (Kim, 2009). Teachers can undergo training that makes them aware of schoolwide and national disparities. Teachers also need resources when they witness or may inadvertently participate in bullying or harassment. LGBT staff and teachers need to feel supported and valued. Finally, curricular changes that are inclusive and resources for teachers and students that are LGBT inclusive need to be available throughout the school environment. The NEA Safety, Bias and LGBT Issues Training Program contains the following components in its modules (Kim, 2009):

- Ground rules or operating norms
- Explanation of LGBT terms
- Distinguishing professional role from personal or private religious beliefs or values
- Contextual information: why LGBT issues relate to student health, safety and achievement
- Statistics on bullying, harassment, discrimination
- Activities and discussion on bias, stereotypes and myths about LGBT people
- Activities on connection between sexual orientation and gender/gender identity/gender expression
- Videos on bullying and diversity
- Demonstration on lessons and activities for the classroom
- Responding to community concerns
- Legal considerations
- Resources for school employees
- Creating an action plan

Community organizing also improves school climate. Schools, as we have heard many times, are microcosms of the communities in which they reside. Schools need to gauge how receptive their communities are to LGBT youth, what resources exist for LGBT individuals in their communities, and what barriers there are for inclusion of LGBT individuals in their communities. National organizations are helpful in assessing these issues and most communities have community wide organizations that promote LGBT issues of equality.

Resources should be provided to enhance the ability of schools and administrators to address the barriers to improving school climate.

Parents are encouraged to be engaged, especially the parents of victims and perpetrators. There is evidence that worksite programs that teach parents to talk to their children about sex have been effective in improving overall communication between youth and their families. Schools should promote these efforts in the community (Schuster, et al., 2008). Parents are often the best avenue for community change and organizing. It has been shown that LGBT youth who do not have open connection with their parents suffer poorer health outcomes than those who do experience a sense of connectedness with their parents (Needham and Austin, 2010).

Parent support groups are good avenues for addressing the ability of a community to enhance gender diversity and inclusiveness. Parents, Families and Friends of Lesbians and Gays (PFLAG), a national nonprofit organization with over 200,000 members and supporters and over 500 affiliates in the United States has been a very valuable resource for many schools and communities. PFLAG promotes the health and well-being of LGBT persons, their families and friends in an overall effort to end discrimination against LGBT individuals (www.community.pflag.org).

Ongoing evaluation of these concurrent steps to improve schools for LGBT youth is a necessary component of any successful effort. Culture changes rapidly and young people continue to have mixed messages about issues relating to sex and gender. Social media has made it more difficult for educators to teach consistent messages of equality. Broad comprehensive approaches such as those described above are necessary so that one area of changes does not carry the entire burden of problems that may arise.

In summary, LGBT youth continue to be at high risk for deleterious outcomes in education. Harassment and bullying continue to plague our schools, in spite of a more tolerant society at large, and more access to proactive forums for youth. Programs to support LGBT youth are in place, with several schools and states implementing policies and practices to address the needs of LGBT youth in schools. Yet these efforts have yet to be implemented nationwide and many areas, especially poor rural areas, have been slow to implement these practices.

The persistence of bullying of LGBT youth, in spite of anti-harassment legislation, is not well studied. Further research needs to be developed on why certain districts are successful and others continue to struggle. Students of color who identify as LGBT have consistently reported school environments as hostile. There is inadequate research available that allows us to understand the specific factors that lead to these differences.

Research that focuses on questioning youth and sexual development among young children needs to occur. While we have a clearer understanding of sexual development and practice among heterosexual individuals, persistent homophobia has prohibited effective research on sexual development in LGBT youth. Questioning youth appear to be at higher risk for school failure and this raises a concern about issues we may not understand in sexual development among this group of young people.

School climate is improved when there is schoolwide support for LGBT youth. Studies that examine barriers to implementing these policies need to occur. There is extensive research on the programs that are successful but less research on school districts that are unsuccessful in their ability to improve. Schools are local phenomena and schools that have not made changes in their curriculum to promote tolerance and implement anti-bullying campaigns have no incentive to do so if there is little community or local support.

Nationwide efforts to protect LGBT youth have continued to grow. Fourteen states and Washington, D.C. have laws that address discrimination, harassment, and/or bullying of students based on sexual orientation and gender identity. Twenty-two states prohibit bullying in schools but offer no specific categories of protection. Comparison studies that address the successes of LGBT youth in these environments have yet to occur.

We have achieved much in the way of civil liberties over the past century in our schools. The provision of a safe and healthy school environment for all students has been an essential part of this progress. The experience of LGBT youth remind us that we have much yet to accomplish.

Resources

Resources for Developing Cultural Competence in Schools for LGBT Youth

1. *Advocates For Youth* (www.advocateforyouth.org): This organization has multiple fact sheets and information about implementing services for LGBT youth in schools. The material has been peer reviewed by experts in the field of adolescent health and young people.
2. *Gay Lesbian and Straight Education Network* (www.glsen.org): GLSEN has provided essential research on discrimination among LGBT in school settings.
3. *Human Rights Campaign* (www.hrc.org): The HRC has up-to-date research and develops advocacy to promote human rights for LGBT individuals. The HRC website http://www.welcomingschools.org/ is a valuable resource in developing programs in schools to promote equality for LGBT youth.

Resources for Support of Successful Interventions in Schools

1. *The Federation of Parents and Friends of Lesbians and Gays* (www.pflag.org): PGLAG is a valuable resource to engage parents in schools.
2. *The Safe Schools Coalition* (www.safeschoolscoalition.org) and *The Melissa Institute for Violence Prevention and Treatment* (www.teachsafeschools.org): Both of these organizations have materials to promote curriculum in schools for the implementation of anti-bullying programs.
3. *The Gay Straight Alliance Network* (www.gsanetwork.org): An essential resource for developing Gay and Straight Alliances in schools.

References

Allensworth, D., & Kolbe, L. (1987). The comprehensive school health program: Exploring an expanded concept. *Journal of School Health, 57*(10), 409–412.

American Psychiatric Association. (2000). *Diagnostic and statistical manual of mental disorder* (4th ed., Text Revision.). Washington, DC: Author.

Bearss, N. (2010). Gay, Lesbian, Bisexual, Transgender (GLBT). In C. S. Clauss-Ehlers (Ed.), *Encyclopedia of cross-cultural school psychology* (pp. 465–471). New York, NY: Springer.

Birkett, M., & Espelage, D. (2009). Lesbian, gay, bisexual and questioning students in schools: The moderating effects of homophobic bullying and school climate on negative outcomes. *Journal of Youth and Adolescence, 38*(7), 989–1000.

Bridges, E. (2007). *Impact of homophobia and racism on Gay, Lesbian, Bisexual, Transgender and Questioning (GLBTQ) Youth of Color*. Washington, D.C.: Advocates for Youth.

Bronfenbrenner, U. (1977). Toward an experimental ecology of human development. *American Psychologist, 32*(7), 513–531.

Centers for Disease Control and Prevention. (2011). Sexual identity, sex of sexual contacts, and risk behaviors among students in grades 9-12-youth risk behavior surveillance, selected sites, United States, 2001–2009. *Morbidity and Mortality Weekly Report, 60*(7), 1–133.

Centers for Disease Control and Prevention. (2001). School health guidelines to prevent unintentional injuries and violence. *Morbidity and Mortality Weekly Report, 50*(RR-22), 1–73.

Chesir-Teran, D., & Hughes, D. (2009). Heterosexism in high school and victimization among lesbian, gay, bisexual, and questioning students. *Journal of Youth and Adolescence, 38*(7), 963–975.

Espelage, D. L., Aragon, S. R., Birkett, M., & Koenig, B. (2008). Homophobic teasing, psychological outcomes, and sexual orientation among high school students: What influence do parents and schools have? *School Psychology Review, 37*(2), 202–216.

Gay, Lesbian and Straight Education Network (GLSEN), & Harris Interactive. (2008). *The principal's perspective: School safety, bullying and harassment, a survey of public school principals*. New York: GLSEN.

Gilliam, J. (2002). Respecting the rights of lesbian, gay, bisexual, transgender and questioning (LGBTQ) youth, a responsibility of youth-serving professionals. *Transitions, 14*(4).

Griffin, P., & Ouellett, M. (2002). Going beyond gay-straight alliances to make schools safe for lesbian, gay, bisexual and transgendered students. *Angles, 6*(1), p. 2.

Haffner, D. (1999). *From diapers to dating: a parent's guide to raising sexually healthy children*. New York: Newmarket Press.

Health Resources and Services Administration.(2008). *Bullying among children and youth on perceptions and differences in sexual orientation.* Retrieved February 5, 2011 from www.stopbullyingnow.hrsa.gov.

Horn, S., Kosciw, J. G., & Russell, S. (2009). Special issue introduction: New research on lesbian, gay, bisexual, and transgender youth: Studying lives in context. *Journal of Youth and Adolescence, 38*(7), 863–866.

Hurwitz, L. H., & Weston, L. (2010). *Using coordinated school health to promote mental health for all students.* Washington, DC: National Assembly on School-Based Health Care.

Just the Facts Coalition. (2008). *Just the facts about sexual orientation and youth: A primer for principals, educators, and school personnel.* Washington, DC: American Psychological Association. Retrieved December 26, 2010 from www.apa.org/pi/lgbs/publications/justthefacts.html.

Kim, R. (2009). *A report on the status of gay, lesbian, bisexual and transgender people in education: stepping out of the closet, into the light.* Washington. D.C.,: National Education Association.

Kosciw, J., & Diaz, E. (2008). *Involved, invisible, ignored: the experience of lesbian, gay, bisexual and transgender parents and their children in our nation's K-12 schools.* New York: GLSEN.

Kosciw, J., Greytak, E., Diaz, E., & Bartkiewicz, M. (2010). *The 2009 National School Climate Survey: The experiences of lesbian, gay, bisexual and transgender youth in our nation's schools.* New York: GLSEN.

Lawrence, R., Appleton Gootman, J., & Sim, J. (Eds.). (2009). *Adolescent health services: Missing opportunities.* Washington, DC,: National Academies Press.

Meyer, I. (2003). Prejudice, social stress, and mental health in lesbian, gay, and bisexual populations: Conceptual issues and research evidence. *Psychological Bulletin, 129*(5), 674–697.

National Guidelines Task Force. (2004). *Guidelines for comprehensive sexuality education: Kindergarten—12th grade.* New York, NY: National Guidelines Task Force, Sex Information and Education Council of the U.S.

Needham, B., & Austin, E. (2010). Sexual orientation, parental support, and health during the transition to young adulthood. *Journal of Youth and Adolescence, 39*(10), 1189–1198.

Ray, N. (2006). *Lesbian, gay, bisexual and transgender youth: An epidemic of homelessness.* New York: National Gay and Lesbian Taskforce Policy Institute.

Russell, S., Muraco, A., Subramaniam, A., & Laub, C. (2009). Youth empowerment and high school gay-straight alliances. *Journal of Youth and Adolescence, 38*(7), 891–903.

Savin-Williams, R. (2005). *The new gay teenager: Adolescent lives.* Cambridge, MA: Harvard University Press.

Schuster, M., Corona, R., Elliott, M., Kanouse, D., Eastman, K., et al. (2008). Evaluation of talking parents, healthy teens, a new worksite based parenting programme to promote parent-adolescent communication about sexual health: Randomised controlled trial. *British Medical Journal, 337,* a308. doi:10.1136/bmj.39609.657581.25.

Stiegler, K., & Lever, N. (2008). *Summary of recognized evidence-based programs implemented by the expanded school mental health (ESMH) programs.* Baltimore, Maryland: University of Maryland School of Medicine Center for School Mental Health.

Toomey, R., Ryan, C., Diaz, R., Card, N., & Russell, S. (2010). Gender-nonconforming lesbian, gay, bisexual, and transgender youth: School victimization and young adult psychosocial adjustment. *Developmental Psychology, 46*(6), 1580–1589.

Unks, G. (1995). *The gay teen: Educational practice and theory for lesbian, gay, and bisexual adolescents.* New York: Routledge.

Advancing School-Based Mental Health for Asian American Pacific Islander Youth

Matthew R. Mock

Introduction

As the mental health needs of children, adolescents, and families continue to grow, so do appropriate settings to provide prevention, early intervention, and clinical treatment. The increase of cultural, ethnic, racial, and linguistic diversity of children and teenagers creates additional challenges as well as unique opportunities. In recent years, schools have come into sharper focus in part due to high-profile incidents including bullying, suicides, and student-on-student violence such as the shootings at Columbine High School and the Virginia Tech massacre. These incidents are not necessarily new. Violence is an everyday occurrence for some, especially in urban areas of poverty, blight, unemployment, and social fragmentation. What may be striking for many are the heightened levels of violence turned toward oneself or others.

The Asian American Pacific Islander (AAPI)* community is one of the fastest growing in the U.S. The purpose of this chapter is to:

- Understand the "fit" of schools, education, and AAPI students.
- Emphasize schools and educational institutions as important settings for meeting some AAPI mental health needs.
- Acknowledge important cultural characteristics and influences to better serve AAPI youth.
- Describe culturally competent, responsive, and effective mental health practices for AAPI students.
- Advance research, training, practice, and policies essential for addressing AAPI family needs in schools.

The Virginia Tech shooting on April 16, 2007, was a tragedy of multiple dimensions. In all, 33 people died and countless others were seriously wounded. Now known as the "worst school shooting in American history," the perpetrator who eventually killed himself was a Korean American immigrant. In the aftermath of these shootings, mental health professionals, school administrators, researchers, policymakers, and politicians theorized why such violence was becoming all too common. Shock and dismay that the shooter was Korean reverberated from Korean American communities to South Korea. The myth of the "model minority" was raised once more as was the question of could this tragedy have been prevented with different mental health intervention (Hong, Cho, & Lee, 2010). Caution was raised to not use Virginia Tech as an event summarizing AAPI needs. This would be single-minded and limiting. Instead, for many, this was yet another unavoidable wake-up call that some AAPI youth and families have less than ideal lives. Like other

---

*Throughout the text, Asian American Pacific Islander, AAPI as an abbreviation, Asian Americans and Asians will be used interchangeably.

M.R. Mock, Ph.D. (✉)
John F. Kennedy University, Pleasant Hill, CA, USA
e-mail: mmock@jfku.edu

students, AAPI youth have identity struggles, family conflicts, educational disappointments, and worries about growing up (Hong, 1993; Lee & Mock, 2005a, 2005b; Tewari & Alvarez, 2009). They experience many sources of familial, social, and mental stress.

Throughout this chapter, the voices of AAPI children and adolescents will be provided as examples. These sample comments not only serve as a reminder of diverse AAPI mental health needs but also emphasize the urgency of culturally competent, school-based approaches specific to this population.

The Challenges of Stereotypes for Asian American Pacific Islander Youth

> My friends know me as smart and studious, a good student. What they don't see is that I have doubts about myself, feel lonely sometimes, and my parents put pressure on me. I am successful on the outside, but at what cost on the inside? (13-year-old Chinese American girl)

> I was happy to be here in a new school, an exciting place where I had the world to explore. I even learned English pretty quickly. When I heard that I would have to go back home to Japan after my parents finished their work, it was so painful. That's why I took all of those pills. I eventually told my teacher (16-year-old visiting Japanese high school student).

The "model minority" myth continues to plague AAPI youth contributing to stereotypes they are in less need of mental health services than others. Along these same lines, the image of Asian American students as "whiz kids" is harming them and contributing to hesitancy to seek help. Simplistic, even stereotypical, portrayals of Asian American students as "overachievers," "overrepresented" in higher education, and as overcoming racial obstacles still faced by other racial and ethnic groups, conveys an incorrect and distorted picture of Asian youth (Lee, 1996; Sue & Okazaki, 1990; Umemoto & Ong, 2006).

An additional challenge is acknowledging that Asian American and Pacific Islander youth in schools are very diverse. In order to advance school-based mental health for AAPI youth and work effectively with them, service providers and policymakers must recognize their different cultural identities, backgrounds, and social influences. In order to provide effective mental health services in schools, cultural complexities must be taken into account. Summarizing a description of current AAPI communities is in order followed by a snapshot of educational successes and concerns.

Asian American Pacific Islanders as a Diverse and Growing Population

The term "Asian American Pacific Islander" (AAPI) refers to a diverse population with origins from over 50 countries. Recent 2010 US census analyses underscore the significant demographics of the Asian American population. In July 2006, the estimated number of US residents who said they were Asian or Asian in combination with one or more other races was 14.9 million. As of 2010, the number of AAPI residents increased to 16.6 million or approximately 5.4% of the total US population. This significant increase in AAPI communities is projected to continue in the future. Nearly two-thirds of AAPIs are foreign-born. Of the foreign-born from Asian countries, 52% are naturalized US citizens (Census Bureau, 2010). Asian American Pacific Islanders are different by geographic origin, histories, languages, customs, beliefs, traditions, values, and generations in the United States. On the west coast, initial immigrants in the early 1900s were primarily Chinese, Japanese, and Filipino. In recent years, the dramatic change in population is attributed to large increases in Korean, Southeast Asian, East Indian or South Asian, and Indochinese migration.

Household income is often cited as one source of Asians being "the model" for others, i.e., studying, achieving in education, then working hard to climb the employment ladder leads to success and the "American Dream." While the median household income for Asians ($64,238) is higher than other groups, 12.6% of Asians are at or below the poverty rate. Southeast Asian families are overrepresented among these households with Hmong (37.8%), Laotian (18.5%), and Vietnamese (16.6%) struggling with poverty (National Commission on Asian American and Pacific Islander Research in Education, 2008). Economic and resource limitations for AAPI families and others have a profound impact on educational pursuits, and mental and social stress. This will also be described later in this chapter.

It has been noted that some AAPI groups share notable cultural similarities. For example, Chinese, Japanese, Koreans, and Vietnamese share the influences of ancient traditions, though to differing degrees. Buddhism, Taoism, Confucianism, and Shintoism convey generations of beliefs and ways of conducting one's life. In contrast, Cambodians, Laotians, and to some degree, Thais are influenced by Indian Civilization and Theravada Buddhism. Filipino, Samoan, and other Pacific Islander groups are influenced by histories connected to Polynesian and Melanesian cultures. These common groupings form *inter*ethnic differences or ways AAPIs differ from other ethnic, racial, and cultural communities (Chan, 1994; Lee & Mock, 2005a, 2005b; Uba, 1994). This understanding of some common AAPI influences among groups is further complicated by *intra*ethnic differences. *Intra*ethnic refers to contrasts within AAPI communities such as written or oral communication differences, rural or urban origins, immigrant or refugee family status, and first, third, or fifth generation US resident. There are different reasons Asian newcomers left their homelands and different ways they felt received in America.

Asian American Pacific Islanders can often identify at least one common major language spoken within their country-of-origin or region. Over 100 different languages are spoken among AAPI groups. Beyond the official language there are also several dialects that may be similar or sometimes totally distinct from one another. Following Spanish, Chinese is the most widely spoken non-English language in the United States. Vietnamese and Tagalog speakers total more than one million (Hune & Takeuchi, 2008; Census Bureau, 2010). Children of an immigrant or refugee family raised in a monolingual, English-only, or bilingual home have unique experiences that shape their identity. Residing in a homogenous, segregated community versus one that is diverse and multi-racial further contributes to different courses of identity development.

Asian students and their families are also diverse by social and cultural histories in the United States. Early immigrant Chinese were initially brought as temporary workers and laborers with the intent that they would be sent back home. South Asian and Filipino men arrived to temporarily work in farms, and with exposure to Mexican female workers sometimes formed early interracial relationships. The Japanese gained a foothold to American shores through the sugar cane fields of Hawaii. Some would take on picture brides, forming families with females who they only met initially by correspondence and photographs. For some families, their histories and narratives in the United States are rich with generations of textured experiences. Painful stories of racism, sexism, classism as well as other treatment as "undesirables" or depictions as "constant foreigners" contrast with triumphant stories of resilience, tenacity, cultural survival, familial, and community strengths. The cultural tapestries of AAPI families are often colorfully woven and should be acknowledged in educational settings. The past of AAPI families and communities influence present strivings and behaviors of current students in schools (Lee & Mock, 2005a, 2005b; Wong & Mock, 1997). With a consideration for AAPI diversity as a backdrop, AAPI student achievement in schools will now be described.

Asian American Pacific Islanders and the Pursuit of Education

My parents are both academically successful and have jobs to prove it. My interests are just different. I like theater, music and even the arts. I was even encouraged to try out for the varsity basketball team. How do I tell this to my parents who have done so much for me? I feel so much pressure, don't sleep much and even recently lost some weight. My teacher made me promise that I would come see you (Chinese-Japanese biracial male, high school senior to a school mental health counselor).

As long as I could remember we were supposed to be the "model minority," the "brainiac" in classes.

But model for what and by who? My brother and I live in the projects and take three buses through some of the worst neighborhoods to go to school. How does learning in school help me when I go home every night to this? My teacher thinks I have attention problems. I do because she doesn't know what I always have to contend with at home then at school (Vietnamese middle school female student during a home visit).

Educational attainment varies among different AAPI groups. The percentage of Asians 25 years or older who have an advanced degree is 20% or double that of all Americans 25 or older. Among Asians, 68% of Asian Indians have a Bachelors degree compared to 24% of Vietnamese. The education concerns for AAPIs break the often portrayed, stereotypical picture. Nearly one out of four AAPI students is Limited English Proficient (LEP) or living in a linguistically isolated household with parents who are LEP. Opposite to being "whiz kids," the high school drop out rate continues to be of major concern, especially for certain AAPI groups. The drop out rate of Southeast Asian youth is staggering with 40% of Hmong, 38% of Laotian, and 35% of Cambodian students not completing high school. It has also been reported that only 14% of Native Hawaiians and Pacific Islanders 25 years or older have at least a Bachelors degree compared with 27% of the total general population (Hune & Takeuchi, 2008; Umemoto & Ong, 2006).

While a cultural explanation has often been proposed for Asian American academic achievement, it does not explain why some AAPI students do well while others do not. It also does not explain why some AAPIs do not emphasize academic accomplishments in their home countries. An argument having salience here is relative functionalism (Suzuki, 1980). By this it is meant that Asian American immigrants find that education in the United States contributes significantly to future success. Education directly contributes to self-improvement and social mobility. American schools also reward some common existing, valued cultural traits such as respect for authority, obedience, and self-discipline (Lee, 1996; Sue & Okazaki, 1990; U.S. Department of Health and Human Services, 2001).

Asian American Pacific Islander Families: Child and Adolescent Presentation in Schools

(Waverly): "I wish you wouldn't do that, telling everyone that I am your daughter...why do you have to use me to show off!" (Mother): "Embarrassed to be my daughter?... This girl not happy concerning for us, this family not concerning this girl! (From the film The Joy Luck Club (Stone & Yang, 2003), book by Amy Tan)

I don't think anyone will truly understand my culture and what it has meant as a student. Sure I am big and tough. I have to uphold my Samoan culture. We are like native people who have roots that have been cut off. Unless we work hard to maintain our histories our family tree will topple. Only my other homeboys understand this. This was never discussed in school (Young adult in lockup to his probation officer).

Teachers, school administrators, and school mental health providers should be aware of shared cultural influences and characteristics specific for AAPI parents and their children. These are significant for understanding behaviors related to schooling. With exposure to similar values of childrearing and parenting, the importance of family as a central concept often informs expectations and relationships between family members. Reciprocity or the importance of give and take between family members throughout the lifespan may be the valued norm. Rather than focus on individualism or goals of ultimate family separation or waning of relationships, AAPI students are often raised with values of connection, obligation to family across generations, awareness of how behaviors impact others, and successes including academically and in school performance as public reflections on one's upbringing and being parented (Chung, 1997; Lee & Mock, 2005a, 2005b).

Educators, mental health service providers, and school administrators should also be aware that cultural influences play a significant role in AAPI individual and social identity development. Beginning with the centrality of family in conducting one's life, AAPI families are often organized and operate in a hierarchical manner, from parents or elders to the youngest child. Roles and relationships are often conducted along lines of hierarchical respect, with parents speaking then children listening and obeying. Elders are generally to be revered and given respect. Egalitarianism is not necessarily preferred. The often continued dominance of patriarchy plays out in gender development, identity, and relationships. Studies have shown that AAPI males may be afforded more opportunities than females (Abelmann, 2009; Huang, 1997). Gender role stereotypes culturally passed down generations may contribute to subtle or overt messages that schooling and academic achievement for AAPI girls may be secondary to eventually raising a family or caring for fragile elders. Speaking readily about one's own issues or concerns runs against lessons of not standing out; to do so may translate into being self-centered or selfish due to a need for attention. While experiencing similar joys, pains, fears, and triumphs as is the human experience, AAPI students may hold back in showing emotional expression.

As in so many cultures, heterosexuality is considered the norm with homosexuality often viewed as a deviance from expectations. For AAPI parents, sex is often still considered a topic not to be directly discussed with their teenagers. While sexual orientation is more than sex, for traditional parents they are often linked. As is the case with other cultures, coming out as gay, lesbian, or bisexual may be extremely difficult, perhaps additionally so given some Asian family expectations. An AAPI teenage male might come out to his father, only to have the father question how he failed to convey masculine traits or turned his son away from taking on the culturally traditional masculine, heterosexual role (Mock, 2008).

For Asians, there has been an increased interest on concepts of "face," face-saving behaviors and how they relate to family dynamics (Zane & Mak, 2003). "Face" relates to how others see you. With an orientation toward upholding family honor and respect, there should be no interactions that bring shame or embarrassment on oneself as this reflects directly on one's family. Intra-familial differences play a significant role in family health and social-emotional well-being. Cultural values brought from the homeland have different ways of being transmitted and adhered to with subsequent generations trying to fit into current contexts. For some AAPI families with painful or traumatic histories including those from primary immigration and secondary relocation, there may be family secrets or emotional cutoffs. These intergenerational conflicts often show up in current lives. Different rates of acculturation impact AAPI youth adjustment and mental health. In summary then, in the school context, educators and service providers should be aware of Asian-influenced cultural values of:

- Importance of and central organizing nature of the family.
- Respect and interactions based on status and roles.
- Emphases on hierarchy in relationships and interrelating.
- Dominance of patriarchy inter-generationally conveyed.
- Orientation toward the group or collective.
- Sense of duty and obligation through the life span.
- Shame, guilt, and the concept of maintaining a positive "face."
- Different styles of interpersonal communication.
- Restraint of self-expression, particularly with strangers.
- Expectations following from different, sometimes multiple roles.
- An orientation toward achievement and socially sanctioned measures of success (Lee & Mock, 2005a, 2005b; Uba, 1994).

While cultural values may be taught or carried forward within Asian American families and communities, their meaning and depth of being valued across generations may differ. For some AAPI youth, there may be relevancy of culture in their home life but seemingly less so in their classroom or school environments. For example, traditional foods from home packed as a child's lunch may be a source of unwanted curiosity or embarrassment among peers unfamiliar with Asian cultures. Unless the environment is one of proactive cultural inclusion, the traditional garb or even ceremonial dress of one culture may be misconstrued as an oddity or open to "exotic curiosity" or "othering" without acceptance. From an historical, relational perspective, often because of physical appearance, a history of discrimination, colonialism, racialization, and racism, AAPIs may be unconsciously or overtly viewed as "foreigners" on some level. While cultural differences are at least tolerated, "fitting in" with others in schools is often a child's desire. Without significant others "reflecting" or endorsing their cultural, racial, and ethnic identities, AAPI students may be challenged in forming an early positive identity. Classrooms and schools are excellent environments for proactively teaching and practicing social inclusion and acceptance of diversity. Films are excellent sources of rich dialogue affirming Asian American cultural identity (Mock, 2008; Xing, 1998).

The Importance of Schools in the AAPI Socialization Process

Academicians, educators, mental health professionals, and policymakers have contributed to the rich role that schools play in the lives of Asian American youth and families. Given the diverse cultural backgrounds described earlier, the school context is an important one for "testing the waters" along social, intellectual, and emotional lines. For families who grow up more insulated from mainstream culture, schools may represent an early foray into larger society and future possibilities. The learning experience for Asian Americans goes beyond grades, textbooks, and exams.

The importance of education is commonly emphasized among AAPI families and communities. Educational achievement is a tangible source of pride, respect, and accomplishment. For newcomer families, schools are a primary source for learning English, Western-based values, and to acculturate. Learning English fluently is often the goal of AAPI immigrants. Negotiating relationships and daily activities in English is often an indication of adjustment and social acceptance. Good grades and academic achievements are identifiable markers of success not only in the realm of academics but also socially (Lee & Mock, 2005a, 2005b). Graduating to attend a prominent university is climbing the ladder in social standing and class in the community.

For some AAPI families, schools are the primary source for socializing their children in a larger context. Parents often look to teachers in the classroom to instruct their children on ways of behaving, negotiating of challenges in daily living, and teaching successful ways in being with others. For immigrant families, schools also represent an interface between prior home and American cultures (Canino & Spurlock, 1994). Even for Asian American families that have strong, multigenerational roots of being in the United States, they inherit the strong influence of what education means to the family. The book Battle Hymn of the Tiger Mother written by Amy Chua stirred controversy after excerpts were shared depicting some of her practices raising her daughters. For some readers, her dictatorial-like music lessons, physical discipline for lack of adequate studying, and critiquing her daughter with friends using strong, verbal admonishments were viewed as abusive. For others, including the author, husband, and her children, this was viewed as being earnest in the importance of achievement and ways of showing care and investment in a child's or adolescent's future (Paul, 2011). Because children are viewed as directly connected to parents through a relational lens, AAPI children or youth that are not successful to a point of needing remediation or summoning of parents may viewed by some as a direct result of parents falling short of giving parental instruction, guidance, or modeling. In other words, children in the school context may be seen as direct reflections of their parents at home. This has ramifications for contacting parents to give consent to mental health treatment for their minor children.

The impact of racialization and the experience of it by AAPI students with others are significant. For acculturated and immigrant AAPI families, schools are a primary component of a liberal ideal that working hard, achieving academically, and thriving in personal development will be rewarded with meeting dreams only imagined by parents or elders. In her ethnographic study and analysis of Korean American students, Abelmann (2009) concludes that ideals of an inclusive modern, American university, in her case the University of Illinois in the Midwest, are compromised by stereotyping and racial segregation. She writes that it is overly simplistic to conclude that the social segregation of Korean American students is self-imposed but more accurately reflects the narrowness of the university experience in expanding issues of race, ethnicity, class, and gender. Rather than inspired and elevated for future possibilities, students Abelmann (2009) interviewed reflected disappointments, identity questions rather than answers and even future doubts about self, family, faith, and community. Opposite from being prepared globally, some students felt in some ways more constrained by their race, ethnicity, and class status at the university. She concluded that the new "family" portrayed in the mission statement of the specific mid-west university under study was a reflection in values and process of a specific type of "family." In other words, the overall mental health of AAPI students, in this case Korean Americans, may be directly connected to the environment of the school in which they participate.

Asian American Pacific Islander Mental Health Issues and Concerns in Schools

> My parents used to fight and my mom even called the police one time on my dad after he hit her. But it is not okay for Asians to divorce. Still, I wish my parents would physically separate because they live separate lives anyway. Sometimes I go right to my room after school because I can't deal with the tension. And they wonder why I can't seem to concentrate on my studies (Chinese-American high school student speaking to his counselor).

> I am grateful to be here. They won't talk about our home country much because it was terrible during the war. But I just can't always tell my parents in English what they only understand in Vietnamese. When I try to help my dad in his new business he used to get frustrated. Now that I am a little older, I think he looks more mad. Who can I talk to? (9-year-old girl with parents from Vietnam)

> I don't know what's wrong with me. I study twice as much as others. It takes me much longer to read things. My brothers and sisters do well. My parents think I just need to concentrate more. My mother's parents from the home country think it has to do with the war and my spirit. I saw a brochure in the office about being evaluated for learning needs. What should I do? (15-year-old Hmong teenager in a rural school)

Ongoing research has shown that AAPIs tend to show mental health problems in specific, common ways. Compared to other cultural groups, there is relatively limited information regarding the mental health needs of AAPI youth. Common diagnoses have often included adjustment disorders, post traumatic stress, anxiety, depression, and other mood disorders. Interestingly, more behavioral concerns such as behavioral addictions (e.g., gambling, internet addiction) have been recently identified among AAPI groups. From a culturally competence perspective, it is important to utilize the DSMIV-TR (American Psychiatric Association, 1994; Kramer, Wang, Kwong, Lee, & Chung, 2002) cultural formulation in therapeutic assessment, engagement, ongoing, dynamic hypothesis generating and treatment for continuous, successful outcomes. For some, it may be important to identify culturally bound syndromes which are presentations of problems contextually grounded in a cultural frame. For example, there have been descriptions of Hmong youth having problems due to their spirit not being firmly planted in their physical bodies. Traditional Hmong often turn to elders or shaman to reconnect spirits jeopardized by war, trauma, and ongoing migration stress. As noted previously, the conflicts between traditional family values and more mainstream culture may lead to additional stress, confusion, social fragmentation, and exacerbate anxiety for some AAPI youth.

Longstanding research and multiple studies have indicated that prevalence of mental health problems among AAPI children and youth may be similar to that of other cultural and ethnic groups and minors, in general. However, manifestation and identification of problems may only occur when symptoms and behaviors are more severe (Lee & Mock, 2005a, 2005b; Tewari &

Alvarez, 2009). Immigration problems including not only traumas experienced *prior* to leaving the home country but also *after arriving* can have a direct impact on the physical and mental health of children and teenagers. Family therapists are quite well versed in understanding how unresolved traumas and losses can be continued in future generations. Between parents and their children there may be intergenerational problems. There may be culture conflicts and disagreements with the previously listed common values and norms of AAPI behaviors. There can be culturally based conflicts in attitudes and lifestyles. Behavioral styles in prior contexts (e.g., home country, rural village, small town) may differ with current situations (e.g., school playground, urban setting, large city, student high school organization) (Chung, 1997; Mock, 1998). Developmentally there are common challenges in becoming a teenager, then young adult. Resolving one's ethnic, cultural, and racial identity brings additional challenges. The importance of family issues or individual issues viewed through a family frame of reference is critical. Differences in language and even accented English are important to negotiate socially for AAPI children and teenagers.

Awareness of specific problems identified among AAPI children and teenagers such as body image, self esteem, and eating disorders such as bulimia or anorexia, risk of suicide are significant (Huang, 1997; Wong & Mock, 1997). In the fact sheet "Suicide Among Asian American/Pacific Islanders" (Suicide Prevention Action Network, 2007), between 1999 and 2004, suicide ranked as the second leading cause of death for AAPIs between ages 15 and 24 years old. Domestic violence has been identified as a significant issue through several AAPI community service centers. Some AAPI youth groups have formed to intervene early in potential cycles of violence. Learning problems in school for AAPI students must be more accurately and appropriately identified. Some studies have shown that AAPI learning needs and evaluation for learning support are under-identified (Chan, 1994).

Effective Mental Health Service Strategies for Asian American Pacific Islander Students

There are several service strategies that educators, school administrators, and mental health counselors need to acknowledge to effectively serve AAPI students. The first are recognition of barriers. Some of these include language differences, mistaken labeling of achievement problems as solely problems in learning English, and unconscious beliefs the student should be a "model for other minorities" leading to hesitancy in making a service referral. Among parents, issues of shame, stigma, and embarrassment in front of strangers may also be contributors. Eventually, the problems may be viewed as greater than the family can hold private or within the home with a crisis erupting. With a value on saving face, the approaching of problems may need to be identified by a source outside of the family and come from a place of authority.

Familial belief systems rooted in culture have important ramifications for understanding physical, emotional, and mental health needs and ways of help seeking. The different ways one may understand or attribute sources of problems have significant impact on seeking assistance. Early discussions on working with Asian Americans often focused on the importance of understanding somatic complaints. While this still tends to be true, a focus on a more holistic perspective in viewing one's life may be more instructive. From a holistic perspective, mind, body, spirit, and soul are not separate entities but interact within a larger, whole person. Physical and mental health is often seen as connected. In some AAPI families, a student's sadness may be attributed to nutritional deficits or being out of physical balance. For some families, hyperactivity may not be pathologized but viewed as a norm reflecting the child's natural personality and tendencies. Undesirable or unacceptable thoughts may be seen as lack of concentration or inadequate training at home. These beliefs and points of view should be considered in any school-based interventions.

Given some of the described cultural norms and values of many AAPI children, adolescents, young adults, and their families, the school context may be an ideal setting for primary prevention, early intervention, and behavioral health care intervention and treatment. For some AAPI students, mental health concepts are not readily understood or valued within the culture. Tangible physical signs of health may be more understandable or acceptable. Students may reveal emotional, psychological, or familial and relationship concerns to teachers through headaches, stomach problems, or trouble concentrating.

While racism and the experience of power differentials including oppression may be hard to talk about, thinking about these sources of stress while providing service initiation, engagement, and ongoing services can make the relationship more meaningful. Rather than just being culturally competent, the service provider should also be aware of cultural humility and professional compassion. As written elsewhere, cultural competence is best understood as not a final endpoint but an ongoing process of learning. Cultural humility refers the clinician's acknowledgment that when it comes to culture, we do not know everything and instead continuously strive to respectfully know more. We can never absolutely know another's experience, but if we listen with an open heart and mind, our expressed compassion can contribute to healing (Mock, 2008).

While a primarily psychologically based problem may be more complex, understanding how the individual and their support system (family, friends, and community) view the situation has important ramifications for interventions in schools. Young AAPI children experiencing stress in their initial classes may find a group for making friends as newcomers as less stigmatizing than being in a remedial classroom. Students identified as having difficulty socializing on the playground or connecting with peers may have some of their needs addressed through a class teaching study skills or supporting cultural ways of communicating and interacting. For AAPI families adjusting to being in America as immigrants, an English-as-a-Second-Language (ESL) class that integrates mental health wellness perspectives in the classroom can be an effective strategy. In other words, a more psychoeducational approach may be more in keeping with cultural norms as well as be less stigmatizing.

Innovative Approaches, Evidence-Based, Effective, and Best Practices in School Mental Health for AAPI Students

Several recommendations emerge for providing school-based services to AAPI youth. I directed mental health services for children, adolescents, and their families in the diverse context of Berkeley, California, for twenty years. We launched comprehensive mental health and related health services for minors from kindergarten through high school. I also led projects to address mental health disparities for multicultural communities throughout California for several years. I have served as an administrator, direct service provider, researcher, and professor throughout my career. There should be a comprehensive network of referral agencies and providers that wraparound and provide an array of services with cultural competence integrated, infused, and integrated throughout service provision. Administrators, teachers, academic counselors, probation officers, juvenile justice providers, social service workers, are important sources of referrals, intervention, and networks of support. Filipino and Korean families, for example, may rely on their religious or faith institutions for support. Research has shown how religious institutions have played important roles in each of these communities (Abelmann, 2009; Tewari & Alvarez, 2009). More recent AAPI immigrants may utilize community leaders or traditional healers. To involve cultural brokers in educational services can be a culturally responsive community intervention.

Due to continuing stigma in directly discussing mental or emotionally related problems by going to a stranger, the school setting poses a culturally appropriate setting for addressing potential problems. Ongoing research, studies, and interviews with AAPI youth and families have yielded important promising, effective, and evidence-based mental health practices. The author managed a project at the California Institute for Mental Health (CiMH), reviewing and collating effective practices specific for different cultural communities (see resources in the Appendix). Titled the Adopting Culturally Competent Practices (ACCP) Project (2006), therapeutic practices were reviewed in the psychological research and practice literature. These practices were demonstrated to be effective for AAPI youth through scientific research testing the actual interventions. Levels of practice evidence were designated as either "effective," "efficacious," or "promising." It has been demonstrated, for example, that many AAPI youth may respond to a more cognitive-behavioral approach to treatment. This seems to fit with a more intellectual emphasis of schools. In contrast, some AAPI communities such as Korean Americans place spirituality at the center of identity along with culture. In Merced, a rural community in central California, Hmong shaman now work collaboratively with medical doctors. Youth are involved in garden projects for the well-being of elders connected to nature and spirits. This reciprocally impacts the well-being of children, youth, and their families. Evidence-based practices have also been adapted for the specific case of Asian Americans. LaFromboise (1995) has researched and promoted an evidence-based curriculum called American Indian Life Skills to address suicide risk among Native American youth. This has led to adaptations and curriculum in Asian American communities. For example, an anti-violence, anti-drug curriculum based on this model has been utilized in Hawaii. Teenage anti-violence programs for AAPIs have been tailored to meet the needs of Samoans, Filipinos, and Vietnamese (Ida & Ja, 2007; Mock, 1998).

In the ACCP Matrix, the list of identified practices culturally responsive to the needs of AAPI youth include: Incredible Years (effective for disruptive disorders); Functional Family Therapy and Multidimensional Treatment Foster Care (each effective for mixed emotional and behavioral problems); Multisystemic Therapy and Wraparound (each promising for serious mixed emotional and behavioral problems); Group Cognitive Behavioral Therapy (effective for depression and anxiety); and Psychoeducational Family Intervention (promising for severe mental health problems like schizophrenia). For more details about each practice and others, the level of research evidence for AAPI populations, recommendations for cultural adaptations and accommodations, staffing potentially needed for school implementation, availability in different Asian languages, refer to the ACCP Matrices on the CiMH website at www.cimh.org. Each of these specific interventions and more are carefully referenced in the matrices provided online. It is significant to note that while there have been studies conducted using AAPI samples, there continues to be a high need in researching therapeutic practices effective for different AAPI groups including those to be implemented in school-based settings. For children and teenagers of diverse cultural backgrounds, policymakers must not only be aware of evidence-based practices but also therapeutic practices that are community-defined, promising, and practice-based evidence (Mock, 2003; U.S. Department of Health and Human Services, 2001). Culturally sensitive research must continue targeting the specific needs, help seeking behaviors and relevance of interventions for the Asian community of interest. For Asian at-risk youth, programs and services that reflect contemporary ways of learning and interacting socially can be very beneficial in schools. In the San Francisco Bay Area, a longstanding program that addresses substance use and abuse, Asian American Recovery Services (AARS) incorporates dramatic role play for teenagers returning to wellness. Another program, Community Health for Asian Americans (or CHAA, formerly known as Asian Pacific Psychological Services) incorporates hip-hop and the sharing of cultural narratives in ways that teenagers speak and relate. Titled BEATZ, the program is described as follows:

> BEATZ is a program that seeks to promote youth leadership and development through music, and is housed in the STEP AHEAD building along with

Southeast Asian Youth Leaders (SEAYL). With instruction from DJ professionals, students devise, lead, and execute projects promoting community wellness. The BEATZ team recently wrote, produced, and recorded an original album speaking out against violence, and is currently providing DJ training on site at the RYSE Center in Richmond.

Yet another program of CHAA is the Health and Wellness anchor at RYSE, a collaborative in Richmond providing programming and leadership opportunities for youth aged 14–24. In addition to providing traditional counseling services, CHAA offers personalized wellness plans, which all RYSE members are encouraged to complete. Wellness plans provide youths the opportunity to analyze various areas of their lives and pick an area for improvement, such as fitness, school, sexual health, career plans, relationships, and academic progress, among others. Finally, for substance abuse concerns, CHAA has a school involved program Substance Abuse Treatment and Empowering Youth (SATAEY). The program description is as follows:

Community Health for Asian Americans (CHAA) will provide early intervention outpatient Alcohol and Other Drug (AOD) treatment program that targets adolescents age 18 and under with substance abuse issues that affect major areas of functioning. Moreover, SATAEY emphasizes the association of AOD abuse and multicultural issues, especially to recent immigrants and other API youth. The services will be provided in schools and at the clinic in order to promote a healthy community and reduce the harmful effects associated with alcohol and drug use.

The author has talked with his teenage daughter, an accomplished Taiko (Japanese) drumming performer, regarding music embodying cultural traditions as contemporary learning processes for positively embracing cultural identity, a source of strength and resilience. In the face of familial adversity such as domestic violence, being a member of a campus club like Taiko drumming can provide an avenue for belonging, connecting, and sense of cultural sharing further contributing to positive self-identity and esteem. Research is being formulated in this regard.

With the popularity of different social media, curricula reflecting Asian American life and experiences can be quite powerful. Rather than promote usual AAPI stereotypes, a dynamic, carefully crafted class specifically focusing on the needs of students attending can be a powerful, deep, and lasting learning experience. Anecdotally, the author has conducted years of trainings and workshops involving storytelling by AAPI students. Students often reflect on the power this has had in their lives in terms of helpful critique, deep analysis, reflection, and rich, shared experiences. The overall message has often been one of feeling validated in their experiences. Some of these positive comments have been shared even several years after the actual class experiences.

Psychoeducation can be an effective community intervention strategy as well as a primary component of school initiatives. After a serious of consecutive crises and school-related deaths of different Asian identified youth, the author proposed and articulated a prevention curriculum for Asian American middle and high school students. A set of culturally specific workshops were prepared and provided for AAPI students and their families at the beginning of each academic year. Topics were of a practical nature including adjusting to a new school environment, effective study habits, balancing home and school life, making friends, immigration, and foreign status student issues and more. The involvement of students with their families proactively at the beginning of the year before school problems arose seemed to set a healthy tenor for investment and school involvement by Asian families in their child's lives. The importance of engaging cultural communities in a bi-directional, shared manner is extremely important. In other words, culturally competent approaches for mental health prevention, promotion, and intervention in school contexts are best informed by continuously asking families and communities themselves (Mock, 2003). This keeps services relevant and accountable to the community and may further empower families in the process. From a collective perspective often framed by Asian American and Pacific Islander families and their children, solutions that emanate from families may provide best "fit" in schools.

Conclusion: A Call to Action for AAPI Youth

This chapter initially framed some of the stereotypes and myths perpetuating a false image that AAPI youth have few mental health needs in school contexts. Research and events involving AAPI reported in the media and actual narratives reflected throughout underscore a great need to better understand the mental health and related health needs of the AAPI community. AAPI communities are not monolithic but diverse and complex. As a call to action, there is enough documented information in the educational and psychological fields to argue that AAPI youth need more services responsive to the specific AAPI cultural group. More research documenting effective cultural interventions in schools must be continuously conducted. Direct interventions tied to educational outcomes can reduce stigma and shame, known barriers for help seeking among AAPIs. AAPI families and communities have strong historical legacies of surviving and thriving amid multiple sources of adversity including racism, classism, oppression, anti-immigration, and other forms of social marginalization. Culturally competent interventions that actually work for AAPI children and adolescents are best informed by involving AAPI families and the community. With a group or "we" identity as central to understanding AAPI families, relational and systemic perspectives to mental health intervention and prevention in schools are invaluable. Interventions sensitive to cultural values carry greater credibility for being successful. Lastly, trusting and forming ongoing relationships with AAPI communities can lead to mutual identification and ownership of not only problems but also cultural solutions and experiences of empowerment contributing to overall better mental health.

Acknowledgment

The author wishes to acknowledge his daughter Rachel E. Mock for the inspiration of sample narratives reflecting AAPI home and school experiences. She is at the University of California, Irvine, majoring in Asian American Studies and Psychology. While these are actual narratives, some of the information has been changed to maintain anonymity and confidentiality.

Appendix

Specific Asian American Pacific Islander (AAPI) Mental Health Resources:
American Psychiatric Association
1000 Wilson Blvd., Suite 1825
Arlington, VA 22209–3901
703-907-7300
www.healthyminds.org
Asian American Psychological Association (AAPA)
of the American Psychological Association
PMB#527
5025 North Central Avenue
Phoenix, AZ 85012
www.aapaonline.org
California Institute for Mental Health (CiMH)
Center for Multicultural Development (CMD)
2125—19th Street, 2nd Floor
Sacramento, CA 95818
(916) 556–3480
www.cimh.org
Center for Asian American Media (CAAM)
145 Ninth Street, #350
San Francisco, CA 94103
(415) 863–0814
www.caamh.org
National Asian American Pacific Islander Mental Health Association (NAAPIMHA)
1215—19th Street, Suite A
Denver, CO 80202
(303) 298–7910
www.naapimha.org
National Asian Pacific American Families Against Substance Abuse (NAPAFASA)
340 East Second Street, Suite 409
Los Angeles, CA 90012
(213) 625–5795
www.napafasa.org

References

Abelmann, N. (2009). *The intimate university: Korean American students and the problems of segregation.* Durham, NC: Duke University Press.

American Psychiatric Association. (1994). *Diagnostic and statistical manual of mental disorders* (4th ed.). Washington, DC: Author.

California Institute for Mental Health (2006). *Adopting culturally competent practices.* Available online under the Center for Multicultural Development from www.cimh.org.

Canino, I., & Spurlock, J. (1994). *Culturally diverse children and adolescents: Assessment, diagnosis, and treatment.* New York, NY: Guilford.

Chan, S. (1994). Families with Asian roots. In E. Lynch & E. M. Hanson (Eds.), *Developing cross-cultural competence: A guide for working with young children and their families* (pp. 181–257). Baltimore, MD: Brookes.

Chung, W. (1997). Developmental and life cycle issues of Asian Americans: Asian American children. In E. Lee (Ed.), *Working with Asian Americans: A guide for clinicians* (pp. 165–174). New York, NY: Guilford Press.

Hong, J., Cho, H., & Lee, A. (2010). Revisiting the Virginia Tech shootings: An ecological systems analysis. *Journal of Loss and Trauma, 15*(6), 561–575.

Hong, M. (1993). *Growing up Asian American.* New York, NY: Avon Books.

Huang, L. (1997). Developmental and life cycle issues of Asian Americans: Asian American adolescents. In E. Lee (Ed.), *Working with Asian Americans: A guide for clinicians* (pp. 175–195). Guilford Press: New York, NY.

Hune, S., & Takeuchi, D. (2008). *Asian Americans in Washington State: Closing their hidden achievement gaps.* Seattle, WA. Available from www.capaa.wa.gov: University of Washington.

Ida, D. J., & Ja, D. (2007). Research and evaluation on programs for Asian American, Native Hawaiian, and other Pacific Islander populations. *Focal Point, 21*(2), 28–31.

Kramer, E., Wang, C., Kwong, K., Lee, E., & Chung, H. (2002). Culture and medicine: Cultural factors influencing the mental health of Asian Americans. *Western Journal of Medicine., 176*(1), 227–231.

LaFromboise, T. (1995). *American Indian life skills development curriculum.* Madison, WI: University of Wisconsin Press.

Lee, E., & Mock, M. (2005a). Asian families: An overview. In M. McGoldrick, J. Giordano, & N. Garcia-Preto (Eds.), *Ethnicity and family therapy* (pp. 269–289). New York, NY: Guilford.

Lee, E., & Mock, M. (2005b). Chinese families. In M. McGoldrick, J. Giordano, & N. GarciaPreto (Eds.), *Ethnicity and family therapy* (pp. 302–318). New York, NY: Guilford.

Lee, S. (1996). *Unraveling the "model minority" stereotype: Listening to Asian American youth and teachers.* New York, NY: College Press.

Mock, M. (2008). Visioning Social Justice: Narratives of diversity, social location and personal compassion. In M. McGoldrick & K. Hardy (Eds.), *Re-visioning family therapy: Race, culture, and gender in clinical practice* (2nd ed.). New York: Guilford.

Mock, M. (2003). Cultural sensitivity, relevance, and competence in school mental health. In M. Weist, S. Evans, & N. Lever (Eds.), *Handbook of school mental health: Advancing practice and research* (pp. 349–362). New York, NY: Plenum.

Mock, M. (1998). Clinical reflections on refugee families: Transforming crises into opportunities. In M. McGoldrick (Ed.), *Revisioning family therapy: Race, culture and gender in clinical practice* (pp. 347–369). New York, NY: Guilford.

National Commission on Asian American and Pacific Islander Research in Education (2008). *Asian Americans and Pacific Islanders—Facts, notification: Setting the record straight.*, available from the College Board on the Web. www.collegeboard.com.

Paul, A. M. (2011). The roar of the tiger mom. *Time Magazine, 177*(4), 34–41.

Stone, O., Yang., J. (Executive Producers). (2003), *The Joy Luck Club* (DVD).

Sue, S., & Okazaki, S. (1990). Asian-American educational achievements: A phenomenon in search of an explanation. *American Psychologist, 45*(8), 913–920.

Suicide Prevention Action Network. (2007). *Suicide among Asian Americans/Pacific Islanders*, Washington, DC: SAMHSA, U.S. Department of Health and Human Services. Retrieved June 17, 2012 from www.sprc.org.

Suzuki, R. H. (1980). Education and the socialization of Asian Americans: A revisionist analysis of the "model minority" thesis. In R. Endo, S. Sue, & N. Wagner (Eds.), *Asian-Americans: Social and psychological perspectives* (pp. 155–175). Ben Lomond, CA: Science and Behavior Books.

Tewari, N., & Alvarez, A. (2009). *Asian American psychology: Current perspectives.* New York: NY: Taylor & Francis.

Uba, L. (1994). *Asian Americans: Personality patterns, identity, and mental health.* New York, NY: Guilford.

Umemoto, K., & Ong, P. (2006). Asian American and Pacific Islander youth: Risks, challenges and opportunities. *Aapi Nexus, 4*(2), v–ix.

U.S. Census Bureau (2010) *U.S. Census Bureau news: Facts for features – Asian/Pacific heritage month.* Retrieved May 2010 from www.aapi.gov.

U.S. Department of Health and Human Services. (2001). *Mental health: Culture, race and ethnicity—A supplement to mental health: A report of the surgeon general.* Washington, DC: Office of the Surgeon General.

Wong, L., & Mock, M. (1997). Developmental and life cycle issues of Asian Americans: Asian American young adults. In E. Lee (Ed.), *Working with Asian Americans: A guide for clinicians* (pp. 196–207). New York, NY: Guilford.

Xing, J. (1998). *Asia America through the lens: History, representations, and identity.* Oxford: Altamira.

Zane, N., & Mak, W. (2003). Major approaches to the measurement of acculturation among ethnic minority populations: A content analysis and an alternative empirical strategy. In G. Marin, P. Balls Organista, & K. M. Chun (Eds.), *Acculturation: Advances in theory, measurement, and applied research* (pp. 39–60). Washington, DC: American Psychological Association.

Raising Consciousness: Promoting Healthy Coping Among African American Boys at School

Keisha L. Bentley-Edwards, Duane E. Thomas, and Howard C. Stevenson

While African American boys make up only a small percentage of the overall primary and secondary school student populations, they account for a staggering proportion of students who experience significant and consistent negative outcomes at school. According to recent national estimates (U. S. Department of Education, 2010), African American males constituted less than 10% of the public school population, yet accounted for approximately 26% of students who were retained and 49% and 17% of those suspended or expelled, respectively. The last decade has witnessed a surge in discourse on comprehensive school-based mental health reform efforts to address these problems and promote more positive outcomes for African American males (Caldwell, Sewell, Parks, & Toldson, 2009; Gregory, Skiba, & Noguera, 2010; Noguera, 2003; Thomas & Stevenson, 2009). As part of these efforts, there has been a call for professionals providing mental health services in schools to help address the ecological risk and protective factors confronting African American males.

This chapter examines the racially and gender-charged contexts of African American boys as a foundation for developing healthy coping in school settings. By addressing school policies that disproportionately punish and even criminalize African American boys, the authors suggest that researchers and practitioners utilize culturally relevant theoretical frameworks and research-based evidence as the basis for strategies to promote successful outcomes. Theoretical models that utilize identity-based resilience (Spencer, 1995) and racial/ethnic socialization (Stevenson, 2012) are reviewed as well as culturally relevant assessments and interventions. Implications for practice are discussed, particularly training for teachers and school-based mental health providers on how to appraise their own race and gender-based beliefs and interactions with African American boys, and to use contextually relevant strategies specific to this youth population.

Healthy Coping Among African American Males

Despite a good amount of research and intervention, a disproportionately large number of African American boys continue to encounter significant problems at school and this may be attributable, in part, to the lack of focus on "coping." We define coping as healthy or maladaptive behavioral and emotional responses to situations and environments. Spencer, Fegley, Harpalani, and

K.L. Bentley-Edwards (✉)
University of Texas at Austin,
Austin, TX, USA
e-mail: kbentleyedwards@austin.utexas.edu

D.E. Thomas
University of Virginia, Charlottesville, VA, USA
e-mail: det5r@virginia.edu

H.C. Stevenson
University of Pennsylvania, Philadelphia, PA, USA
e-mail: howards@gse.upenn.edu

Seaton (2004) were among the first of a cadre of researchers to draw attention to cultural coping strategies arising from within the ethos of the African American male experience that might adversely affect these students' emotional and behavioral outcomes in school. They posited that particular coping strategies evidenced in these students' responses to perceived or actual race-based hostility by teachers and/or peers might negatively impact African American male students' ability to successfully negotiate interpersonal situations in schools. As such, promoting the development of healthy culturally-based coping is vital for African American boys' success at school, and an important consideration for school mental health.

School Contexts as Uniquely Problematic for African American Males

African American boys face racial discrimination that often preempts the acquisition of many of the gender-based privileges that can result from living in a male-dominated American culture (Thomas & Stevenson, 2009). For example, while male students in primary and secondary education are afforded privileges (Beaman, Wheldall, & Kemp, 2006; Croll, 1985) that can result in subsequent employment, earnings, and access to higher education and wealth, this is not the case for African American males (U.S. Census Bureau, 2010).

In their critical review on gender equity and schooling, Thomas and Stevenson (2009) documented findings from seminal work across multiple disciplines showing that African American boys remain the most at-risk relative to other groups for disparities in education. According to their findings, African American boys, especially those in urban public schools, are overrepresented in remedial classes while underrepresented in advanced classes and receive lower grades and standardized tests scores compared to their White and Asian American counterparts. Moreover, these boys tend to garner more biased and erroneous accusations of wrongdoing from teachers and experience more heightened levels of friction with those and other adults in the school setting from the early elementary years through high school (Epstein, March, Conners, & Jackson, 1998; Farkas, 2003; Neal, McCray, Webb-Johnson, & Bridgest, 2003; Thomas, Coard, Stevenson, Bentley, & Zamel, 2009). As such, African American male students tend to experience challenges that are different from those experienced by males from other ethnic and racial groups. Thus, African American boys are placed in a Catch-33 situation where they are not just "damned if they do" or "damned if they don't," they're "just damned" (Cassidy, Davis, & Stevenson, 2003). African American boys encounter these Catch-33's in multiple situations in the home, neighborhood and school. They navigate these situations, often without success, as they are often conflated with hypermasculinity (Spencer et al., 2004) or invisibility (Franklin & Boyd-Franklin, 2000).

Finally, African American boys receive less critical research analysis, and school policies and counseling interventions fail to consider their developmental status as children and adolescents (Edwards, 2010). For example, challenging authority figures—a normative and transitory behavior commonly associated with adolescence—is oftentimes viewed as a persistent and developmentally aberrant personality characteristic associated with adulthood when exhibited by African American boys (Stevenson, Herrero-Taylor, Cameron, & Davis, 2002). This "adultification" of young African American male students often leads to overly punitive responses and practices by school personnel. This process has been shown to begin as early as preschool (Gilliam & Shahar, 2006) and elementary school (Browne, Losen, & Wald, 2002; Ferguson, 2003; Wald & Losen, 2007) and predisposes African American boys to school failure, and, in some cases, future incarceration.

School Policies and Practices that Predispose African American Male Students to Negative Educational, Social, and Emotional Outcomes

Research consistently shows that African American boys receive more suspension and expulsion discipline, despite the lack of evidence that they have more problems with misbehavior than other males (Gilliam & Shahar, 2006; Gregory et al., 2010; Skiba, Michael, Nardo, & Peterson, 2002; The Advancement Project, 2005, 2010). African American boys are more likely than their White counterparts to be displaced from school for both minor and serious offenses (Skiba et al., 2002). There is also an enduring misconception that African American youth are prone to drug addiction despite the fact that African American males are less likely than white males in their teen years to take drugs, such as cocaine (Centers for Disease Control and Prevention, 2006). African American males are also more likely to be arrested and incarcerated based on violations at school. This gateway has increased since "culture-fair" zero tolerance policies began after the Columbine School shooting incident in 1999. While this legislation was instituted in reaction to White male gun violence in schools, it remains now a racially discriminatory policy that efficiently ushers African American and Latino males from schools to penal institutions (The Advancement Project, 2005, 2010). Zero-tolerance policies often take precedence over research evidence and practitioner expertise in managing developmentally appropriate problem behaviors exhibited in school (Casella, 2003). These policies focus on maintaining order at all costs, and do not consider the best interest of African American boys (Gregory et al., 2010).

Significant Lack of Knowledge and Training Within Adult Support Systems

Compounding the discriminatory experiences African American boys face in school, is the lack of availability, acquisition and application of the skill sets required to successfully navigate and transcend them (Cassidy et al., 2003). There is growing recognition that deficits in African American boys' repertoire of skills to negotiate perceived or actual racialized and gender disparities in classroom encounters may be attributable, in part, to insufficiencies in teacher training, but also to the lack of integration of race matters into routine curricula that guide classroom practices; interpersonal interactions, and academic and behavioral supports (Neal et al., 2003; Thomas & Stevenson, 2009; Thomas et al., 2011). Even educators and counselors who have a track record of excellence in their craft, but who have little exposure, training and knowledge of the lives of African American boys can be inadequate in providing the necessary support to these students (Krovetz & Arriaza, 2006).

Parents, teachers, and school counselors are often overwhelmed at how to tackle the educational imbalances that result in African American boys' lower graduation and higher suspension and expulsion rates. Racial stereotyping or unconscious bias are major challenges even for well-intentioned authority figures, and without training, can contribute to damaging psychological effects for African American boys (Stevenson et al., 2003). As with most youth, the boys themselves do not understand the long-term impact of momentary or repeated lapses in judgment. The coping mechanisms utilized by African American boys depend on the available support systems they have, and skill set to recast stereotyped expectations. It is also critical to take into consideration that each life transition brings unique racial and gender crises (Cross & Cross, 2008; Erikson, 1968) which require specific racial and gender negotiation knowledge and skill sets. Despite early physical maturation and hypermasculine behaviors, African American boys must first and foremost be interacted with as children, not men (Stevenson et al., 2003).

The Need for New Theoretical Lenses

To develop successful school-based policies, programming, and practices researchers and practitioners must first consider the unique racial and gender experiences of African American boys within schools. One approach is to explicitly target racial and gender discrimination using racial socialization-focused interventions. Educational and legal systems are reticent to identify racial discrimination as a culprit for obvious reasons of "egalitarianism of treatment or application of the law." The problem is that while we have a democratic system that idealizes egalitarianism, by in large African American boys do not receive the same treatment as boys of other races and this results in disparate outcomes. African American boys' unique experiences may not be sufficiently addressed by a universal approach to behavioral assessment and control in the classroom. Understanding African American boys' behavioral expressions, and employing appropriate techniques to manage problem behavior requires a consideration of preexisting stigma and bias inherent in the classroom.

A key first step is to identify and analyze the depth of racial discrimination in the systems and contexts in which African American boys engage as explicitly as possible. Researchers must reconsider customary racial comparison studies between African Americans and other groups, which are essentially comparisons of skin color differences. Instead, they must recognize that possessing a racial status is not racial discrimination. Counselors and administrators who attempt to interpret African American versus White differences without considering the daily racialized experiences and policies at their schools cannot adequately influence the achievement and coping of African American boys (Johnson & Avelar La Salle, 2010).

The second step is to identify and assess how racial stress and socialization permeate the racialized experiences of educators, counselors, and students. Often, unconscious and insidious racial stress in both school personnel and African American boys undermines the positive perceptions and potential of African American boys. The research on racial stress reveals that it may lead to stereotype threat and the internalization of academic inferiority (Steele, 1997, 1998; Steele & Aronson, 1995). This is a disturbing outcome of unchecked racial stress that cannot be left to school cultures that promote "niceness" or attempt to curb fighting, but do not target the root stress and its multiple dimensions directly. For example, an increase in altercations after Black History Month-related activities may be an indicator of underlying racial tensions on campus. Insensitive or disparaging remarks by classmates after these events are often downplayed while administrators focus on the ensuing fight or conflict. School counselors may feel that an African American boy's reaction may outweigh the racial slight, however, preventing recurrences must address the underlying causes not just the student's behavioral response.

A final critical step is to teach students and educators the skills to appraise, recast, and reduce racial stress so that it does not interfere with emotional, academic, or professional functioning in the school. Educators and clinicians have to be able to both learn the skills to personally negotiate racial stress and to teach these skills to African American youth in tandem to academic instruction (Arriaza, 2003). Parents, as the first teachers, can be an important source of information regarding how to teach African American boys coping skills. However, educators must provide this teaching as well, as they spend a great deal of time socializing students. An important consideration is how teachers can teach something of which they themselves have little knowledge (Howard, 1999). Successfully negotiating racial stress in one's interactions with African American male youth is a key component of teaching them how to succeed in school. Unfortunately, schools of education and teacher training do not address these matters well and very few theoretical models address racial conflict and tension between African American male students and school personnel.

Theoretical Frameworks for Promoting Effective Coping in African American Boys

Two theoretical frames are applied in promoting the healthy coping of African American boys: Phenomenological Variant of Ecological Systems Theory (PVEST)—a phenomenological ecological systems model developed by Margaret Beale Spencer and her colleagues (Spencer, 1995, 1999; Spencer, Dupree, & Hartmann, 1997; Spencer, Noll, Stoltzfus, & Harpalani, 2001), and RECAST—a racial stress and socialization model developed by Howard Stevenson (Stevenson, 2012). These models offer developmentally appropriate explanations and guidance for moving African American boys from being typecasts in stereotyped and disparaged roles, to roles they redefine and re-script for themselves.

PVEST. Spencer's PVEST is a cyclic, recursive model of development for youth that requires African American students' experiences to be examined within various contexts, taking into account both risk and protective factors for their behavioral functioning and academic outcomes (Spencer, 1995, 1999; Spencer et al., 1997). An integral concept in this developmental model is that strong identity formation is essential in helping African American youth develop coping strategies necessary for emotional well-being and efficacy in schools and other social contexts (Spencer, Fegley, & Harpalani, 2003). This assertion is supported by longstanding research associating positive racial identity with higher academic achievement (Altschul, Oyserman & Bybee, 2006; Ford & Harris, 1997) and, self-esteem (Spencer et al., 2001) and, decreased problem behaviors (Wong, Eccles, & Sameroff, 2003).

Spencer's PVEST identifies five components that contribute to their cyclical model of identity-based resilience (Spencer et al., 2003; Spencer, Swanson, & Edwards, 2010). The model begins with the *Net Risk/Vulnerability Level*, which includes contextual factors that may provide support or interfere with positive development or safety. The balance between risk contributors and protective factors is the *Net Stress Engagement Levels*, or what someone must deal with personally as they face the world. For example, even after a parent provides a safe home environment with appropriate supervision, a young boy may still have to deal with the solicitation of local drug dealers who want them to run errands as they walk to school. The way the child responds to the repeated solicitations is a result of his *Reactive Coping Strategies*, which may be positive/adaptive (declining and taking a different route to school), or negative/maladaptive (taking on a dangerous errand). After repeated responses to various contexts, the coping methods utilized transition from a reaction to a situation into an *Emergent Identity*, or an integral part of how that child sees himself or is perceived by others. This stable coping response is a function of actions merging into who they are. In this case, the student may self identify, or be perceived by adults as a "good kid" or a "thug." The consequences of the reactive coping methods used, and the emergent identity that develops, puts into motion *Life-Stage Specific Coping Outcomes*-which are either productive (ex. finishing school) or unfavorable (expulsion or incarceration) (Cunningham, Hurley, Foney, & Hayes, 2002; Spencer et al., 2003, 2010). Spencer's PVEST focuses on the interactions within and between processes that influence a child's perceptions of self-efficacy, social challenges, and outcomes.

Using PVEST as a framework requires that African American youth are appraised at an individual level, while recognizing the shared experiences of this population, both at school and in society (Spencer, 1995). Within this framework, supportive academic environments, racial socialization and appropriate supervision can serve as protective factors that shape more favorable net stress, and healthy reactive coping mechanisms. Conversely, high delinquency, disruptive classmates and aggressive school environments can function as risk contributors. For example, as a result of teacher stereotyping, an adolescent may react with behavior that would be considered oppositional, and this may perpetuate the bias-negative coping cyclical pattern which in turn impacts that child's identity, overall academic achievement and social competency. Therefore strong identity formation is considered essential for developing effective coping strategies and ensuring emotional well-being, future orientation, and efficacy.

RECAST. Stevenson (2012) proposed a culturally relevant theoretical model that considers the mediating role that racial/ethnic socialization (R/ES) plays in buffering or promoting the effects of racial stress on racial, academic, and emotional coping. R/ES processes have four functions—to buffer and promote racial identity development by resolving racial stress and conflict using (1) *protection,* (2) *affirmation,* (3) *reappraisal, and* (4) *negotiation* strategies. As individuals develop racial/ethnic stress reduction and negotiation skills through practice and explicit instruction in problem-solving strategies, they can approach racial/ethnic conflicts in classrooms, street corners, and public spaces with confidence.

Moreover, resolution does not leave students of color at risk for stigmatization or worse, criminalization. As such, African American boys' coping behaviors increase as they receive racial/ethnic socialization that leads to the development of racial negotiation skills that counter stereotyping processes visible within the societal and cultural institutions they inhabit.

Culturally-Responsive Approaches to Promoting Coping

As more researchers reveal the positive relationships between cultural strengths and academic achievement and behavioral outcomes (Franklin & Pack-Brown, 2001; Hudley & Graham, 1995; Stevenson, 2002), various practitioners and program developers have attempted to incorporate racial/cultural components in their curricula. Several programs have successfully implemented programs for African American boys utilizing strategies that promote racial/ethnic pride and agency with improved achievement (Bass & Coleman, 1997) and decreased externalizing behaviors (Franklin & Pack-Brown, 2001; Stevenson, 2003). However, there remains an abundance of programs seeking to improve academic or social outcomes for African American boys that make several key errors, leading to unsuccessful and frustrating results.

Successful interventions incorporate the following strategies in their development and implementation; they:
- Clearly define, document and measure the specific adversity, program strategies and outcomes the program is designed to address. This satisfies the requirement of many funding agencies for evidence-based outcomes, and allows for replication with future cohorts and sites
- Utilize key informants and reliable sources (research, community input, and participants) to ascertain programming strategies
- Consider developmentally appropriate strategies and resources in program implementation. Programs designed for adolescent African American boys are not likely to be effective for their elementary-school counterparts
- Use culturally-relevant measurement in the assessment process[1]

Preventing Long-term Anger and Aggression in Youth (PLAAY; Stevenson, 2003*).* The PLAAY project is a culturally relevant intervention project that uses RECAST theory to assess and influence the emotional functioning of youth. A key aspect of this intervention is the use of movement (e.g., basketball) as a means to understand emotional strengths and limitations, bond with youth through stress awareness and negotiation of interpersonal conflicts, and lead youth toward more prosocial interactions. The program emphasizes the reduction of aggression and understanding one's own anger. PLAAY emphasizes that anger management is not anger reduction, and acknowledges that many youth walk into classrooms, neighborhoods and relationships with unresolved trauma from having witnessed tragedy and experienced significant loss of loved ones and friends. These events are often hidden and undisclosed but are an opportunity for emotional healing. Many African American boys are hypervulnerable and respond with hypermasculine behaviors in order to protect themselves from emotional and physical assaults (Cassidy & Stevenson, 2005).

The racial components of these "reactive coping" interactions can be explained through PVEST's focus on how individuals are shaped by the multiple contexts they inhabit (Cunningham et al., 2002). Since African American boys are often alone to make meaning of their lives within invisible racial and gendered contexts, they are at risk of inaccurately interpreting the source of these assaults. Authority figures and educators often do not understand the unique life experiences and stereotyping of African American boys, and may wrongfully define the boys' trauma

---

[1] Jones's (1996) extensive compilation of tests that utilize both mainstream (ex., self-esteem and coping) and culture specific (racial identity, racism stress) psychological constructs, serves as an excellent starting point for practitioners seeking baseline and post-intervention assessments.

reactions as indicating inferiority or confirming stereotypes, rather than a mechanism for coping.

In PLAAY, keys to challenging the reactive coping of African American boys include: (1) identifying that students behaviors be interpreted first from a child development lens ("Boys, not Men"); (2) explicitly socializing the boys to develop skills to identify, negotiate, and resolve gender and racial/ethnic politics; and (3) use play and movement as alternative vehicles to assess and intervene with their "in-the-moment" stressful reactions and interactions.

Outcomes of a randomized field trial of PLAAY with over 300 boys over the course of a 5-year span, indicate the intervention was successful at reducing anger and increasing healthy coping (Davis, Zamel, Hall, Espin, & Williams, 2003; Stevenson, 2003). Important to note is that many of the most aggressive boys were also the most responsive to the PLAAY intervention, even though their expression of anger did not subside. Additionally, as compared to a control group, the PLAAY participants appeared to be more aware of their anger and to what it was related. Participants were also better able to recognize the racial and gender politics within their schooling and neighborhood contexts that endanger them if they chose to express their anger too forcefully. Further, the boys in the PLAAY group also did a better job of using multiple definitions of manhood in lieu of a definition that relied heavily on aggression. Other research shows that the boys who were aware of their racial socialization experiences were also less likely to be targeted by teachers as maladjusted and aggressive (Thomas et al., 2009), thus demonstrating how racial socialization can support effective coping in schools. Future research using PLAAY principles and strategies should consider how to influence authority figures to bond more competently with African American boys by using counter-stereotyping knowledge and skills training.

Got Skillz? Managing and Negotiating Racial Stress in the Classroom

In an attempt to understand the subtleties of racial stress, conflict and negotiation beyond the basketball court, recast theory is being applied to the dynamics of peer- and teacher-African American student relationships in the classroom (Thomas et al., 2011). The *Can WE Talk? (CWT)* project endeavored to understand how African American youth can be taught racial stress awareness and negotiation skills (also described as racial/ethnic literacy) to increase their voice and achievement in academic matters in the classroom. Both racial and academic stresses are challenges for many African American males who to avoid humiliation withdraw from schoolwork.

Strategies to reverse these stress reactions include a curricular frame of five racial/ethnic (R/E) literacy goals (1) R/E self-awareness; (2) R/E stress appraisal; (3) R/E stress reappraisal; (4) R/E conflict management; (5) R/E Resolution. Each of these goals has corresponding skill sets and expectations. *R/E self-awareness* for African American boys is developed through R/E socialization teaching of African American history, psychology, politics and how this knowledge illuminates the strengths and limitations of African American masculinity development. The R/E stress-awareness skills expectations for African American boys, for example, would be to demonstrate the ability to tell their life story inclusive of racial and gender experiences in the classroom. *R/E stress appraisal* for African American boys is developed through personal story-telling elements of their talented or ineffective coping with stress. They are asked to honestly rate how stressful these obstacles are. The recounting and reexamination of one's strengths and weaknesses involves R/E cognitive-behavioral processing which must be accomplished within "safe" contexts with caring facilitators, where the skills expectations of self-efficacy are paramount.

R/E stress reappraisal for African American boys involves taking the most challenging moments of their coping and confronting them to see these "mountains" differently. Through the use of cognitive-behavioral re-socialization of academic and racial "tsunami"-level stressors to become "mountain-climbing" excursions (Lazarus & Folkman, 1987). By role-playing specific stressful situations, African American boys can begin to develop mindfulness skills that are generalizable to multiple school contexts beyond the classroom (performance on athletic teams, leadership in extracurricular activities). R/E *conflict management* and *resolution* are attainable for African American boys once they can rebut the psychological debilitation of stereotyping in their own minds and in the discourses of classroom pedagogy and banter. The previous strategies of storytelling, cognitive-behavioral restructuring, and role-playing are combined with stereotype debating exercises where the boys have to verbally argue their positions with facts, style, personal wit and all forms of cultural expression. The difference between R/E conflict management and resolution is twofold: conflict management focuses on the development of listening skills since the boys need to hear opposing viewpoints in order to battle those viewpoints, while conflict resolution focuses on applying all previous skills learned into actual classroom conflicts that bring them the most challenge. In R/E conflict resolution, African American boys learn to not just listen and debate the academic stressors and conflicts before them, but negotiate them toward self-preservation through academic achievement.

CWT is designed to (1) improve students' and teachers' capacity to reappraise schoolwork and racial relationship conflicts as workable obstacles rather than menacing statements of inferiority; (2) enhance academic and racial negotiation self-efficacy and competence; and (3) track the impact of any changes in threat reappraisals on teacher–student and African American male student–student relationships, and student academic engagement and achievement.

Culturally-Relevant Measurement and Assessment

It is critical that intervention and prevention programs that use strategies that promote racial or cultural strengths, employ measures that assess racial/ethnic socialization (Bentley & Stevenson, 2012; Brown & Krishnakumar, 2007; Hughes & Chen, 1997; Stevenson, 1994; Stevenson et al., 2002). Using the RECAST theoretical framework, the Cultural and Racial Experiences of Socialization (CARES; Bentley & Stevenson, 2012) is a new measure of R/ES that examines the frequency, belief and source (including family, peers, teachers, & media) of these messages. Utilizing the CARES allows researchers and practitioners to ascertain the prevalence of R/ES messages, but to also discover what their students believe about race and racial hierarchies. Research with the CARES instrument (Bentley & Stevenson) shows that specific sources more strongly predicted what African American students believed, even if they were less frequently cited sources. More specifically, hearing both empowering messages around cultural heritage, and diminishing messages that promoted stereotyped beliefs about African American people from teachers best predicted African American student beliefs around these constructs. As a multifaceted assessment, CARES enables practitioners to understand African American boys' exposure and meaning-making around race and racial hierarchies.

The Racial Investment Questionnaire (RIQ) and the Black Racial Dissonance Inventory (BRDI) (Bentley, 2012) assess the intersections of racial identity, altruism and social cohesion or racial ambivalence and disconnect, respectively. Bentley (2012) found a positive relationship between positive psychological racial cohesion and grades. It was also revealed that African American students that scored high on the BRDI were less likely to be involved in any form of community service or social justice activities, even those unrelated to race. Thus, African American students demonstrating high racial dissonance may have an overall apathy that may represent a desire to remain disassociated with any vulnerable or stereotyped population. This ambivalence must be addressed to empower those from disenfranchised communities and support leadership development in African American boys. Measurements that acknowledge cultural strengths provide empirical evidence of African American youth's racial coping strategies and emerging identity that will inevitably be confronted in some fashion in intervention and prevention programs tailored for this population.

Implications for Promoting Coping in Schools

This chapter highlights the need to consider the intricate and inextricable linkage between racialized gender socialization processes, the various contexts and situations that engender these processes, and the individual reactive coping strategies of African American boys. This has important implications for applied efforts to promote adaptive outcomes for this population across multiple domains of development. Given the momentous challenges faced by African American boys in schools from their initial transition into formal schooling throughout their primary and secondary school year experiences (see Farkas, 2003; Noguera, 2003; Thomas & Stevenson, 2009) efforts to promote coping should be undertaken in schools. Whether schools are dealing with social rebuffs, low expectations, or excessive suspensions, initiatives should address the personal attitudes and practices of teachers directly through training about race and racial stress operating within classrooms between themselves (and/or colleagues) and students of color.

Formal teacher education programs and/or continued professional development/service learning opportunities should include considerable self-exploration around issues of race. This is unchartered territory in educational research. There is a natural tendency to skirt around the scrutinization of teachers' personal attitudes about race (with respect to their own referent group and to different racial groups) and the role these attitudes may (or may not) play in the maintenance of racial inequities in school policies and practices that grossly disadvantage African American boys (Stevenson, 2008). There is an inherent vulnerability to teachers' processing and coming to terms with their beliefs about and attitudes towards African American boys. However, acquiring knowledge about and/or learning particular technical skills to work with this population should be but are not fundamental components of multicultural training in teacher-education programs. Racial self-awareness is essential because teachers are not impervious to racial stereotypes and are susceptible to bringing overgeneralizations, preconceived notions, and fears concerning African American boys with them into the classroom (Thomas & Stevenson, 2009). When teachers are challenged to examine their attitudes about race, it helps minimize bias and opens the door to pedagogical techniques that draw upon the inherent strengths and talents of African American boys. This in turn, supports teacher practices that help foster adaptive coping strategies and positive outcomes among these students.

It is important to note that culturally informed practices for African American boys do not require same-race leadership. Non-African American practitioners can implement programs like PLAAY and CWT as these programs help practitioners address personal race-based discomforts, and promote trust building and informed regard for African American boys' contexts and experiences. Ultimately, African American boys and their parents need to believe with certainty that their teachers and mental health providers have their best interest at heart. Regardless of race, these practitioners should make it clear to their students that they are a consistent ally and advocate for African Americans—this is particularly important for African American boys in predominantly White settings.

There are also important implications for mental health service providers working with and developing interventions germane to the cultural experiences of African American boys. Effective acquisition and interpretation of culturally relevant research and assessment must be a high priority and driving influence in promoting coping strategies. Interventions that target African American boys' preoccupation with and reactions to racial stereotypes (Steele, 1997; Steele & Aronson, 1995; Steele, Spencer, & Aronson, 2002), emotional distress, and behavioral adjustment problems linked to racial dynamics in classrooms are of great value. Given the demonstrated utility of this approach with both clinical (Hudley & Graham, 1995; Stevenson, 2003) and normative (Franklin & Pack-Brown, 2001; Thomas et al., 2011) samples of African American male student populations, programs with a joint goal of enhancing healthy racial identification and social problem-solving skills through racial socialization-based principles may be of particular benefit. The infusion of student racial negotiation skills to address tense interactions with teachers (and peers) may also equip African American boys with strategies to effectively cope with and respond to classroom situations, leading to outcomes that culturally neutral interventions have failed to consider.

Taken together, a critical step in promoting the academic success and wellbeing of African American boys in schools is training teachers, counselors, and other school-based clinicians to attend to the significant and unique challenges confronting these boys face in their daily racialized gender experiences. Helping teachers and practitioners develop and utilize different cultural-based competencies may, in turn, instill in African American boys rich repositories of skills to successfully negotiate racial dynamics operating within classrooms and broader contexts in schools.

As we consider strategies to promote healthy coping in African American boys, we must also veer away from the concept of exceptionalism as a form of encouragement. In other words, teachers and other adults should not tell children that they are special because they are African American and smart, thus implying that being a high achiever serves as an exception to the rule of African American underachievement. Educators often reinforce individualistic academic paradigms and success endeavors (Sankofa, Hurley, Allen, & Boykin, 2005; Tyler, Boykin, & Walton, 2006) despite the research that demonstrates that communalism and culturally based common-fate orientations engender student learning (Hurley, Boykin, & Allen, 2005), peer acceptance (Tyler et al., 2006) and more well-rounded resilience (American Psychological Association, 2008).

In sum, enhanced competencies may serve as the bedrock for strategies that develop healthy coping in schools. Given the ever-widening gaps in achievement and school disciplinary policies that disproportionately shortchange African American male students (Gregory et al., 2010) and forecast their unparalleled residence in the school-to-prison pipeline (The Advancement Project, 2005, 2010), the consequences for not addressing these and other contemporary issues facing African American boys may be calamitous.

References

Altschul, I., Oyserman, D., & Bybee, D. (2006). Racial-ethnic identity in mid-adolescence: Content and change as predictors of academic achievement. *Child development, 77*(5), 1155–1169.

American Psychological Association. (2008). *Resilience in African American children and adolescents: A vision for optimal development* (p. 134). Washington, DC: American Psychological Association Task Force on Resilience and Strength in Black Children and Adolescents.

Arriaza, G. (2003). Schools, social capital and children of color. *Race Ethnicity and Education, 6*(1), 71–94.

Bass, C. K., & Coleman, H. L. K. (1997). Enhancing the cultural identity of early adolescent male African Americans. *Professional School Counseling. Special Issue: Exemplary Practices from the Field: Elementary and Middle School Counselors Sharing What Works for Them, 1*(2), 48–51.

Beaman, R., Wheldall, K., & Kemp, C. (2006). Differential teacher attention to boys and girls in the classroom. *Educational Review, 58*(3), 339–366.

Bentley, K. L. (2012). Hope, agency or disconnect: The impact of racial experiences on the racial cohesion of Black college students [Submitted].

Bentley, K. L., & Stevenson, H. C. (2012). Beyond pride and mothers: Recasting racial/ethnic socialization measurement for multidimensional processes and informants [Submitted].

Brown, T. L., & Krishnakumar, A. (2007). Development and validation of the adolescent racial and ethnic socialization scale (ARESS) in African American families. *Journal of Youth and Adolescence, 36*, 1072–1085. doi:DOI 10.1007/s10964-007-9197-z.

Browne, J. A., Losen, D. J., & Wald, J. (2002). Zero tolerance: Unfair, with little recourse. In R. J. Skiba & G. G. Noam (Eds.), *Zero tolerance: Can suspension and expulsion keep school safe? new directions for youth development* (pp. 73–99). San Francisco, CA: Jossey-Bass.

Caldwell, L. D., Sewell, A. A., Parks, N., & Toldson, I. A. (2009). Guest editorial: Before the bell rings: Implementing coordinated school health models to influence the academic achievement of African American males. *Journal of Negro Education, 78*(3), 204–215.

Casella, R. (2003). Zero tolerance policy in schools: Rationale, consequences, and alternatives. *Teachers College Record, 105*(5), 872–892.

Cassidy, E. F., Davis, G. Y., & Stevenson, H. C. (2003). "If we must die": CPR for managing catch-33, alienation and hypervulnerability. In H. C. Stevenson (Ed.), *Playing with anger: Teaching coping skills to African American boys through athletics and culture* (pp. 89–114). Westport, CT: Praeger.

Cassidy, E. F., & Stevenson, H. C. (2005). They wear the mask: Hypervulnerability and hypermasculine aggression among African American males in an urban remedial disciplinary school. *Journal Aggression, Maltreatment & Trauma, 11*(4), 53–74. doi:10.1300/J146v11n04_03.

Centers for Disease Control and Prevention. (2006). Youth risk behavior surveillance 2005 *Surveillance summaries* (pp. 112). Atlanta, GA: Centers for Disease Control and Prevention.

Croll, P. (1985). Teacher interaction with individual male and female pupils in junior-age classrooms. *Educational Research, 27*(3), 220–223. doi:10.1080/0013188850270309.

Cross, W. E., & Cross, T. B. (2008). Theory, research, and models. In S. M. Quintana & C. McKown (Eds.), *Handbook of race, racism, and the developing child* (pp. 154–181). Hoboken, NJ US: Wiley.

Cunningham, M., Hurley, M., Foney, D., & Hayes, D. (2002). Influence of perceived contextual stress on self-esteem and academic outcomes in African American adolescents. *Journal of Black Psychology, 28*(3), 215–233. doi:10.1177/00998402028003003.

Davis, G., Zamel, P. C., Hall, D., Espin, E., & Williams, V. (2003). Life after PLAAY: Alumni group and Rites of Passage Empowerment (ROPE). In H. C. Stevenson (Ed.), *Playing with anger: Teaching coping skills to African American boys through athletics and culture* (p. 203). Westport, CT: Praeger.

Edwards, M. C. (2010). Understanding adolescence: A policy perspective. In D. P. Swanson, M. C. Edwards, & M. B. Spencer (Eds.), *Adolescence: Development during a global era* (pp. 477–498). Burlington: Academic.

Epstein, J. N., March, J. S., Conners, C. K., & Jackson, D. L. (1998). Racial differences on the Conners Teacher Rating Scale. *Journal of abnormal child psychology, 26*(2), 109–118.

Erikson, E. H. (1968). *Identity: youth and crisis*. Oxford, England: Norton & Co.

Farkas, G. (2003). Racial disparities and discrimination in education: What do we know, how do we know it, and what do we need to know? *Teachers College Record, 105*(6), 1119–1146.

Ferguson, R. F. (2003). Teachers' perceptions and expectations and the Black-White test score gap. *Urban Education. Special Issue: Educating African American males, Volume 1, 38*(4), 460–507.

Ford, D. Y., & Harris, J. J., III. (1997). A study of the racial identity and achievement of Black males and females. *Roeper Review, 20*(2), 105–110.

Franklin, A. J., & Boyd-Franklin, N. (2000). Invisibility syndrome: A clinical model of the effects of racism on African-American males. *American Journal of Orthopsychiatry, 70*(1), 33–41.

Franklin, R. B., & Pack-Brown, S. (2001). Team brothers: An Africentric approach to group work with African American male adolescents. *Journal for Specialists in Group Work. Special Issue: The use of groups for prevention, 26*(3), 237–245.

Gilliam, W. S., & Shahar, G. (2006). Preschool and child care expulsion and suspension: Rates and predictors in one state. *Infants & Young Children, 19*(3), 228–245. doi:10.1097/00001163-200607000-00007.

Gregory, A., Skiba, R. J., & Noguera, P. A. (2010). The achievement gap and the discipline gap: Two sides of the same coin? *Educational Researcher, 39*(1), 59–68. doi:10.3102/0013189x09357621.

Howard, G. R. (1999). *We can't teach what we don't know: White teachers, multiracial schools* (2nd ed.). New York: Teachers College Press.

Hudley, C., & Graham, S. (1995). School-based interventions for aggressive Africa-American boys. *Applied & Preventive Psychology, 4*(3), 185–195.

Hughes, D., & Chen, L. (1997). When and what parents tell children about race: An examination of race-related socialization among African American families. *Applied Developmental Science, 1*(4), 200–214.

Hurley, E. A., Boykin, A. W., & Allen, B. A. (2005). Communal versus individual learning of a math-estimation task: African American children and the culture of learning contexts. *Journal of Psychology: Interdisciplinary and Applied, 139*(6), 513–527.

Johnson, R. S., & Avelar La Salle, R. (2010). *Data strategies to uncover and eliminate hidden inequities: The wallpaper effect*. Thousand Oaks, CA: Corwin Press.

Jones, R. L. (1996). *Handbook of tests and measurements for black populations* (1 & 2nd ed.). Hampton, VA: Cobb & Henry Publishers.

Krovetz, M. L., & Arriaza, G. (2006). *Collaborative teacher leadership: How teachers can foster equitable schools*. Thousand Oaks, CA: Corwin Press.

Lazarus, R. S., & Folkman, S. (1987). Transactional theory and research on emotions and coping. *European Journal of Personality, 1*(3, Spec Issue), 141–169.

Neal, L. V. I., McCray, A. D., Webb-Johnson, G., & Bridgest, S. T. (2003). The effects of African American movement styles on teachers' perceptions and reactions. *Journal of Special Education, 37*(1), 49–57.

Noguera, P. A. (2003). The trouble with Black boys: The role and influence of environmental and cultural factors on the academic performance of African American males. *Urban Education. Special Issue: Educating African American males, Volume 1, 38*(4), 431–459.

Sankofa, B. M., Hurley, E. A., Allen, B. A., & Boykin, A. W. (2005). Cultural expression and black students' attitudes toward high achievers. *Journal of Psychology: Interdisciplinary and Applied, 139*(3), 247–259.

Skiba, R. J., Michael, R. S., Nardo, A. C., & Peterson, R. L. (2002). The color of discipline: Sources of racial and gender disproportionality in school punishment. *Urban Review, 34*(4), 317–342.

Spencer, M. B. (1995). Old issues and new theorizing about African American youth: A phenomenological variant of ecological systems theory. In R. L. Taylor (Ed.), *African American youth: Their social and economic status in the United States* (pp. 37–69). Westport, CT: Praeger.

Spencer, M. B. (1999). Social and cultural influences on school adjustment: The application of an identity-focused cultural ecological perspective. *Educational Psychologist. Special Issue: Social influences on school adjustment: Families, peers, neighborhoods, and culture, 34*(1), 43–57.

Spencer, M. B., Dupree, D., & Hartmann, T. (1997). A phenomenological variant of ecological systems theory (PVEST): A self-organization perspective in context. *Development and Psychopathology, 9*(4), 817–833.

Spencer, M. B., Fegley, S. G., & Harpalani, V. (2003). A theoretical and empirical examination of identity as coping: Linking coping resources to the self processes of African American youth. *Applied Developmental Science, 7*(3), 181–188.

Spencer, M. B., Fegley, S., Harpalani, V., & Seaton, G. (2004). Understanding hypermasculinity in context: A theory-driven analysis of urban adolescent males' coping responses. *Research in Human Development, 1*(4), 229–257.

Spencer, M. B., Noll, E., Stoltzfus, J., & Harpalani, V. (2001). Identity and school adjustment: Revisiting the "acting White" assumption. *Educational Psychologist. Special Issue: The schooling of ethnic minority children and youth, 36*(1), 21–30.

Spencer, M. B., Swanson, D. P., & Edwards, M. C. (2010). Sociopolitical contexts of development. In D. P. Swanson, M. C. Edwards, & M. B. Spencer (Eds.), *Adolescence: Development during a global era* (pp. 1–27). Burlington: Academic.

Steele, C. M. (1997). A threat in the air: How stereotypes shape intellectual identity and performance. *American Psychologist, 52*(6), 613–629.

Steele, C. M. (1998). Stereotyping and its threat are real. *American Psychologist, 53*(6), 680–681.

Steele, C. M., & Aronson, J. (1995). Stereotype threat and the intellectual test performance of African Americans. *Journal of Personality and Social Psychology, 69*(5), 797–811.

Steele, C. M., Spencer, S. J., & Aronson, J. (2002). *Contending with group image: The psychology of stereotype and social identity threat*. San Diego, CA: Academic.

Stevenson, H. C. (1994). Validation of the scale of racial socialization for African American adolescents: Steps toward multidimensionality. *Journal of Black Psychology, 20*(4), 445–468.

Stevenson, H. C. (2002). Wrestling with destiny: The cultural socialization of anger and healing in African American males. *Journal of Psychology & Christianity, 21*(4), 357–364.

Stevenson, H. C. (2003). *Playing with anger: Teaching coping skills to African American boys through athletics and culture*. Westport, CT: Praeger.

Stevenson, H. C. (2008). Fluttering around the racial tension of trust: Proximal approaches to suspended black student-teacher relationships. *School Psychology Review, 37*, 354–358.

Stevenson, H. C. (2012). *Recasting racial-ethnic encounters: Theorizing the stress reappraisal role of racial/ethnic socialization*. Submitted for Publication. Philadelphia, PA.

Stevenson, H. C., Cameron, R., Herrero-Taylor, T., & Davis, G. Y. (2002). Development of the teenager experience of racial socialization scale: Correlates of race-related socialization frequency from the perspective of Black youth. *Journal of Black Psychology, 28*(2), 84–106.

Stevenson, H. C., Davis, G. Y., Herrero-Taylor, T., & Morris, R. (2003). Boys not men: Hypervulnerability in African American Youth. In H. C. Stevenson (Ed.), *Playing with anger: Teaching coping skills to African American boys through athletics and culture* (pp. 3–20). Westport, CT: Praeger.

Stevenson, H. C., Herrero-Taylor, T., Cameron, R., & Davis, G. Y. (2002). "Mitigating instigation": Cultural phenomenological influences of anger and fighting among "big-boned" and "baby-faced" African American youth. *Journal of Youth and Adolescence, 31*(6), 473–485.

The Advancement Project. (2005). *Education on lockdown: The schoolhouse to jailhouse track* (p. 64). Washington, DC: The Advancement Project.

The Advancement Project. (2010). *Test, punish and push out: How "zero tolerance" and high-stakes testing funnel youth into the school-to-prison pipeline* (p. 56). Washington, DC: The Advancement Project.

Thomas, D. E., Coard, S. I., Stevenson, H. C., Bentley, K. L., & Zamel, P. C. (2009). Racial and emotional factors predicting teachers' perceptions of classroom behavioral maladjustment for urban African American male youth. *Psychology in the Schools, 46*(2), 184–196. doi:10.1002/pits.20362.

Thomas, D. E., & Stevenson, H. C. (2009). Gender risks and education: The particular classroom challenges for urban low-income African American boys. *Review of Research in Education, 33*, 160–180. doi:10.3102/0091732x08327164.

Thomas, D. E., Stevenson, H. C., Bentley, K. L., Thompson, C. I., Miller, G., Li, Z., et al. (2011). Got skillz? recasting and negotiating racial tension in teacher-student relationships [Submitted for Publication].

Tyler, K. M., Boykin, A. W., & Walton, T. R. (2006). Cultural considerations in teachers' perceptions of student classroom behavior and achievement. *Teaching and Teacher Education, 22*(8), 998–1005.

U.S. Census Bureau. (2010). Current Population Survey, 2009 Social and Economic Supplement. *Educational attainment of the population 18 years and over, by age, sex, race, and hispanic origin.* Washington, DC: U.S. Census Bureau.

U.S. Department of Education. (2010). Status and trends in the education of racial and ethnic minorities: Retention, suspension, and expulsion rates (NCES 2010–015). Retrieved July 30, 2011 from http://nces.ed.gov/pubs2010/2010015/indicator4_17.asp

Wald, J., & Losen, D. J. (2007). Out of sight: The journey through the school-to-prison pipeline. In S. Books (Ed.), *Invisible children in the society and its schools* (pp. 23–37). Mahwah, NJ: Lawrence Erlbaum Associates Publishers.

Wong, C. A., Eccles, J. S., & Sameroff, A. (2003). The influence of ethnic discrimination and ethnic identification on African American adolescents' school and socioemotional adjustment. *Journal of Personality, 71*(6), 1197–1232.

Working with Forced Migrant Children and their Families: Mental Health, Developmental, Legal, and Linguistic Considerations in the Context of School-Based Mental Health Services

Caroline S. Clauss-Ehlers and Adeyinka M. Akinsulure-Smith

Defining Forced Migration

While many understand the meaning of the term immigration generally, individuals are often less aware of what is meant by *forced migration*. In addition to fleeing from their home countries and experiencing harrowing journeys, upon arriving in a safe country, forced migrants often endure a lengthy, complicated legal process to gain residency in their host countries. The forced migratory experience is frequently compounded by post migration stressors similar to those faced by other immigrants, such as learning a new language and culture, adjusting to new gender and familial roles, educational systems, accessing services, and learning new skills (Akinsulure-Smith, Ghiglione, & Wollmershauser, 2009; Blanch, 2008; Drachman, 1995; Miller, Worthington, Muzurovic, Tipping, & Goldman, 2002; Sue & Sue, 2008; van der Veer, 1998). While many refugees and asylum seekers are able to adjust to life in the United States (U.S.) without significant stress, some are at risk for emotional difficulties that can have devastating consequences such as posttraumatic stress disorder (PTSD), depression, and anxiety. In addition, forced migrants may also experience intense grief as a result of multiple losses experienced, even after resettling in a safe environment (Athey & Ahearn, 1991; Fazel, Wheeler, & Danesh, 2005; Keyes, 2000; Lustig et al., 2004; Porter & Haslam, 2005; Rousseau, 1995).

This distressing process can be particularly challenging for forced migrant children and their families. To ethically provide competent clinical services, mental health professionals who work with this growing population must familiarize themselves with the impact this process has on the emotional well-being of forced migrant children and their families. This chapter provides a framework to understand the stressful nature of forced migration on children and their families. In so doing, it highlights how school mental health professionals are important resources for positive mental health promotion.

Unlike many immigrants who choose to leave their homelands in search of better economic or educational opportunities and who embark upon organized and planned journeys to do so, forced migrants are typically forced out of their countries due to armed conflict, human rights abuses, civil and political instability, persecution, and torture. In their search for safety, their departures are often sudden, unplanned, and under life-threatening circumstances, forcing them to flee with few or no belongings (Akinsulure-Smith & O'Hara, 2012; Akinsulure-Smith et al., 2009;

C.S. Clauss-Ehlers, Ph.D. (✉)
Rutgers, The State University of New Jersey,
New Brunswick, NJ 08901-1183, USA
e-mail: cc@gse.rutgers.edu

A.M. Akinsulure-Smith
City University of New York, New York, NY, USA
e-mail: aakinsulure-smith@ccny.cuny.edu

Bemak & Chung, 2008; Blanch, 2008; Drachman, 1995; Gorman, 2001; Pope & Garcia-Peltoniemi, 1991; van der Veer, 1998).

According to the United Nations High Commission on Refugees (UNHCR, 2009), by the end of 2008 there were approximately 15.2 million refugees and 827,000 asylum seekers worldwide. The U.S. is among the world's largest resettlement countries (UNHCR). Those immigrants who come to the U.S. as forced migrants often face the biggest hurdles. These challenges are largely due in part to a traumatic experience in the family's homeland that leads to a quick departure coupled with the unplanned traumatic arrival in a new sociocultural environment. This process has a huge impact on children. In the U.S., for instance, children make up more than 40% of all refugee admissions. Further, the U.S. Department of State Refugee Processing Center (2009a) reports that between 2004 and 2008, an average of 21,842 refugee children were admitted to the U.S. annually.

Forced migrant children arrive in the U.S. accompanied by parents, caregivers, or on their own (i.e., see unaccompanied minors below). As mentioned, many have lived through multiple traumatic events, losses, and difficult circumstances prior to and during their journey to the U.S. (Lustig et al., 2004). Forced migrant children also arrive with varying of immigration statuses: as refugees, asylum seekers, unaccompanied minors, or as undocumented (i.e., a person from another country who has come to the U.S. without obtaining lawful status, or who has stayed beyond expired visas). Depending upon their immigration status, forced migrants are either eligible or ineligible for a range of benefits and social services. Having an understanding of the different categories of immigration status can help school mental health professionals address some of the pressing concerns that forced migrant children confront in school settings. These varying statuses are described below as a general introduction.

Refugees. The United Nations Refugee Convention (1951) defines a *refugee* as: "a person who owing to well-founded fear of being persecuted for reasons of race, religion, nationality, membership of a particular social group or political opinion, is outside the country of his nationality, and is unable to or, owing to such fear, is unwilling to avail himself of the protection of that country; or who, not having a nationality and being outside the country of his former habitual residence [as a result of such events], is unable or, owing to such fear, is unwilling to return to it" (Article 1, The 1951 Convention Relating to the Status of Refugees, Center for the Study of Human Rights, 1994, pp. 57–58).

The quota of people who can obtain refugee status in the United States is set each year by the President. Typically, those seeking to obtain refugee status in the U.S. are referred by the office of the United Nations High Commissioner for Refugees (UNHCR) for interviews with an immigration officer. Once the application is approved after a lengthy referral and screening process, the refugee is connected to an American resettlement organization. All refugee applications to the U.S. are approved outside the country, enabling the individual or family to migrate with lawful status. Upon arrival to the U.S., refugees are eligible for numerous social service benefits including medical care, food stamps, housing assistance, food, and clothing (American Psychological Association (APA), 2010; Wilkinson, 2007). According to the American Psychological Association (2010), 43.5% of refugees who resettled in the U.S. between 2005 and 2008 were under 18 years of age. Currently, most refugee children enter the U.S. with caregivers.

Unaccompanied minors. Some refugee children, however, arrive to the U.S. as *unaccompanied minors.* This means they arrive without adult guardians or caregivers. According to the U.S. Department of Health and Human Services, Office of Refugee Resettlement (2009), approximately 13,000 minors have entered the Unaccompanied Refugee Minors program. Many of these children are placed in licensed foster homes. Those unaccompanied minors who have not received official sanction from the U.S. government are often detained by immigration officials (Byrne, 2008).

Asylum seekers. Usually, refugee status is determined and granted to the individual (and his/her family) while outside the U.S. The process is different, however, for an *asylum seeker* who comes to the U.S. first and then applies for asylum. This process is based on the grounds of the asylum seekers persecution in his/her home country. Children who become involved in this process are either unaccompanied minors or the dependents of parents seeking refuge in the U.S. The process of seeking asylum is ongoing and emotionally stressful. Asylum seekers live in constant fear of deportation, and face daunting legal challenges, along with limited or no access to work, education, and social welfare benefits (Drachman, 1995, Wilkinson, 2007). Stressors faced by asylum seekers include unemployment, little or no access to educational systems, and no access to social welfare benefits. The emotional stressors, along with limited or no resources, presents a highly stressful situation that leaves the asylum seeker with very limited formal means to cope.

Those who are eventually granted asylum obtain *asylee* status. An asylee is granted asylum after his or her arrival in the U.S., by an immigration official or immigration judge. Asylee status acknowledges that the individual has now met the definition of a refugee. This person can now remain in the U.S. legally, become eligible for refugee assistance and services, and eventually, like refugees, become eligible for citizenship (Blanch, 2008; Drachman, 1995; Sue & Sue, 2008; Wilkinson, 2007).

Undocumented children. Children and their families who live in the U.S. without any legal status fall into the undocumented category. As noted by the APA Taskforce (2010), typically, these children do not have access to adequate medical care, housing, or government benefits. This group is particularly vulnerable to immigration detention and deportation. Immigration detention is defined as "an administrative process by which the federal government holds people it wants to deport in prisons and prison-like 'detention facilities' throughout the country" (Guskin & Wilson, 2007). These authors state that immigration detention "exists to facilitate 'removal' (deportation). In other words, the immigration agency detains immigrants so that it can more easily deport them" (Guskin & Wilson).

Clearly there are many ways that youth immigrate to the United States. The lengthy and often traumatizing forced migratory experience is further compounded by post- migration stressors similar to those faced by other immigrants (Akinsulure-Smith et al., 2009; Blanch, 2008; Drachman, 1995, Miller et al., 2002; Sue & Sue, 2008; van der Veer, 1998).

While many forced migrants are able to adjust to life in the U.S. without significant difficulties, some are at risk for emotional difficulties that can have devastating consequences on their psychosocial functioning (Athey & Ahearn, 1991; Fazel et al., 2005; Keyes, 2000; Lustig et al., 2004; Porter & Haslam, 2005; Rousseau, 1995). The paragraphs that follow discuss mental health, developmental, legal, and linguistic considerations for school personal who work with youth who had a forced migratory experience. Implications of each area within the school context are discussed.

Mental Health Considerations

Indeed, much of the literature highlights the multiple mental health challenges faced by children and adolescents who have been exposed to armed conflict. Substantial research has found that youth exposed to war and those who are refugee children experience "elevated symptoms of PTSD, depression, anxiety, somatic complaints, sleep problems, and behavioral problems" (APA, 2010, p. 26). What is often described as the "dose-effect" refers to the view that greater exposure to trauma results in greater depression, anxiety, and behavior problems (APA, 2010; Ellis, MacDonald, Lincoln, & Cabral, 2008; Garbarino & Kostelny, 1996). According to the dose hypothesis, the more a child is exposed to trauma, the more likely the child will experience mental health problems.

While initially the dose effect sounds like a rational configuration of the relationship between the experience of forced migratory youth and mental health outcomes, research actually demonstrates a much more complex picture. Questions raised include, but are not limited to, notions such as: If two siblings are exposed to the same levels of traumatic experience will their mental health outcomes be similar? If a child is exposed to the effects of war as an infant, is the impact of that experience the same as the infant's neighbor who is 8-years-old? How do we explain differences in adaptation and coping among children who have a shared experience of consistent and ongoing trauma? What is the role of development and implications for developmental stage in mental health outcomes?

These questions speak to the role of other factors in children's mental health outcomes when faced with war, armed conflict, and forced migratory status. The potential for such variability is documented in the literature. For instance, research has found wide ranging prevalence rates of PTSD among children affected by war span a range from 7 to 75%. Similarly, research has documented prevalence rates for depression as ranging from 11 to 47% (Allwood, Bell-Dolan, & Husain, 2002; APA, 2010). The range in prevalence rates implies that other variables play a role in the mental health outcomes among youth affected by war (Clauss-Ehlers, 2006). Some researchers have found that factors such as postwar stress, resettlement stress, family functioning, and discrimination can influence the clinical picture presented (Ajdukovic & Ajdukovic, 1993; APA, 2010).

The American Psychological Association formed a task force to specifically examine the impact of war on children and families with refugee status. This working group, formally called the Task Force on the Psychosocial Effects of War on Children and Families Who Are Refugees from Armed Conflict Residing in the United States, published a report entitled *Resilience and Recovery after War: Refugee Children and Families in the United States* (APA, 2010). The key theme of this report is that children affected by war demonstrate immense resilience. The report states that wide ranging prevalence rates highlight the many ways children actively cope with their surrounding environments.

The report continues to state that a focus on PTSD is too narrow and does not address the complexity associated with individual differences in response to trauma that can occur at different developmental phases. Rather, it is argued that resilience plays a tremendous role in reactions and mental health outcomes. More research is needed to identify factors that promote resilience.

However, existing research does begin to identify protective factors that help children cope with trauma. In their study that explores resilience factors that help children cope with sexual abuse, Newberger and Gremy (2004) found that parents who responded with a combination of early intervention (i.e., psychotherapy), parental support, and parental belief that their child's report of sexual abuse was true helped children cope and recover from sexual abuse trauma.

Clauss-Ehlers (2004) discusses the concept of cultural resilience as a way that individuals can tap into the sociocultural context to overcome the hardship they face. At its most basic term, resilience refers to the ability to overcome adversity. An individual is resilient when s/he is able to "bounce back" from a given situation, here a trauma, and return to the day-to-day functions of his or her life. Clauss-Ehlers has extended this individual notion of resilience to examine how the sociocultural environment promotes resilience. She defines cultural resilience as aspects of one's culture that help the individual overcome adversity (Clauss-Ehlers, Yang, & Chen, 2006). Cultural resilience attempts to locate factors that promote resilience beyond those located in the individual (i.e., motivation, intelligence) to examine aspects of the individual's sociocultural environment that promote coping in the face of adversity.

The question of cultural resilience is: What are those factors in the individual's sociocultural environment that promote resilience? (Clauss-Ehlers, 2004; Clauss-Ehlers 2008a, 2008b; Clauss-Ehlers et al., 2006). This definition makes resilience much more about the child in interaction with the environment rather than focusing solely on individual character traits within the child. This framework for resilience is particularly relevant for children affected by war who may experience a sense of depletion of internal resources as it suggests that the surrounding environment (i.e., what happens in the school) can promote resilience. The aforementioned range of prevalence further supports the notion that the child in interaction with his/her environment leads to varying mental health outcomes.

While not linked to the experience of children affected by war per se, there is some existing trauma research that supports the notion of sociocultural factors being responsive to resilience promotion. For instance, a study of college-aged women found there were racial/ethnic differences in specific cultural factors that promoted resilience in response to adverse circumstance (Clauss-Ehlers, 2008b). Three major cultural factors reported to promote resilience among the White women in the study included family, religion, and identifying a new objective, with religion identified as the most prevalent cultural component of resilience. These findings were thought to indicate that for the White women in the study, religious faith was a critical component in dealing with adversity. In addition, it was thought that identifying a new objective fit with the mainstream American cultural value of doing/engaging in activities (Kluckhohn & Strodtbeck, 1961). As such, identifying a new objective appeared to be a cultural response to stress. Cultural factors were reported as promoting resilience among the women of color in the sample. Women of color identified family, pride in one's cultural heritage, personal strength, and meeting with people from the same culture as primary contributors to resilience. These findings demonstrate cultural aspects of resilience and the varied factors that support resilience among diverse groups of women (Clauss-Ehlers).

Developmental Considerations

Similar to the complex picture presented with regard to the mental health outcomes described above, the impact of forced migration on children's development presents a complicated picture. Much of the current research shows that living through war as a child "is a complex developmental process with multiple influential variables" (APA, 2010, p. 28). This complexity is further underscored by the need for longitudinal research that examines developmental outcomes for children over a period of time, rather than at one interval or data point (APA). A longitudinal approach would be best served by examining the experience of children over time and across cultures (APA). Despite these limitations, areas of stress and vulnerability can be surmised based on what we know about standard developmental processes throughout childhood. The experience of forced migrant children, however, must be understood in the context of multiple factors that influence developmental processes.

Having stated these limitations, developmental themes for forced migrant children include, but are not limited to: separation, attachment, and mastery. A key developmental task during infancy includes developing a sense of trust with a caregiver (Erikson, 1959). This attachment is critical for a sense of consistency, routine, and nurturance. The possibility of caregiver attachment being ruptured either due to war, separation because of political conflict, or the immigration process, is a huge risk factor for this age group (Punamäki, 2002).

For children aged 2–5, key developmental tasks among some cultures include physical control over one's body, an increasing sense of independence, and a greater sense of control and assertion over one's environment (Erikson, 1959). Disruptions in these tasks due to an experience of war, immigration, and/or forced migration can interfere with the developmental achievement of mastery (Erikson). Indeed, research has found that young children who have lived in war torn areas are vulnerable to enuresis, physical destruction of objects, and separation anxiety (Chimienti, Nasr, & Khalifeh, 1989). Moreover, much of the toddler's transition towards greater autonomy during this time includes caregiver supervision. For instance, the toddler attempts walking and falls down, only to be picked up by his mother and encouraged to try again. The disruption in this process if the caregiver is not able to be present is another critical point to consider.

Erikson (1959) presents industry vs. inferiority as the key developmental task for children aged 6–11. Industry is achieved when children are able to cope with school and the pressure of an academic environment. Failure to do so results in a sense of inferiority. Adjustment to school is challenging in and of itself during this stage. The process of adjustment is even more difficult when stressors faced by forced migrant children are taken into account. War can interfere with developing connections to school and relationships with peers (APA, 2010). Resettlement means that children leave their school communities, often going to a new educational system within a new cultural and linguistic context. The learning process may likely be quite different for the child (see School responsiveness to linguistic considerations) and academics and peer relationships may suffer during the transition. Further, if the child is separated from his/her parents, the lack of parental presence and school involvement can have a negative impact on school success (Clauss-Ehlers, 2006).

Finally, the adolescent years are characterized by identity vs. role confusion (Erikson, 1959). A key task during this stage is to develop a sense of one's identity. Social relationships are a critical vehicle to identity development and a hallmark of this stage. The stressors experienced by forced migrant children and those who have experienced war can interfere with the ability to develop a sense of trust in others (Punamäki, 2002). Additionally, the process of resettlement may include leaving behind close friends, mentors, and a social network upon which the adolescent has come to rely.

Legal Considerations

While it is beyond the scope of this chapter to discuss all the legal implications for the varying immigration statuses among forced migrant children and their families, several points are noteworthy. It is critical that school mental health professionals are aware that the children and families they serve, particularly those who are asylum seekers or undocumented, may be dealing with the legal system. As children and their families go through a lengthy and often stressful immigration process, school personnel may be approached by the family's legal representative to obtain information about the child's experience to support their asylum case.

Unfortunately, limited attention has been paid to the experience of children who are caught up in the legal process to gain asylum. As Bhaba and Schmidt (2006) have observed, when children are involved in the asylum process they are either unaccompanied minors or dependents of parents seeking refuge in the U.S. The sad reality is that the process is extremely lengthy and costly, and shows little regard to the needs and rights of children. Children and adolescents entangled in lengthy immigration processes may need a range of culturally and linguistically appropriate supportive services to promote their well-being, including basic daily living, education, and positive physical and mental health across the various domains in which they function. Given that all children attend school, the school system can become an important resource for families while also providing information about the impact of forced migration on children's behavioral and psychological functioning.

Linguistic Considerations

Overview of languages spoken at home. Linguistic diversity plays a critical role in the fabric of our nation. The 2009 U.S. Census Bureau American Community Survey identified a vast array of languages spoken at home as documented in their report entitled *Language Spoken at Home by Ability to Speak English for the Population 5 Years and Over* (U.S. Census Bureau, 2009). The outcome of this survey was the identification of 40 language categories. In reality, however, the actual number of languages spoken is much higher given the category function under which more than one language was housed. For instance, while some categories include Italian, German, and Yiddish, others incorporated more than one language. Language categories such as Other

Asian Languages and African Languages are two such examples. Moreover, given that these numbers reflect participants in the U.S. Census, and, as such, were identified by the government, the numbers might look very different among forced migrant children and their families. Schools may struggle to provide instruction and support in the child's language of origin. Being able to communicate, inform, and involve parents may also be a challenge related to language barriers.

Specific issues that arise for youth. Youth are confronted with a range of changes and cultural shifts upon arrival to a new country. This transition may be more challenging among forced migrant children who come to the U.S. with a history of trauma and loss, have limited resources, and are faced with the uncertainty of their immigration status. While younger children may not grasp the concept of immigration and its implications, they may very well be attuned to the stress experienced by their parents who must also cope with the change.

Children who come to the U.S. speaking a language other than English face an additional layer of adjustment in the life of the school (Javier & Camacho-Gingerich, 2004). Children may feel isolated from their peers given the language barrier and an inability to communicate verbally as well as through the written word. These language differences may translate into decreased academic standing such as demotion to a lower grade. Such changes can introduce other developmental considerations such as not being with one's developmental peer group as well as losing the academic standing gained in one's country of origin. These shifts can be devastating for a child who is already coping with major shifts in his/her environment.

Language also incorporates culture. The loss of the use of one's language of origin in the classroom constitutes a loss of one's culture. Losing the ability to express oneself in the cultural ways one expresses language as a means of learning cuts back tools of skill acquisition that are familiar to the child (Clauss, 1998).

Interpreters. Effective and culturally competent interpreters can facilitate effective services in the school setting, assess children's needs, and provide effective school based services. Scholars in the field have reported that clients who are unable to communicate effectively are less satisfied with the client-provider relationship, have a poorer understanding of their diagnosis and treatment, are misdiagnosed, or receive inappropriate care (Baker, Hayes, & Fortier, 1998; Flores, Rabke-Verani, Pine, & Sabharwal, 2002; Hornberger, Itakura, & Wilson, 1997; Lee, 1997; Marcos, 1979; Pöchhacker, 2000; Sabin, 1975). For forced migrant children and families who struggle with language barriers, the inability to communicate in English can serve as a significant barrier for accessing supportive services (Akinsulure-Smith, 2007; Gong-Guy, Cravens, & Patterson, 1991; O'Hara & Akinsulure-Smith, 2011). Interpreters can help bridge this gap by enhancing service provision.

School Responsiveness to Mental Health, Developmental, Legal, and Linguistic Considerations

School responsiveness to mental health considerations. The notion that contextual factors can promote positive mental health outcomes (i.e., resilience) for children is excellent news for schools. Schools have a unique opportunity to support children with a forced migratory experience through the natural environment in which the child is seen regularly. In fact, the mere routine of going to school to learn on a daily basis can provide a sense of normalcy for children and their families. Children feel more secure when they are aware of expectations and have consistency. Simply attending school can facilitate a sense of security and routine. Simultaneously, school personnel can play an active role in identifying signs and symptoms of mental health problems and provide intervention as needed (APA, 2010). School-based mental health services can provide children and adolescents with treatment in an environment that is part of their day-to-day experience. Services provided can include individual and group therapy, creative arts counseling, and mentoring support, among others (Clauss-Ehlers, 2008a).

School responsiveness to developmental considerations. Schools provide a unique opportunity to be responsive to developmental considerations among forced migrant children. School personnel spend a great deal of time with the children in their institution (APA, 2010). As such, school personnel get to know children well and can hopefully notice significant changes in a child's social, emotional, and academic functioning. Similarly, through an awareness of the child, school personnel can develop a sense of when a child appears stuck or is not growing in developmentally expected ways. Thus, one overall aspect of responsiveness is for school personnel to actively engage students in the life of the school, noting any important changes that may arise.

In addition to this ongoing, informal assessment stance, schools address developmental considerations by the stability and sense of community they provide. A sense of routine and expectation can provide a safe, stable environment for children and adolescents who have experienced major upheavals. The opportunity to connect with teachers, mentors, coaches, and others, allows for the development of connection and trust that underscores much of Erikson's (1959) theory. That schools are learning environments suggests that they are places that encourage students to learn and master new material. This function directly corresponds with the tasks of mastery that arise during toddler and early childhood years as well as a sense of industry characterized by middle childhood.

For children across various developmental stages, schools can provide a new sense of community. As such, schools can help children adjust to a new culture and environment. Connections with peers in school can enhance social networks, decrease isolation, and provide youth with a new normative framework. This process may be particularly important for adolescents who are actively engaged in identity development while also looking to peers as a reference group. School personnel can facilitate social connections through classroom assignments that connect children, after school activities with peers, and linkages with school-based mental health services such as group therapy.

School responsiveness to legal considerations. A key learning for school personnel faced with a child's legal status is to be aware that the child and his/her family may be involved with the legal system as they navigate their immigration experience. This awareness translates into responsiveness when school personnel understand the child's situation from a perspective that takes this reality into account. For instance, a child's absences may be due to having to attend court as part of the family's immigration process. Here a responsive intervention is to support students in their academic lives by reaching out to the family to send work home, review homework, and in general, work with the child so that s/he does not miss out on access to learning skills due to court-related absence.

An additional legal consideration concerns the request from the family's legal representative for information about the child's functioning in asylum seeking cases. Here it is important that schools have a protocol in place to address the legal request while also honoring ethical codes of confidentiality, getting consent to release information, and consultation with the family about the request.

School responsiveness to linguistic considerations. In their document entitled, *Supporting Linguistically and Culturally Diverse Learners in English Language*, The National Council of Teachers of English (NCTE) present eight ways to support linguistically and culturally diverse learners in English education within the classroom (NCTE, n.d.; see http://www.ncte.org/cee/positions/diverselearnersinee). The first tenet states that the classroom be a place that respects the cultural identities of all participants. The second tenet acknowledges that all students bring a *fund of knowledge* to the classroom. Both points underscore the importance that the student's linguistic and cultural knowledge are incorporated into the life of the classroom. Building on this foundation, the third component calls on teachers to "empower students who have been traditionally disenfranchised by public education" to "learn about and know their students in more complex ways." Educators are encouraged to take an "anthropologically and ethnographically informed teaching stance" (NCTE, n.d.). At the same time, the fourth tenet discusses the importance of exposing students to a range of educational experiences that mirror the student's world.

The next two principles focus on the teacher's approach. Teachers are encouraged to model culturally and linguistically responsive practice. As such, teachers are invited to be active participants and learners within the classroom community. Similarly, the sixth tenet acknowledges that classrooms include both native speakers of English as well as those where English is a second language. This principle states that teachers are to teach English learners the new language while also honoring the language of their home country. The point highlighted here is that English language learners know the rules of their language of origin by the time they are 5 or 6. As a result, immersion rather than instruction is the focus for English learners. Finally, tenets 7 and 8 focus on the need for teachers to recognize inequity, advocate for the learning of all students, and act as models of social justice.

Conclusion

School mental health professionals, by virtue of their role in schools, play a potentially critical role in being responsive to the immigration process experienced by forced migrant children and adolescents. School mental health providers can be leaders in this arena, engaging teachers, school psychologists, and school counselors as vital resources to assist children and adolescents in school adjustment as well as emotional and learning challenges (APA, 2010). School mental health professionals can play a major role in identifying forced migrant children who need "mental health services, evaluating educational or trauma-related needs, and consulting with school administration and staff (p. 28)." They can also work to support vulnerable young people and their families who are going through the asylum seeking process through sensitivity and understanding about the complexities of this legal maze. In addition, the school environment, by virtue of being in a school, provides the opportunity for a non-stigmatizing setting in which therapeutic supports can be implemented (Akinsulure-Smith, 2009; Lustig et al., 2004).

References

Ajdukovic, M., & Ajdukovic, D. (1993). Psychological well-being of refugee children. *Child Abuse & Neglect, 17*, 843–854.

Akinsulure-Smith, A. M. (2007). Use of interpreters with survivors of torture, war, and refugee trauma. In H. E. Smith, A. S. Keller, & D. W. Lhewa (Eds.), *Like a refugee camp on first avenue. Insights and experiences from the Bellevue/NYU program for survivors of torture* (pp. 82–105). New York: The Bellevue/NYU Program for Survivors of Torture.

Akinsulure-Smith, A. M. (2009). Brief psychoeducational group treatment with re-traumatized refugees and asylum seekers. *Journal for Specialists in Group Work, 34*, 137–150.

Akinsulure-Smith, A. M., Ghiglione, J. B., & Wollmershauser, C. (2009). Healing in the midst of chaos: Nah We Yone's African women's wellness group. *Women & Therapy, 32*(1), 105–120.

Akinsulure-Smith, A. M., & O'Hara, M. (2012). Working with forced migrants: Therapeutic issues and considerations for mental health counselors. *Journal of Mental Health Counseling, 34*(1), 38–55.

Allwood, M. A., Bell-Dolan, D., & Husain, S. A. (2002). Children's trauma and adjustment reactions to violent and non-violent war experiences. *Journal of the American Academy of Child and Adolescent Psychiatry, 41*, 450–457.

American Psychological Association. (2010). *Resilience and recovery after war: Refugee children and families in the United States*. Washington, DC: Author. Retrieved May 12, 2011 from http://www.apa.org/pubs/info/reports/refugees.aspx

Athey, J. L., & Ahearn, F. L. (1991). *Refugee children: Theory, research and services*. Baltimore, MD: Johns Hopkins University Press.

Baker, D. W., Hayes, R., & Fortier, J. P. (1998). Interpreter use and satisfaction with interpersonal aspects of care for Spanish-speaking patients. *Medical Care, 36*(10), 1461–1470.

Bemak, F., & Chung, R. C.-Y. (2008). Counseling refugees and migrants. In P. B. Pederson, J. G. Draguns, W. J. Lonner, & J. E. Trimble (Eds.), *Counseling across cultures* (6th ed., pp. 307–324). Thousand Oaks, CA: Sage.

Bhaba, J., & Schmidt, S. (2006). *Seeking asylum alone: United States*. Retrieved May 12, 2011 from http://www.childtrafficking.com/Docs/seek_asylum_alone_us_0108.pdf

Blanch, A. (2008). *Transcending violence: Emerging models for trauma healing in refugee communities*. Alexandria, VA: National Center for Trauma Informed

Care. Retrieved May 12, 2011 from http://www.theanainstitute.org/RefugeeTraumaPaper_Biography_July212008.pdf

Byrne, O. (2008). *Unaccompanied children in the United States: A literature review.* New York, NY: Vera Institute of Justice. Retrieved from http://www.vera.org/publication_pdf/478_884.pdf

Chimienti, G., Nasr, J., & Khalifeh, I. (1989). Children's reactions to war-related stress: Affective symptoms and behavior problems. *Social Psychiatry and Psychiatric Epidemiology, 24*, 282–287.

Clauss, C. S. (1998). Language: The unspoken variable in psychotherapy practice. *Psychotherapy: Theory, research, practice, training, 35*, 188–196.

Clauss-Ehlers, C. S. (2004). Re-inventing resilience: A model of "culturally-focused resilient adaptation". In C. S. Clauss-Ehlers & M. D. Weist (Eds.), *Community planning to foster resilience in children* (pp. 27–41). New York, NY: Kluwer Academic Publishers.

Clauss-Ehlers, C. S. (2006). *Diversity training for classroom teaching: A manual for students and educators.* New York, NY: Springer.

Clauss-Ehlers, C. S. (2008a). Creative arts counseling in schools: Toward a more comprehensive approach. In H. L. K. Coleman & C. Yeh (Eds.), *Handbook on school counseling* (pp. 517–530). Newbury Park, CA: Sage.

Clauss-Ehlers, C. S. (2008b). Sociocultural factors, resilience, and coping: Support for a culturally sensitive measure of resilience. *Journal of Applied Developmental Psychology, 29*, 197–212.

Clauss-Ehlers, C. S., Yang, Y. T., & Chen, W. J. (2006). Resilience from childhood stressors: The role of cultural resilience, ethnic identity, and gender identity. *Journal of Infant, Child, and Adolescent Psychotherapy, 5*, 124–138.

Drachman, D. (1995). Immigration statuses and their influence on service provision, access, and use. *Social Work, 40*(2), 188–197.

Ellis, B. H., MacDonald, H. Z., Lincoln, A. K., & Cabral, H. J. (2008). Mental health of Somali adolescent refugees: The role of trauma, stress, and perceived discrimination. *Journal of Consulting and Clinical Psychology, 76*, 184–193.

Erikson, E. H. (1959). *Identity and the life cycle.* New York, NY: International Universities Press.

Fazel, M., Wheeler, J., & Danesh, J. (2005). Prevalence of serious mental disorder in 7000 refugees resettled in western countries: a systemic review. *Lancet, 265*, 1309–1314.

Flores, G., Rabke-Verani, J., Pine, W., & Sabharwal, A. (2002). The importance of cultural and linguistic issues in the emergency care of children. *Pediatric Emergency Care, 18*(4), 271–284.

Garbarino, J., & Kostelny, K. (1996). The effects of political violence on Palestinian children's behavior problems: A risk accumulation model. *Child Development, 67*, 33–45.

Gong-Guy, E., Cravens, R. B., & Patterson, T. E. (1991). Clinical issues in mental health service delivery to refugees. *American Psychologist, 46*, 642–648.

Gorman, W. (2001). Refugee survivors of torture: Trauma and treatment. *Professional Psychology: Research and Practice, 32*(5), 443–451.

Guskin, J., & Wilson, D. L. (2007). *Immigration detention: Questions and answers.* Retrieved January 23, 2012 from http://www.immigrantsolidarity.org/Documents/detq&aflier).

Hornberger, J., Itakura, H., & Wilson, S. R. (1997). Bridging language and cultural barriers between physicians and patients. *Public Health Reports, 112*(5), 410–417.

Javier, R. A., & Camacho-Gingerich, A. (2004). Risk and resilience in Latino youth. In C. S. Clauss-Ehlers & M. D. Weist (Eds.), *Community planning to foster resilience in children* (pp. 65–82). New York, NY: Kluwer Academic Publishers.

Keyes, E. (2000). Mental health status in refugees: An integrative review of current research. *Issues in Mental Health Nursing, 21*, 397–410.

Kluckhohn, F. R., & Strodtbeck, F. L. (1961). *Variations in value orientations.* Evanston, IL: Row, Peterson.

Lee, E. (1997). Cross-cultural communication: Therapeutic use of interpreters. In E. Lee (Ed.), *Working with Asian Americans: A guide for clinicians* (pp. 477–489). New York, NY: Guildford Press.

Lustig, S., Kia-Keating, M., Knight, W. G., Geltman, P., Ellis, H., Kinzie, J. D., et al. (2004). Review of child and adolescent refugee mental health. *Journal of the American Academy of Child & Adolescent Psychiatry, 43*, 24–36.

Marcos, L. R. (1979). Effects of interpreters on the evaluation of psychopathology in non-English-speaking clients. *American Journal of Psychiatry, 136*(2), 171–174.

Miller, K. E., Worthington, G., Muzurovic, J., Tipping, S., & Goldman, A. (2002). Bosnian refugees and the stressors of exile: A narrative study. *American Journal of Orthopsychiatry, 72*, 341–354.

Newberger, C. M., & Gremy, I. (2004). The role of clinical and institutional interventions in children's resilience and recovery from sexual abuse. In C. S. Clauss-Ehlers & M. D. Weist (Eds.), *Community planning to foster resilience in children* (pp. 197–215). New York, NY: Kluwer Academic Publishers.

O'Hara, M., & Akinsulure-Smith, A. M. (2011). Working with interpreters: Tools for clinicians conducting psychotherapy with forced immigrants. *International Journal of Migration, Health, and Social Care, 7*(1), 33–43.

Pöchhacker, F. (2000). Language barriers in Vienna hospitals. *Ethnicity & Health, 5*(2), 113–119.

Pope, K. S., & Garcia-Peltoniemi, R. E. (1991). Responding to victims of torture: Clinical issues, professional responsibilities, and useful resources. *Professional Psychology: Research and Practice, 22*, 269–276.

Porter, M., & Haslam, N. (2005). Predisplacement and post displacement factors associated with mental health of refugees and internally displaced persons: A meta-analysis. *Journal of the American Medical Association, 294*(5), 602–612.

Punamäki, R. (2002). The uninvited guest of war enters childhood: Developmental and personality aspects of war and military violence. *Traumatology, 8*(3), 45–63.

Rousseau, C. (1995). The mental health of refugee children. *Transcutural Psychiatric Research Review, 32*, 299–331.

Sabin, J. E. (1975). Translating despair. *The American Journal of Psychiatry, 132*(2), 197–199.

Sue, D. W., & Sue, D. (2008). *Counseling the culturally diverse: Theory and practice* (5th ed.). Hoboken, NJ: Wiley.

United Nations High Commissioner for Refugees. (1951). *Article 1, The 1951 Convention Relating to the Status of Refugees* (United Nations General Assembly A/CONF.2/2/Rev.1). Retrieved May 12, 2011 from http://unhcr.org.au/unhcr/images/convention%20and%20protocol.pdf

United Nations High Commissioner for Refugees. (2009). *Global trends: Refugees, asylum- seekers, returnees, internationally displaced, and stateless persons.* Retrieved January 30, 2012 from http://www.unhcr.org/4c11f0be9.html

United States Census Bureau. (2009). *American community survey, B16001, "Language spoken at home by ability to speak English for the Population 5 years and over."* Retrieved May 12, 2012 from http://www.census.gov

United States Department of Health and Human Services, Office of Refugee Resettlement. (2009). *Unaccompanied refugee minors program.* Washington, DC: Author. Retrieved May 12, 2011 from http://www.acf.hhs.gov/programs/orr/programs/unaccompanied_refugee_minors.htm

United States Department of State, Bureau of Population, Refugees, and Migration, Office of Admissions, Refugee Processing center (RPc). (2009a). *Aggregate data on refugee minors by state, country of origin, and age: Fiscal years 2004 to 2008.* Unpublished raw data. Washington, DC: Author.

Van der Veer, G. (1998). *Counselling and therapy with refugees and victims of trauma* (2nd ed.). New York, NY: Wiley.

Wilkinson, J. (2007). Immigration dynamics: Processes, challenges, and benefits. In H. Smith & A. Keller (Eds.), *Like a refugee camp on first avenue: Insights and experiences from the Bellevue/NYU program for survivors of torture* (pp. 65–81). New York, NY: Bellevue/NYU Program for Survivors of Torture.

Mental Health and Rural Schools: An Integrated Approach with Primary Care

Jody Lieske, Susan Swearer, and Brandi Berry

Introduction

According to the *Mental Health: A Report of the Surgeon General* an estimated 21% of children and adolescents aged 9–17 in the U.S. have a diagnosable mental health or addictive disorder. However, according to the same report approximately 70% of children and adolescents who need mental health services do not receive them (U.S. Department of Health and Human Services, 1999). These numbers translate into a significant challenge that our nation's schools and communities face. Where do these afflicted youth and their families receive services? In rural settings, these services are typically delivered by physicians in primary health care settings and staff in the child's school.

In the early 1990s, in an effort to coordinate prevention of mental disorders in the U.S., the Senate Appropriates Committee of the U.S. Congress mandated the National Institute of Mental Health (NIMH) to work with the Institute of Medicine (IOM) to review the research on mental illness, provide recommendations on federal policy, and to prepare a final report that would encourage collaboration on prevention research between universities, colleges, hospitals, and federal agencies (Mrazek & Haggerty, 1994). In this chapter, the IOM framework for reducing risks for mental disorders is used as a framework for our understanding of mental health service delivery in rural schools.

The IOM framework was established in response to limitations in the original public health classification system (i.e., primary, secondary, and tertiary) and with Gordon's, 1987 alternative classification system (i.e., universal, selective, and indicated). In order to address the limitations in the aforementioned classification systems, the IOM devised a new framework, "the mental health intervention spectrum for mental disorders" (Mrazek & Haggerty, 1994, p. 23). In this spectrum, the prevention area includes Gordon's nomenclature, "universal, selective, and indicated"; however, the term prevention is reserved for interventions that are delivered before the initial onset of a disorder. The second area is "treatment" and includes "case identification" and "standard treatment for known disorders." The third area in the spectrum is "maintenance" and includes "compliance with long-term treatment" and "after-care." Thus, the IOM spectrum for mental disorders is broad, is influenced by public health, and can be applied to our conceptualization of mental health prevention, treatment, and maintenance in rural schools.

In this chapter we review the research on prevalence of mental health disorders in rural settings,

J. Lieske, Ph.D. (✉)
Children and Adolescent Clinic, P.C. Munroe Meyer Institute-UNMC, Hastings, NE, USA
e-mail: jlieske@unmc.edu

S. Swearer, Ph.D. • B. Berry, M.A.
University of Nebraska—Lincoln, Lincoln, NE, USA

discuss an integrated approach of service delivery in rural schools, and end with a case example of mental health service delivery in a rural community. The focus will be on an integrated mental health service delivery model that is currently on the cutting edge of research and practice. The integrated approach involves integrating a mental health provider into a primary care setting, thus affording better continuity of care among children in rural schools and communities. The approach is one that focuses on the mental health provider closely collaborating with multiple school systems in small rural communities, as the provision of mental health services within schools are often constrained by issues related to resources and rural culture.

Prevalence of Mental Health Disorders in Rural Samples

In order to apply the mental health intervention spectrum for mental disorders in rural communities, the first step is to review the research on the prevalence of mental health disorders in rural areas.

Few studies have examined the prevalence rates of psychological disorders among children and adolescents in purely rural areas (Costello, Mustillo, Erkanli, Keeler, & Angold, 2003), but the findings from mixed studies have been largely consistent. Compared with urban samples, it appears as though rural youth are at similar risk for experiencing anxiety, depression, conduct disorder, and substance abuse. A study that compared the prevalence rates of different types of psychopathology for boys and girls 6–11 years of age living in large cities versus rural areas found no significant differences in the prevalence of internalizing problems, such as anxiety and depression (Zahner, Jacobs, Freeman, & Trainor, 1993). While there were also no significant differences in the prevalence of externalizing problems (e.g., conduct disorder) between boys living in large cities or rural areas, girls living in large cities had significantly higher rates of externalizing problems than girls living in rural areas. Studies comparing the use of various substances among rural and urban samples have also found few differences; most notably the use of illicit substances (i.e., alcohol and tobacco) tends to be higher for rural students (Cronk & Sarvela, 1997; Gfroerer, Larson, & Colliver, 2007). Thus, with few exceptions, youth in rural areas experience a number of psychological disorders at similar rates as their urban peers. When urban versus rural differences do emerge, these differences are likely a result of SES, cultural, and other factors and not the level of urbanization or rurality (Angold et al., 2002; Zahner et al., 1993) of communities.

Thus, from the IOM perspective, we use the above prevalence data to suggest that mental health disorders are just as prevalent in rural communities as they are in non-rural communities and prevention, treatment, and maintenance efforts for anxiety, depression, conduct disorders, and substance use disorders are equally important in these communities. However, there are additional challenges that rural communities face in coordinating mental health interventions.

Challenges Faced By Rural Schools

Nearly one in three of America's school-aged children attend public schools in rural areas or small towns (Beeson & Strange, 2003). Rural schools face many difficulties when it comes to meeting the mental health needs of their children and youth. Most students are in school for eight hours a day and schools tend to be the settings where students receive mental health services (Burns et al., 1995; Hoagwood & Erwin, 1997). However, rural schools and communities are faced with unique challenges. Families in rural areas generally have a lower socioeconomic status and educational level compared to families in urban areas (McCracken & Barcinas, 1991). Since rural schools are often geographically isolated and the cost of program delivery is higher, rural communities often experience problems with limited resources (Deewes, 1999). For example, compared to urban schools, rural schools are more likely to have fewer teachers, teacher's aides, support staff (e.g., counselors and psychologists), administrators, as well as fewer curricular and extra-curricular activities (McCracken & Barcinas, 1991). In public schools, the average number of students per counselor, social worker, school psychologist, and special education instructional aide in the elementary and secondary schools has been found to be higher in rural areas than in urban cities (Provasnik et al., 2007). Furthermore, rates of help-seeking and service utilization for mental health problems are lower in rural compared with urban communities (Caldwell, Jorm, & Dear, 2004; Parslow & Jorm, 2000).

Solutions

The IOM mental health intervention spectrum for mental disorders is a comprehensive model for prevention, treatment, and maintenance of treatment gains that calls upon schools, medical clinics, community mental health centers, and community agencies to coordinate care. Rural communities, given oft-limited resources, are in an ideal position to put the IOM spectrum into practice, with mental health intervention coordinated across settings.

Mental health integrated into pediatric primary care. One cutting-edge solution to address pediatric mental health is an integrated approach where services are provided in the primary care clinics affording the potential for collaboration with the patient's physician and other community members (Kolko, Campo, Kelleher, & Cheng, 2010). Collaboration utilizes a teamwork approach in which professionals from multiple disciplines come together and share their expertise to create a community in which comprehensive services can be provided seamlessly (Walsh & Fortner, 2002). Collaboration also ensures that services will be efficient (Law & Crane, 2000), cost-effective (Chiles, Lambert, & Hatch, 1999), and have a lasting impact over the course of presenting problems (Miller, 1996; Robin, Siegel, Koepke, Moye, & Tice, 1994). A "chronic care model" suggests that ideal care is accomplished when families are interacting with a collaborative and multidisciplinary team of professionals who provide consistent communication about the patient's care (Bodenheimer, Wagner, & Grumbach, 2002; Rothman & Wagner, 2003; Wagner, 2000).

Given the limited resources available in rural communities, approaches to delivering pediatric mental health services must be innovative and carefully thought out. The psychology department at the Munroe Meyer Institute-University of Nebraska Medical Center, located in Omaha, NE, has pioneered focused training on an integrated mental health care model. Doctoral-level psychologists (mostly doctoral-level school psychologists) have been placed into primary care settings across the state. This type of model provides multiple advantages for small rural communities and schools. Integrated care involves a psychologist working at the same site as a child's primary care physician, increasing continuity of care. Psychologists are trained to implement empirically based assessment and treatment in both the home and school settings for children and their families. Examples of primary referral concerns/disorders that psychologists are trained to assess and treat include: disruptive behavior including noncompliance, temper tantrums, aggression; oppositional behaviors; anxiety, including obsessive-compulsive disorder; depression; adjustment issues including divorce and bereavement; elimination disorders including enuresis/encopresis; attention deficit hyperactivity disorder (ADHD); autism spectrum disorders; issues related to obesity; and substance use disorders.

Advantages of integrated care. It is estimated that 12–27% of pediatric visits involve a behavioral and emotional concern (Cassidy & Jellinek, 1998; Simonian, 2006; Williams, Klinepeter, Palmes, Pulley, & Foy, 2004). The most common concerns raised during pediatric visits are ADHD, noncompliance, depression, and sleep problems (Valleley et al., 2007). The primary care physician has been termed as the "gatekeeper" to pediatric mental health as it has been estimated that approximately 75% of children with psychiatric problems are seen in primary care (Williams et al., 2004). Given that the initial contact is made in the primary care office, there are multiple advantages to having a psychologist providing services in the same setting. This is especially true for families residing in rural settings.

Communication with relevant professionals. When psychologists are co-located in a primary care setting, multiple opportunities are opened up for communication between the professionals in the community and the mental health provider. Given the sharing of space, various aspects about a child's care might be discussed between the primary care physician, psychologist, and parent. This may include the evaluation of problems, diagnoses, treatment planning, and medication management. Given that therapy occurs in a neutral setting and with someone who is not directly involved with the child's school, this affords parents the opportunity to provide relevant information to a mental health provider that parents may not feel comfortable sharing with the child's school. This also allows an opportunity to extend services to other community members such as school staff, speech therapists, physical therapists, and occupational therapists. For example, a school may refer a child and then invite the psychologist to meetings for the child. The school also can then request further evaluation that the school psychologist in the school may not be able to perform. Furthermore, if a child needs individual or family therapy, the psychologist can communicate with the school counselor to ensure that therapy is reinforced not only in the home setting, but also the school setting.

Since a large proportion of parents turn to their primary care physicians for their children's mental health concerns, it is also important to highlight that many professionals do the same. For instance, in many small rural communities, professionals in the school will encourage the family to discuss mental health issues with their primary care physician. Unfortunately, physicians do not have the time and training to deal with many of these concerns. This is especially true in rural communities. When a psychologist is on-site, physicians can immediately and effectively communicate with the psychologist about the presenting problems and then refer as needed. Furthermore, an integrated care model offers the opportunity to collaborate with community members such as school personnel, case workers, guardian ad litem, and other medical professionals. Often times, as the physician is too busy, they will circumvent the problem by asking the psychologist to initiate contact with the school, send out behavior rating scales, and set up/attend school meetings.

Reduced stigma. Many parents in rural communities are hesitant to seek help for mental health problems that they are facing with their children. This is largely due to the stigma that is associated with seeking and receiving such services. When a parent's attention is drawn to their child's misbehavior at school, a parent may be left feeling defensive, alone, and desperate regarding how to best handle their child. In a small community, families may be hesitant to park their car outside a well-known mental health agency due to concerns about the stigma that is attached to receiving such services. When psychologists are located in a primary care setting, this eliminates any stigma that families might feel in a small community as there is a certain level of anonymity provided by primary care settings.

Improved access to care. Physicians in rural communities often face the stress of high caseloads and limited time to devote to specific mental health care needs (Galuska et al., 2002). Physicians report a lack of training and having access to mental health professionals as a barrier to delivering effective services (Jellinek, 1998; Kelleher et al., 1997; Rushton, Bruckman, & Kelleher, 2002). Thus, when they encounter complicated mental health cases, they may feel overwhelmed as these cases take longer to manage and most physicians have limited training on mental health management. They also may not have access to relevant referral resources within their community. When a psychologist is placed in a primary care clinic, it frees up a physician's time to manage medical problems and therefore see more patients. Rather than spending extra time attempting to figure out how to treat patients with mental health concerns, the primary care physician can immediately refer to the on-site psychologist. Physicians who have adopted an integrated model of care in Nebraska report strong agreement that this model helps to improve factors such as: (1) quality and continuity of care for their patients, (2) time that it allows them to spend on medical issues, (3) cost, (4) follow-up, (5) physician confidence with identification/management of problems, and (6) reduced stigma (Lieske, Valleley, & Evans, 2009). Furthermore, physicians report that utilizing a collaborative approach affords expedient referrals, earlier intervention, and the opportunity to capitalize on patients' "sense of urgency" (Todahl, Linville, Smith, Barnes, & Miller, 2006).

Improved identification of mental health problems. An additional result of having a psychologist located in a primary care office is the incidental teaching/education that goes on by constant communication between the primary care provider and the psychologist. For instance, a child may come in with concerns of oppositional behavior, but, upon further evaluation by the psychologist, it appears that the child is actually exhibiting symptoms of depression or anxiety. This scenario provides an opportunity for the psychologist to educate the physician on signs to look for, questions to ask, and screeners to administer in relation to depression and anxiety. Communication is facilitated not only both through progress notes and reports that are provided to the physicians, but also via on-the-spot consultations initiated by either the psychologist or the physician.

Limitations

While the integrated care model shows promising preliminary results and appears to be a cutting-edge approach when it comes to an optimal service delivery model for rural pediatric mental health, there are some limitations. The first is making sure that psychologists are adequately trained to handle the stress of working in rural communities where resources are scarce. This factor can lead to clinicians feeling overwhelmed and burnt out. Fortunately, state and national debt forgiveness plans are available for those who are willing to work in these areas. Additionally, working in rural areas can lead to feelings of isolation since there are fewer mental health professionals in a large geographic space. The use of the internet can help reduce these feelings of isolation as can affiliations with local colleges, universities, and agencies. However, there are fewer resources in rural areas and this can prove to be limiting for some individuals. Additional research is needed to help identify specific program elements that lead to successful outcomes for both families and professionals working in an integrated care model.

Why not provide services in schools? One may pose the question, "why not provide the service directly in schools?" From a rural perspective, it becomes a matter of scarcity in resources coupled with the notion that the physician is the gatekeeper to mental health care for children and their families. For example, in a community with a population of 25,000, there may be anywhere between 8–15 elementary schools, 2–3 middle schools, and 2–3 high schools, and typically, one pediatric primary care setting. As such, the majority of these school children are receiving health services at the pediatric primary care office. If a doctoral-level clinician were to be placed directly in a school, they would not be able to extend services to a wide range of children at other schools unless there was a main location within the schools to provide the services. Because of the materials needed for therapy sessions, it may be difficult for a clinician to travel from one school to the next to provide mental health services. Furthermore, clinicians who are providing services in small communities often also serve other surrounding communities that may be as far as 120 miles away. In the Nebraska outreach clinics, it is common for a family to travel 60–120 miles to receive mental health services. Again, it is logical to have mental and behavioral health providers located in one central location such as the primary care setting.

In addition to the scarcity of services, research supports that follow through may be better in an integrated care setting rather than a school. For example, when parents were referred by school counselors to a school-linked mental health program where the services were provided in the school, only 44% followed through with treatment or successfully completed treatment, and over half left prematurely (Evans, Radunovich, Cornette, Wiens, & Roy, 2008).

Evidence further supports that an integrated approach is especially helpful in a rural setting. For children identified in need of mental health services in urban pediatric practices, only 17% attended that initial appointment with a co-located social worker (Hacker et al., 2006). Evidence suggests that rural citizens may be more likely to follow through with physician recommendations than with mental health recommendations (Greeno, Anderson, Shear, & Mike, 1999; Valleley et al., 2007). When utilizing an integrated behavioral health specialist/psychologist in a rural community, 81% of children and their families who were referred showed up for their initial appointment (Barlow, 2007; Valleley et al., 2007).

Treatment adherence is also generally high among these patients; with the majority of children being rated as demonstrating some type of improvement (Barlow, 2007; Valleley et al., 2008). With an integrated mental health intervention approach, most parents have initially sought out help from their primary care physician to address their child's behavioral and mental health needs and may be more motivated to follow through with recommendations. The maintenance phase of the IOM mental health intervention spectrum is particularly important and the integration of services with primary care settings appears to be one mechanism for increased compliance and coordinating after-care.

A third factor that limits a doctoral-level psychologist to practice in the schools is the collaboration with parents and physicians that is necessary for successful outcomes. When working with young children, the involvement of parents is an essential component of treatment. This could be done in the schools, but with limitations. For example, the integrated model allows for a clinician to easily communicate with the primary care provider about evaluations, medication, and progress. Families who come in may have some minor questions that do not necessitate a scheduled appointment with the physician. The mental health provider has ready access to the physician to discuss concerns that arise. This increases the continuity of care across the mental health intervention spectrum.

Additionally, when a psychologist is providing mental health services in a primary care setting versus the school, the psychologist serves as a neutral and/or mediating party for concerns/problems that the parents are experiencing with the school. In Nebraska, the majority of the clinicians in the behavioral outreach clinics have a doctoral degree in school or clinical psychology and are educated on testing/evaluation in the schools, special education rights, etc. They are able to assist parents with their children's Individualized Education Plan (IEP), collaborate with the schools, and attend school meetings. Information from the school meetings are then communicated by the psychologist to the physician. In some situations, schools staff will attend meetings at the primary care office so that the pediatrician/physician can be present.

Case Example

Ben is an 8-year-old Caucasian boy who attends a small rural Nebraska school. He was referred to the on-site psychologist by his pediatrician, Dr. King. Ben was referred due to concerns that he was exhibiting some oppositional symptoms at home and school. Ben was being prescribed Risperdal for some aggressive behavior and Concerta for his impulsive/hyperactive behavior. Upon meeting Ben, he presented as an eccentric child who was focused on discussing his Yu-gi-oh and Pokeman cards. During the initial evaluation, Ben's parents expressed concern that the staff at his school had a negative view of him and were missing opportunities to see how wonderful of a child he could be. The parents requested that school consultation be done to help resolve these issues. They indicated that Ben was due for his re-evaluation in the next couple of weeks and that an IEP meeting would be scheduled soon after. When the school was contacted, Ben's teacher expressed frustration and the opinion that all Ben needs is some discipline and to be held accountable.

His special education teacher agreed that Ben was simply oppositional. Upon completion of a functional analysis of his behaviors, it was noted that Ben commonly acted up during transitions. When he acted up, his teachers would send him to the "buddy room" where he would sit for several minutes by himself and then rejoin the class. This was occurring every day, multiple times per day.

The psychologist from Ben's primary care office attended Ben's IEP meeting to help assist with Ben's educational planning. During the meeting, Ben's intellectual scores showed that he exhibited above average verbal skills, but that he processed information at a rate that was significantly lower than his peers. Scores also showed that his working memory scores were significantly lower than his peers. Concerns about Ben's social skills were brought up by Ben's special education teacher. She stated that he is one-sided and will only engage with other children if they are playing with something that interests him. A final concern stated by the school nurse at Ben's school was that she noted significant weight gain over the past year. On the basis of the information that was being discussed, the team decided to have Ben evaluated to determine if his symptoms were indicative of an autism spectrum disorder as opposed to oppositional defiant disorder. This information was then relayed back to the child's primary care physician.

The results of Ben's evaluation revealed that Ben was not only exhibiting symptoms of an autism spectrum disorder, but he was also experiencing high amounts of anxiety, mainly in the school setting, that were related to unexpected changes and feeling overwhelmed in highly stimulating, less structured situations. Interventions were immediately put into place and a plan for Ben to "take a short" when his anxiety heightened was implemented. On the basis of the results, Ben's physician changed his medication to one that would address his anxiety. Within several weeks, Ben's aggression had disappeared and his compliance with schoolwork increased. The team met again and cited Ben's social skills as being the next goal to target. This was accomplished by the psychologist providing services both in the primary care clinic and via in vivo exposures at Ben's school. Ben's parents and teachers noted an increase in his overall self-confidence with schoolwork and his peer relationships.

Conclusion

In this chapter we have reviewed some of the challenges and opportunities for mental health intervention in rural schools. The case example illustrates how bridging mental health services between a child's primary care clinic and the school can be implemented effectively in a rural community. As can be seen in Ben's case, a psychologist who is not affiliated with the school can provide a neutral perspective for the school and the family. Collaboration can be done in a non-threatening manner as the psychologist acts as neutral team member for the student, their parents, the school, and the child's physician. While not every case ends with a positive outcome, this type of collaborative model does provide promising results for families living in rural communities.

The IOM framework provides a comprehensive rubric for preventing mental health disorders, effectively treating mental health disorders, and maintaining treatment gains (Mrazek & Haggerty, 1994). In rural areas there may be limited access to health care and mental health care providers; there may be limited access to internet services; and there may be transportation issues to travelling long distances to access educational and health care systems. A collaborative model for integrating mental health and heath care has the possibility to help all Americans reach the Healthy People 2020 goals (http://www.healthypeople.gov/2020/default.aspx).

References

Angold, A., Erkanli, A., Farmer, E. M. Z., Fairbank, J. A., Burns, B. J., Keeler, G., et al. (2002). Psychiatric disorder, impairment, and service use in rural African American and White youth. *Archives of General Psychiatry, 59*, 893–901. doi:10.1001/archpsyc.59.10.893.

Barlow, M. E. L. (2007). *Collaborative care and barriers to treatment: Relationship to parental compliance and* attendance for mental health care services. Doctoral dissertation. Retrieved from EBSCOhost (2007-99014-079)

Beeson, E., & Strange, M. (2003). Why rural matters. The continuing need for every state to take action on rural education. *Journal of Research in Rural Education, 1*, 3–16.

Bodenheimer, T., Wagner, E. H., & Grumbach, K. (2002). Improving primary care for patients with chronic illness. *Journal of the American Medical Association, 288*, 1775–1779. PMid: 7498888.

Burns, B. J., Costello, E. J., Angold, A., Tweed, D., Stangl, D., Farmer, E. M., et al. (1995). Children's mental health service use across service sectors. *Health Affairs (Millwood), 14*, 147–159. doi:10.1377/hlthaff.14.3.147.

Caldwell, T. M., Jorm, A. F., & Dear, K. G. B. (2004). Suicide and mental health in rural, remote and metropolitan areas in Australia. *The Medical Journal of Australia, 181*(7), S10–S14.

Cassidy, L., & Jellinek, M. (1998). Approaches to recognition and management of childhood psychiatric disorder in pediatric primary care. *Pediatric Clinics of North America, 45*, 1037–1052. doi:10.1016/S0031-3955(05)70061-4.

Chiles, J., Lambert, M., & Hatch, A. (1999). The impact of psychological interventions on medical cost offset: A meta-analytic review. *Clinical Psychology: Science and Practice, 6*, 204–220. doi:10.1093/clipsy/6.2.204.

Costello, E. J., Mustillo, S., Erkanli, A., Keeler, G., & Angold, A. (2003). Prevalence and development of psychiatric disorders in childhood and adolescence. *Archives of General Psychiatry, 60*, 837–844. doi:10.1001/archpsyc.60.8.837.

Cronk, C. E., & Sarvela, P. D. (1997). Alcohol, tobacco, and other drug use among rural/small town and urban youth: A secondary analysis of the monitoring the future data set. *American Journal of Public Health, 87*(5), 760–764. doi:10.2105/AJPH.87.5.760.

Deewes, S. (1999). Improving rural school facilities for teaching and learning. Rural education and small schools. ERIC Document Reproduction Service No. ED 438 153, Charleston, WV.

Evans, G. D., Radunovich, H. L., Cornette, M. M., Wiens, B. A., & Roy, A. (2008). Implementation and utilization characteristics of a rural, school-linked mental health program. *Journal of Child and Family Studies, 17*, 84–97. doi:10.1007/s10826-007-9148-z.

Galuska, D. A., Fulton, J. E., Powell, K. E., Burgeson, C. R., Pratt, M., Elster, A., et al. (2002). Pediatrician counseling about preventive health topics: Results from the Physicians' Practices Survey 1998-1999. *Pediatrics, 109*, 83–90. doi:10.1542/peds.109.5.e83.

Gfroerer, J. C., Larson, S. L., & Colliver, J. D. (2007). Drug use patterns and trends in rural communities. *The Journal of Rural Health, 23*, 10–15. doi:10.1111/j.1748-0361.2007.00118.x.

Gordon, R. (1987). An operational classification of disease prevention. In J. A. Steinberg & M. M. Silverman (Eds.), *Preventing mental disorders* (pp. 20–26).

Rockville, MD: Department of Health and Human Services.

Greeno, C., Anderson, C., Shear, K., & Mike, G. (1999). Initial treatment engagement in a rural community mental health center. *Psychiatric Services, 50*, 1634–1637. PMid: 10577887.

Hacker, K. A., Myagmarjav, E., Harris, V., Franco Suglia, S., Weidner, D., & Link, D. (2006). Mental health screening in pediatric practice: Factors related to positive screens and the contribution of parental/personal concern. *Pediatrics, 118*, 1896–1906. doi:10.1542/peds.2006-0026.

Hoagwood, K., & Erwin, H. D. (1997). Effectiveness of school-based mental health services for children: A 10-year research review. *Journal of Child and Family Studies, 6*, 435–454. doi:10.1023/A:1025045412689.

Jellinek, M. (1998). DSM-PC: Bridging pediatric primary care and mental health services. *Journal of Developmental and Behavioral Pediatrics, 18*(3), 173–174. doi:10.1097/00004703-199706000-00007.

Kelleher, K. J., Childs, G. E., Wasserman, R. C., McInerny, T. K., Nutting, P. A., & Gardner, W. P. (1997). Insurance status and recognition of psychosocial problems: A report from PROS and ASPN. *Archives of Pediatrics & Adolescent Medicine, 151*, 1109–1115. PMid: 9369872.

Kolko, D. J., Campo, J. D., Kelleher, K., & Cheng, Y. (2010). Improving access to care and clinical outcome for pediatric behavioral problems: A randomized trial of a nurse-administered intervention in primary care. *Journal of Developmental and Behavioral Pediatrics, 31*, 393–404. doi:10.1097/DBP.0b013e3181dff307.

Law, D., & Crane, R. (2000). The influence of marital and family therapy on health care utilization in a health-maintenance organization. *Journal of Marital and Family Therapy, 26*, 281–291. doi:10.1111/j.1752-0606.2000.tb00298.x.

Lieske, J., Valleley, R., & Evans, J. (2009, June). *Physician satisfaction with an integrated mental health delivery model in pediatric primary care.* Paper presented at the National Association for Rural Mental Health, 35th annual conference, Albuquerque, NM.

McCracken, J. D., & Barcinas, J. D. T. (1991). Differences between rural and urban schools, student characteristics, and student aspirations in Ohio. *Journal of Research in Rural Education, 7*(2), 29–40.

Miller, S. (1996). Family therapy for recurrent diabetic ketoacidosis: Treatment guidelines. *Families, Systems & Health, 14*, 303–314. doi:10.1037/h0089928.

Mrazek, P. J., & Haggerty, R. J. (Eds.). (1994). *Reducing risk for mental disorders: Frontiers for preventive intervention research.* Washington, DC: National Academy Press.

Parslow, R. A., & Jorm, A. F. (2000). Who uses mental health services in Australia? An analysis of data from the National Survey of Mental Health and Wellbeing. *The Australian and New Zealand Journal of Psychiatry, 34*, 997–1008. doi:10.1080/000486700276.

Provasnik, S., KewalRamani, A., Coleman, M. M., Gilbertson, L., Herring, W., & Xie, Q. (2007). *Status of education in rural America* (National Center for Education Statistics No. 2007-040). Retrieved Dec 10, 2010, from http://arsl.pbworks.com/f/Status+of+Education+in+Rural+America+2007.pdf

Robin, A., Siegel, P., Koepke, T., Moye, A., & Tice, S. (1994). Family therapy versus individual therapy for adolescent females with anorexia nervosa. *Journal of Developmental and Behavioral Pediatrics, 15,* 111–116. doi:10.1097/00004703-199404000-00008.

Rothman, A. A., & Wagner, E. H. (2003). Chronic illness management: What is the role of primary care? *Annals of Internal Medicine, 138,* 256–261. PMid: 12558376.

Rushton, J., Bruckman, D., & Kelleher, K. J. (2002). Primary care referral of children with psychosocial problems. *Archives of Pediatrics & Adolescent Medicine, 156,* 592–598. PMid: 12038893.

Simonian, S. (2006). Screening and identification in pediatric primary care. *Behavior Modification, 30,* 114–131. doi:10.1177/0145445505283311.

Todahl, J. L., Linville, D., Smith, T. E., Barnes, M. F., & Miller, J. K. (2006). A qualitative study of collaborative health care in a primary care setting. *Families, Systems & Health, 24,* 45–64. doi:10.1037/1091-7527.24.1.45.

U.S. Department of Health and Human Services. (1999). *Mental health: A report of the Surgeon General—Executive summary.* Rockville, MD: U.S. Department of Health and Human Services, Substance Abuse and Mental Health Services Administration, Center for Mental Health Services, National Institutes of Health, National Institute of Mental Health. Retrieved Jan 1, 2011, from http://www.surgeongeneral.gov/library/mentalhealth/summary.html

Valleley, R. J., Clarke, B., Lieske, J., Gortmaker, V., Foster, N., & Evans, J. H. (2008). Improving adherence to children's mental health services: Integrating behavioral health specialists into rural primary care settings. *Journal of Rural Mental Health, 32,* 18–34.

Valleley, R. J., Kosse, S., Schemm, A., Foster, N., Polaha, J., & Evans, J. H. (2007). Integrated primary care for children in rural communities: An examination of patient attendance at collaborative behavioral health services. *Families, Systems & Health, 25*(3), 323–332. doi:10.1037/1091-7527.25.3.323.

Wagner, E. H. (2000). The role of patient care teams in chronic disease management. *British Medical Journal, 320,* 569–572. PMid: 10688568.

Walsh, S. R., & Fortner, J. (2002). Coming full circle: Family therapy and psychiatry reunite in a training program. *Families, Systems & Health, 20,* 105–111. doi:10.1037/h0089571.

Williams, J., Klinepeter, K., Palmes, G., Pulley, A., & Foy, J. M. (2004). Diagnosis and treatment of behavioral health disorders in pediatric practice. *Pediatrics, 114,* 601–606. doi:10.1542/peds.2004-0090.

Zahner, G. E., Jacobs, J. H., Freeman, D. H., Jr., & Trainor, K. F. (1993). Rural-urban child psychopathology in a northeastern US state: 1986 to 1989. *Journal of the American Academy of Child and Adolescent Psychiatry, 32*(2), 378–387. doi:10.1097/00004583-199303000-00020.

The Racial/Ethnic Identity Development of Tomorrow's Adolescent

Kip V. Thompson, Keshia Harris, and Caroline S. Clauss-Ehlers

Adolescents across racial/ethnic group memberships often experience some degree of confusion and maladaptive symptoms as they sort through the potential components of their personal and ethnic identities (Luyckx et al., 2008; Schwartz, Zamboanga, Weisskirch, & Rodriguez, 2009). The similarities of this process do not end there; research indicates that the structures of both ethnic identity (Roberts et al., 1999) and personal identity (Schwartz, Côté, & Arnett, 2005) are consistent across ethnic groups. Helms (1990) defined racial identity as a "sense of group or collective identity based on the perception that one shares a common racial heritage with a particular group" (as cited by Phelps, Taylor, & Gerard, 2001, p. 210). Ethnic identity, on the other hand, is conceptualized as "the study of attitudes about one's own ethnicity" (Phinney, 1990, p. 499) and may include ethnic group membership self-identification, a sense of belonging, and attitudes one holds toward their ethnic group (Phinney, 1992). As our society becomes more global and welcoming of greater racial/ethnic diversity, the study of racial/ethnic identity development becomes even more salient for adolescents (Berry, Poortinga, Segall, & Dasen, 2002; Schwartz et al., 2009). A major goal of this chapter is to address aspects of both racial and ethnic identity development among adolescents. This goal is accomplished in part by linking theories of adolescent identity development to the experiences of diverse youth.

The following paragraphs highlight the salience of racial/ethnic identity and its development for specific racial/ethnic adolescent groups. This is not meant to be an exhaustive list of the ethnicities represented in today's American schools: several ethnic groups have been omitted or have been otherwise aggregated. This is also not meant to be an exhaustive list of every issue experienced by each racial/ethnic group. In addition, the authors present many strengths associated with each racial/ethnic group—understanding many more can be found in the literature. Our overall goal is to demonstrate the unique processes of racial/ethnic identity development among and within some of the larger ethnic groups in the United States (U.S). We also explore implications of racial/ethnic identity development for work with youth in school-based settings.

American Indian Adolescents

The U.S. Census Bureau (2009) reported that approximately 0.8% of the U.S. population classifies itself as having American Indian or Alaska Native ethnic group membership. There

K.V. Thompson, M.A. (✉)
University of South Carolina, Columbia, SC, USA
e-mail: thompskv@email.sc.edu

K. Harris, Ed.M.
Teachers College, Columbia University,
New York, NY, USA

C.S. Clauss-Ehlers, Ph.D.
Rutgers, The State University of New Jersey,
New Brunswick, NJ, USA

is a significant state by state range in the American Indian population; Alaska has the highest percentage (13.2%), while Pennsylvania has the fewest numbers of citizens who report American Indian descent (0.1%). This community is distinguished as the only ethnic group in the U.S. that either occupies land reservations or chooses to live in more mainstream living situations. These reservations are tribally owned acres of land reserved for American Indians in the wake of the U.S. manifest destiny (Wakeling, Jorgensen, Michaelson, & Begay, 2001).

The American Indian community is represented by over 40 tribal groups across the U.S. territories (U.S. Census Bureau, 2007), and thus, the heterogeneity of this ethnic group cannot be overstated. However, there are a few characteristics that can be found in many American Indian groups, including religiosity and spirituality as major driving forces of the community (Stilling, 1996; West & Newman, 2007). Stilling (1996) further suggested that American Indian adults tend to contribute toward celebratory ceremonies of success for their neighbors and often report considerable involvement in their children's education. The confluence of high participation at school, church, and community centers highlights the communal nature of American Indian racial/ethnic identity and demonstrates how family structure, spirituality, and tribal values are all-encompassing in this community (Red Horse, 1997).

Culture and ethnic identification are key factors in the American Indian's process of acculturation into mainstream society (West & Newman, 2007), quite possibly because of the distinctive risk factor of acculturative stress found in the recent history of this group (LaFromboise, Hoyt, Oliver, & Whitbeck, 2006). Within the American Indian community, this often presents itself as acculturation anxiety which has been characterized as the stressful outcome of blending American Indian beliefs with mainstream paradigms that are seemingly in direct conflict with traditional American Indian life (McNeil, Kee, & Zvolensky, 1999; McNeil, Porter, Zvolensky, Chaney, & Kee, 2000). Incidents and contexts that threaten to elicit acculturation anxiety (e.g., discrimination, racism) have been shown to hinder positive outcomes among American Indian youth (LaFromboise & Medoff, 2004; LaFromboise et al., 2006).

The process of racial/ethnic identity development for American Indian adolescents is a balancing act of fulfilling parental and community expectations that may be contrary to what teachers and other mainstream agents require. Phinney (1989, 1992) asserted that ethnic identity development lies on a double-continuum of exploring the meaning of one's ethnicity and commitment to aspects of the individual's ethnicity, such as religious preferences. As Beauvais (2000) suggests, exploration and commitment for this group includes incorporating American Indian strength with the opportunities of the distal U.S. society. Exposure to inconsistent messages about the value of American Indians in our society, such as the imagery of Native people in the media, make it particularly challenging for American Indian youth to assimilate the cultural patterns they learn within their families into their interaction with the broader society (Newman, 2005). Yet these communities' adolescents are still expected to participate in ritual events as they mature, to demonstrate their acceptance of increased spiritual and community responsibility (Red Horse, 1997).

The ability of American Indian youth to develop resilience and maintain cultural affiliation has been shown to hold constant as long as patterns of interaction with their family and tribal culture that American Indian values demand are sustained (LaFromboise & Medoff, 2004; LaFromboise et al., 2006). The American Indian community can provide resources that support ethnic identification such as peer group and family relations, engagement in culturally relevant activities, and encouraged socialization among one's ethnic group members (Newman, 2005).

Implications for working with American Indian adolescents in school settings. American Indian adolescents face unique struggles in combining their native culture with mainstream American culture. As mentioned above, the inconsistent messages that American Indian adolescents experience can have an impact on their daily social experiences, especially in a school setting. American Indian adolescents may receive negative stereotypical messages about their culture from authoritative figures such as teachers who lack cultural competence and awareness (Newman, 2005). Since adolescents spend much of their time in school, the risk is that these messages will be internalized by American Indian adolescents. LaFromboise et al. (2006) found that reports of discrimination and exposure to racist attitudes and behaviors had a negative relationship to resilience and cultural group pride among the American Indian adolescents who participated in their research.

Mental health professionals working with American Indian adolescents in a school setting may help facilitate the process of racial/ethnic identity development by encouraging them to explore societal messages in comparison with messages received from members within their culture and what this means to them. Newman (2005) identified family support and relationships with community members, such as church leaders, as factors that contribute to resilience among American Indian adolescents. It is important for school counselors to be aware of these potential methods of support within the community when working with American Indian youth.

Arab American Adolescents

There are approximately 17 countries that are considered ancestral Arab homelands (Haboush, 2007) that are clustered in the Middle East and Northern Africa. Arab families with varying levels of socioeconomic status and traumatic experience have migrated to the U.S. in several waves, the last involving the years between the Gulf and Iraq Wars (Erickson & Al-Timimi, 2001). This community established several thriving enclaves across the U.S.; for example, Dearborn, Michigan, is known as one of the largest Arab American populations outside the Middle Eastern region (Goodstein, 2001).

The Arab American Institute, the U.S. Census Bureau's primary information source for this population, estimates that there are approximately 3.5 million individuals of Arab descent living in the U.S. It is important to note that the term *Arab* did not appear on the 2010 U.S. Census form, suggesting that those who identify as Arab American were subsumed under the *White* category (Padgett, 2010). This suggests that a significant number of those classified as White American may in fact represent an ethnic group that has a set of beliefs, values, and customs distinct from traditional White American culture.

Al-Krenawi and Graham (2000) proposed a list of promoting factors for Arab American acculturation, including having lived more years in the U.S., positive diplomatic relations between their country of origin and the U.S., younger age during immigration, and religious affiliation with Christian beliefs. For example, some Arab American activists note that it is sometimes easier for Arab Americans to acculturate into mainstream U.S. society if they were affiliated with Christianity, choosing to anglicize their last names or assume Christian first names (Nagel & Staeheli, 2005). Several ethnic organizations, including the Arab American Institute and the Council on American-Islamic Relations have initiated several campaigns to improve the political climate for all Arab Americans regardless of their religious affiliations. Additionally, education and family income among Arab American immigrants often help to ease the acculturative process (Kulczycki & Lobo, 2002). Presumably native-born Arab American youth with more personal and family resources will have an easier acculturative experience than their foreign-born counterparts; this circumstance, however, is not always the case.

The strong backlash against Arab Americans in the years following September 11, 2001 may have influenced many Arab American adolescents to incorporate Arab culture and values into their identity or risk suffering role confusion with little social support (Erikson, 1968). Even though stereotypes that depict Arab Americans as terrorists existed in the Western media beforehand (Shaheen, 2001), they have proliferated in the decade since and continue to fuel negative perceptions about Arabs and Arab Americans.

Islam is the most commonly endorsed expression of spirituality among Arab American families (Hall & Livingston, 2006) and exerts considerable influence on the family structure of its youth. While Phinney (1992) suggested that all adolescents undertake a process of exploration; Arab American parents might have a different view that does not encourage such explorations if it ventures outside of Islamic values. These views might include high religiosity, collectivism, and emotion concealment (Ajrouch, 2000; Haboush, 2007). These traditional values contrast with predominant Western values, e.g., individualism, liberalism, and self-determination (Chirkov, 2009; Markus & Kitayama, 2003). Inter-generational conflict may occur when Arab American parents believe their children are forsaking family expectations in favor of developing their own coping strategies and are showing other signs of independence (Al-Krenawi & Graham, 2000).

Arab American youth are also likely to feel pressure in school. Sirin and Fine (2007) contend that many Arab American youth are likely to have experienced ethnic- or religious-based discrimination in multiple settings including school. Arab American male youth with high levels of participation in both home and school social activities were less likely to report perceptions of discrimination (Sirin & Fine, 2007). In contrast, Arab American female adolescents were more likely than their male counterparts to have more positive acculturative experiences. One possible explanation is that Arab American young women are more likely to report more fluid movement between their dual identities of being Arab and American in comparison with young men of Arab descent. Thus, the process of racial/ethnic identity development among Arab American youth might be seen as careful exploration (so as to avoid discrimination and other stressors related to acculturation) as the adolescent chooses among any combination of Islamic and Western values to which they may commit (Ajrouch, 2004).

Implications for working with Arab American adolescents in school settings. "I am a Muslim woman wearing a veil and many times in stores and restaurants people will ridicule the way I look," shared a 16-year-old Arab American adolescent (Flanagan, Syvertsen, Gill, Gallay, & Cumsille, 2009, p. 510). In their study on ethnic awareness and experiences of prejudice of Arab American, Latino/a, African American, and European American youth, Flanagan et al. found that Arab American adolescents reported being discriminated against based on group stereotypes of terrorism. It is likely that today's Arab American adolescents have experienced a heightened amount of prejudicial treatment in school.

In addition to experiences of discrimination, Arab American adolescents may experience a conflict between family values and peer relationships. Typically, Arab American parents encourage their children to maintain family honor and cohesiveness; these values may conflict with peer relationships that emphasize the American cultural values of independence and autonomy (Haboush, 2007). It is imperative that mental health practitioners working with Arab American adolescents in school settings examine their own biases about Arab culture and educate themselves on the socialization of this group as well as the cultural clashes that they may encounter in the U.S. in relation to war and terrorist attacks. Researchers found that after September 11, prayer was a method for many Muslims to seek emotional comfort. Incorporating faith may be a beneficial therapeutic intervention for Muslims dealing with turmoil and depression (Ali, Liu, & Humedian, 2004; Inayat, 2002). School counselors can create a safe space for Arab American adolescents by implementing culturally relevant practices that include family values and spirituality.

Asian American Adolescents

According to Barringer, Gardner, and Levin (1993), the term Asian American broadly defines an ethnic group comprised of 28 distinct nationalities with shared Asian origins, physical appearance, and cultural mores. Asian Americans comprise a racial/ethnic group that demonstrates considerable diversity in language, socioeconomic status, religion, occupational skills, and immigration experience (Barringer et al.; Chan, 1991; Ishii-Kuntz, 2000). There are more than 17 million Asian Americans who live in the U.S. (Humes, Jones, & Ramirez, 2011), including individuals with heritage from countries in the Far East, Southeast Asia, or the Indian subcontinent.

Since their arrival over 160 years ago and culminating with the World War II Japanese internment camps, Asian Americans were "portrayed as uncivilized, sinister, heathen, yellow hordes" (Wing, 2007, p. 457) that threatened to defile the White American bloodline (Lee, 1999). However, much of that negative attention was dissipated and transformed by the 1960s Civil Rights era as Asian Americans were finally welcomed into the fabric of American society. This happened in stages: first, the Chinese Exclusion Act was repealed, making it easier for Chinese immigrants to migrate to and live in the U.S. Next, as more U.S. soldiers married Japanese, South Korean, and Filipino women, the number of Asian immigrants increased in the U.S. Finally, the U.S. government passed the Immigration and Nationality Act of 1965, abolishing Asian exclusion and allowing Asian immigrants to more easily become permanent residents (Min, 2006).

Some researchers suggest that acculturation might be a key concept in understanding family life within Asian American communities (Fang, McDowell, Goldfarb, Perumbilly, & Gonzalez-Kruger, 2008) as research has linked this construct to topics like parenting style and identity development within this culture. Asian American fathers may strive to be the primary breadwinner and disciplinarian in their families, while mothers may be expected to facilitate the emotional wellness of their children (Lee & Cynn, 1991). Parental socialization in Asian American families may emphasize familial duty and obligation, and these practices may lead Asian American adolescents to value self-sacrifice in the name of family more than their White American counterparts (Fuligni, Tseng, & Lam, 1999; Vo-Jutabha, Dinh, McHale, & Valsiner, 2009).

The gulf between Asian and American identities can contribute to family obstacles for Asian American youth, such as having to watch younger children despite academic obligations and feeling competing pressures between family obligations and being responsive to the peer group.

Despite these pressures, Umana-Taylor, Bhanot, and Shin (2006) discuss how many Asian American families socialize their children in ways that positively influence racial/ethnic identity achievement for many adolescents. Examples of this family ethnic socialization include consistent exposure to extended family members, attendance at cultural events, and concerted efforts to educate youth about the practices of the family's native culture (Lu, 2001; McLoyd, Cauce, Takeuchi, & Wilson, 2000). Conflicts may arise between Asian American adolescents and their elders when youth do not demonstrate the attitudes and beliefs this ethnic socialization is supposed to provide. Examples of this may include possible isolation of children for behavior that brings perceived shame to the family or when Asian American youth reject the perceived rigid traditional beliefs of their immigrant parents (Hayashino & Chopra, 2009).

Asian nationalities may express this intergenerational conflict differently. For example, some Vietnamese American youth are unaware of the details surrounding their parents' experiences as refugees. Their parents may not know the nuances of navigating relationships with peers and the school setting (Cheung & Nguyen, 2001). Gender roles, displays of affection and respect, and religiosity are other sources of conflict for some Asian American families (Hayashino & Chopra, 2009). Research indicates that social support is an effective protective factor against intergenerational conflict: relying on older offspring and neighbors to teach youth about history and values, socializing with ethnic and religious communities, and maintaining ties with extended family members have been shown to reduce the number of problems within the Asian American parent–child relationship (Agbayani-Siewart, 2002; Bankston, 2006; Hayashino & Chopra, 2009).

Another concept that has an impact on Asian American families is the *Model Minority* stereotype. This stereotype promotes the image of Asian Americans as consistently successful in economic, educational, and social domains of functioning (Lee, Wong, & Alvarez, 2009). This term was first coined in a 1966 *New York Times* article entitled *Success Story, Japanese-American Style* (Petersen, 1966). The term proliferated in the next two decades and beyond to describe the academic achievement of Asian Americans.

While non-Asian Americans might mistakenly believe such a term is flattering, the *Model Minority* stereotype is detrimental to the identity development of Asian American adolescents in at least three distinct ways. First, such a term neglects the diversity among Asian Americans and diminishes the unique histories and victories of each specific nationality. This may result in teachers and school administrators ignoring individual needs in favor of generalized solutions. The second deleterious impact of the *Model Minority* stereotype is that it casts Asian American adolescents as competition for other students of color in the school setting. When the successes of Asian American adolescents are compared to the failures of other youth of color, it creates an environment where Asian American adolescents are socially excluded and even bullied in some cases (Rosenbloom & Way, 2004). The third impact of this harmful stereotype is that it discourages Asian American youth from resisting the *Model Minority* image, leading to potential feelings of shame when one performs less than what is expected and/or inhibits their adaptive-help seeking behaviors (Lee et al., 2009).

As applied to Erikson's (1968) psychosocial model, Asian American racial/ethnic identity development among adolescents involves a process of reconciling positive segments of their identity and culture (e.g., close relationships with extended relatives, cultural event attendance) with negative feelings associated with their identity (e.g., intergenerational obstacles). During this psychosocial stage where the central struggle is between identity and role confusion, Asian American youth (like youth in other ethnicities) may grapple with an identity *moratorium* where they attempt to draw a line between what they will become and what they do not want as part of their identities going forward (Marcia, 1993). This process may be complicated further if the adolescent experiences feelings of incompetence or inadequacy as a result of *Model Minority* bias and feelings that s/he cannot live up to it (Ryckman, 2007).

Implications for working with Asian American adolescents in school settings. Positive strategies include high participation rates among Asian Americans in social activism to deconstruct racist images in the media (Chang & Kwan, 2009). School personnel are encouraged to draw from this finding to engage Asian American students in school activities that proactively promote a positive school climate. The *Model Minority* bias has been associated with high reports of bullying in this population (Hayashino & Chopra, 2009) so school counselors are encouraged to pay close attention when Asian American youth report these experiences. School personnel can help promote positive racial/ethnic identity development by being vigilant against using common stereotypes (e.g., hardworking/academic, compliant/obedient) to describe Asian American youth and to consider using nonverbal means of expression (e.g., journal writing, drawing) that are less likely to seem threatening to Asian American youth who display discomfort in self-disclosing (Yeh, 2001). Yeh suggested that school-based mental health professionals become more familiar with culturally relevant coping methods (e.g., including peer networks, community outreach) to help Asian American youth find more adaptive ways of addressing developmental concerns.

Black American Adolescents

The Black American experience includes first-, second-, and even third-generation Americans with direct African descent, people of color from the Caribbean, and the descendants of U.S. slaves from Africa who reproduced with several ethnic groups in the years since their arrival to the U.S. during the seventeenth century. The U.S. Census (2009) reports that Black Americans comprise 12.4% of the general population. Several generations of racist and discriminatory experiences have engendered varying levels of cultural mistrust among Black American groups that have, in turn, had an impact on adolescent racial/ethnic identity development for this group (Phelps et al., 2001).

Part of the burden of this historical oppression has been the development of obstacles in the process of positive identity for Black American adolescents. *Colorism*, or the internalization of Eurocentric standards of attractiveness, has been shown to inhibit the self-esteem of some Black American adolescents (APA Task Force on the Resilience and Strength in Black Children and Adolescents, 2008; Breland, Coleman, Coard, & Steward, 2002; Ward, 2000). For example, a national survey suggested that skin tone has a direct impact on educational attainment and socioeconomic status among Black Americans (Keith & Herring, 1991). Attitudes and behaviors that suggest the acceptance of negative stereotypes concerning intrinsic worth and ability among racial minorities is known as internalized racism (Jones, 2000). Several researchers have found a positive correlation between racial/ethnic identity and self-esteem among Black Americans so that those with more developed racial/ethnic identities reported higher comfort with their African features and greater self-esteem (Breland, Coleman, Coard, & Steward, 2002; Hesse-Biber, Howling, Leavy, & Lovejoy, 2004; Smith, Burlew, & Lundgren, 1991).

Other forms of internalized racism Black American youth must contend with include a judgment orientation that subjugates other Black Americans and elevates White Americans. An extreme example of this is the "Uncle Ruckus" character from the popular Cartoon Network program *The Boondocks* (McGruder, Barnes, Brooks, Taylor, & Veen, 2008). This Black American cartoon character is known for his disparaging comments about the Black community and glowing praise for all things White American.

Black American adolescents who report well-developed ethnic identities are less likely to demonstrate these internally racialized attitudes (Cokley, 2005). In their predominantly Black American sample, Altschul, Oyserman, and Bybee (2006) found that Black American adolescents who reported feeling connected to their ethnic group and characterized other Black Americans as having achieved high educational attainment, demonstrated higher grade point averages than those who did not share such perceptions. Another benefit of positive racial/ethnic identity development among Black American youth is the construct of critical consciousness, the ability to comprehend the influence of racism and discern stereotypes of others as they navigate their own identity development (Watts, Abdul-Adil, & Pratt, 2002).

Black American families vary in their processes for socializing children and adolescents into their ethnic groups. Some parents and other family members participate in teaching Black American adolescents how to cope with racial discrimination, discuss how their ethnic group membership may have an impact on future opportunities and decision points, and connect them to Black American culture and history (Cooper, McLoyd, Wood, & Hardaway, 2008). The role of family in racial/ethnic identity development is also salient for Black American youth. For instance, Tatum (2004) proposed three approaches adopted by Black families living in White communities: race-conscious family frame (involvement in seeking Black activities and friendships for their children), race-neutral family frame (allowing children to define their own racial group membership), and class-conscious family frame (emphasizing social class status above racial group membership). The Black college students in Tatum's study reported a desire for same-race peer relationships, knowledge and awareness of Black American cultural heritage, access to positive role models within their ethnic group, and the support of significant adults within their lives.

Ethnic socialization has been defined as a two-part process. The first component enhances psychological adjustment for the young person in matters related to ethnicity; the second part involves cushioning the deleterious effects of discrimination on a young person's academic and mental functioning (Cooper et al., 2008). Harris-Britt, Valrie, Kurtz-Costes, and Rowley's (2007) research on perceived racial discrimination experiences among Black American adolescents indicated that in some Black American families, the cushioning Cooper and colleagues (2008) refer to may include messages of Black pride and preparation for bias. In the Black American community, family ethnic socialization often includes discussion about discrimination and appropriate coping strategies, ceremonies designed to instill knowledge and ethnic pride, and brainstorming how to succeed in mainstream society

(Hughes et al., 2006). Research has shown that Black American adolescents who receive this type of socialization from their parents demonstrate higher cognitive coping and adaptive help-seeking than Black American youth from less active families (Newman, 1994; Scott, 2004).

Research indicates that these family ethnic socialization practices also contribute toward lower levels of psychiatric distress and higher levels of psychological wellness for Black American adolescents (Caldwell, Sellers, Bernat, & Zimmerman, 2004; Seaton, Scottham, & Sellers, 2006). Similarly, these ethnic socialization practices have been shown to buffer the negative impact of racial discrimination on the school adjustment experience (Cooper et al., 2008; Neblett, Philip, Cogburn, & Sellers, 2006). Within the context of Phinney's (1989, 1990) model of ethnic identity development, as Black American youth learn from classmates, teachers, and the media what being Black means (*exploration*), their parents employ specific techniques to ensure their children arrive into adulthood with a clear sense of Black racial/ethnic identity (*achieved*).

The Nigrescence model (Cross, 1991) delineates the steps toward racial/ethnic identity development of Black American adults. Cross suggested a four-stage model of racial/ethnic identity development where the individual gradually moves from a place of relative racial/ethnic unawareness toward pride in being Black (Cross, 2001). Progression through the four stages is not a linear process; rather individuals can experience one or more stages multiple times throughout their lifetime. The *Pre-Encounter* stage is distinguished by an unawareness of race and implications for one's identity. Following this is the *Encounter* stage that is characterized by the experiencing of a series of events that induces one to re-examine their race (Vandiver, Cross, Worrell, & Fhagen-Smith, 2002).

If these events resonate deeply enough to move away from the *Encounter* state, then the Black American adolescent will continue matriculating along Cross's hypothesized path toward racial/ethnic identity development to the *Immersion-Emersion* stage. In *Immersion-Emersion*, the individual tends to be idealistic about his/her Black identity and rejects White American culture (Cross, 1991; Vandiver et al., 2002). This is representative of the early part of the stage while the later part of Immersion-Emersion involves a search for less stereotypical symbols of Blackness in an effort to explore what it means to be Black (Tatum, 1997). The final stage of Cross' theory is *Internalization*. This stage refers to the process whereby the individual has established a self-defined racial/ethnic identity and is able to establish meaningful relationships with members of other ethnic groups. Black Americans in this stage have developed a positive racial/ethnic identity and are able to transcend their personal sense of race and ethnicity into a sustainable commitment to Black Americans as a group (Tatum, 2004).

Implications for working with Black American adolescents in school settings. Much of the literature on the school success of Black American adolescents focuses on contextual factors such as poverty, violence, and inadequate health and education services rather than addressing the interaction of race and culture, and the impact these variables have on social and emotional adjustment (Day-Vines, Patton, & Baytops, 2003). Tatum (2004) identified knowledge of Black American heritage and accomplishments, access to positive community role models, and opportunities to connect with same-race peers as components for positive racial identity development of Black adolescents.

School counselors can practice culturally responsive methods by being aware of differences in ethnic socialization and identity development of Black adolescents and exploring personal biases that may influence their ability to work with this group. Wong, Eccles, and Sameroff (2003) found that discrimination experienced from peers and teachers influenced the academic motivation, self-esteem, and psychological health of Black American adolescents. Findings of this study also revealed that connection to racial/ethnic group had an effect on the psychological adjustment of Black American adolescents, serving as a protective factor against perceived discrimination (Wong et al., 2003).

Latino/Latina Adolescents

The term Latino/a refers to people who have heritage in Spanish speaking regions in Latin America, such as Mexico, the Central and South Americas, and the Caribbean (Flores, Cicchetti, & Rogosch, 2005; Javier & Camacho-Gingerich, 2004). Mexican Americans were the first Latino group to be counted in the U.S. Census in the 1930s (Cauce & Domenech-Rodriguez, 2002). At that time, the Latino/a population in the U.S. was estimated at 1.3 million individuals. The U.S. Census Bureau (2009) reports there are now more than 48 million individuals who classify themselves as "Hispanic" or "Latino" in American society. For the past two decades, Cubans, Mexicans and Puerto Ricans have been the three largest subgroups in the U.S. (DeGarmo & Martinez, 2006). It is expected that Latinos/as will account for 44% of all U.S. population growth over the next decade; it has been projected that Latino adolescents alone will account for a quarter of the entire U.S. population by the year 2050 (Ramirez, 2004; Simpkins, O'Donnell, Delgado, & Becnel, 2011).

The Latino experience in the U.S. for many includes residing in predominantly urban districts, living in a household with at least three other people, and having more work experience than other Americans in the same age cohort (Marotta & Garcia, 2003). The family is considered the primary socialization agent for Latinos/as (Cauce & Domenech-Rodriguez, 2002; Garcia Coll, Meyer, & Brillon, 1995), yet it has also been documented that immigrant Latino/a groups (especially adolescents) sometimes report patterns of isolation and interpersonal distance from adults in their family and community networks (Spina, 2002; Stanton-Salazar, 2001). Like many other ethnic groups of color in U.S. society, Latino adolescents must try to construct a positive identity while living in a mainstream culture that often stereotypes and debases the phenotypic, linguistic, and cultural aspects of Latino/a culture (Stanton-Salazar & Spina, 2003; Valenzuela, 1999). The internalization of these negative stereotypes for Latino/a adolescents may result in what Marcia (1993) characterized as an identity crisis period, or *moratorium*. When Latino/a adolescents reconsider past beliefs on ethnicity and replace negative Latino stereotypes with positive messages, this reflects *identity achievement* (Marcia).

Latinos/as account for approximately 11 million students currently enrolled in the U.S. public school system (Kohler & Lazarín, 2007). There are conflicting findings in the research about academic success and racial/ethnic identity for Latino/a adolescents. On the one hand, the pro-acculturation hypothesis is reflected in research that indicates Latino adolescents need to be allowed to create "school identities" apart from their culture to achieve academic success (Cordeiro, 1990; Hébert, 1996). For example, Martinez, DeGarmo, and Eddy (2004) found that greater student acculturation (i.e., U.S. nativity, English proficiency) predicted lower likelihood of high school dropout for a sample of Latino/a adolescents. These results also indicated that discriminatory and otherwise unwelcoming experiences predicted lower grade point averages and a higher risk of high school dropout.

On the other hand, existing research also indicates a lack of alignment with the pro-acculturation hypothesis that promotes academic success among Latino/a adolescents. Perreira, Harris, and Lee (2006), for instance, conducted a study that sought to identify patterns of high school dropout among immigrant and native-born Latinos. These researchers classified four types of capital used to prevent early educational termination. *Human capital* was defined as information, skills, and experiences that increase individual productivity levels, *cultural capital* was conceptualized as family-based core values, *school capital* was defined as expectations of and commitment to activities related to high academic achievement, and *community-level social capital* was described as the conditions within a neighborhood that influence the individual's normative climate and access to future opportunities (Perreira et al., 2006). The absence of community and social capital was found to put Latino/a adolescents at increased risk for dropping out of high school.

These contrasting findings underscore the complexity of the processes being explored.

Additional research is needed to further our understanding of the interaction among such variables. It might be that having a range of strategies to address educational and other challenges, while also valuing one's racial/ethnic identity, promotes positive development among diverse adolescents (Clauss-Ehlers, Yang, & Chen, 2006).

Implications for working with Latino/Latina adolescents in school settings. Much of the research that we have covered illustrates the importance of family in the ethnic socialization and identity development of Latino/a adolescents. Mental health professionals working with Latino/a adolescents in school settings can implement culturally responsive methods of counseling by acknowledging the role that family plays in their lives. Villalba (2007) suggested that counselors encourage Latino/a youth to use their immediate and extended family members as an asset as well as their bicultural skills. Counselors can encourage Latino/a adolescents to seek out mentors within their family and community that will both serve as a positive role model and relate to their ethnic experience. Mental health professionals can also reinforce bilingualism by incorporating dual language capacity into therapeutic work. This can be accomplished through work with a bilingual school mental health professional or via the incorporation of dual languages in counseling (see Clauss, 1998 for specific strategies).

Multiracial/Biracial American Adolescents

Beginning in 2000, the U.S. Census Bureau introduced the multiracial category to their annual reporting form. Currently, 2.4% of the American population self-identifies as multiracial (U.S. Census Bureau, 2009). The term "biracial" indicates an individual born to parents with two distinct sets of phenotypic characteristics associated with race (e.g., skin color, hair texture). "Multiracial" categorizes individuals whose parents possess phenotypic traits representing three or more racial groups. For the purposes of this chapter, we focus on the experiences of multiracial youth. In the last quarter of the twentieth century, interracial marriage rates increased sharply among Asian Americans, Black Americans, and White Americans (Fang et al., 2008; Johnson, 1992; Khanna, 2004; Root, 1995). This social phenomenon is not new, however. Interracial marriage was against the law until the U.S. Supreme Court repealed the last anti-miscegenation laws in 1967 (Root, 2003a).

Multiracial American young children often choose the reference group of their closest primary caregiver (Bowles, 1993). The extended families of each parent are likely to expose the child to the socialization experiences common within respective racial/ethnic groups. For those multiracial adolescents who do not have contact with or have lost their monoracial families, the process of socialization may become more difficult; these youth may have to seek out racial socialization messages from other adults.

There are many reasons why Multiracial American adolescents of European descent might commit to their non-European racial/ethnic identity. Multiracial adolescents with White heritage are believed to enter a period of turmoil when they begin to accept both their minority and majority cultural roots because of a "dual existence." This may lead to questions about where they belong in peer groups and society (Renn, 2008). It may be easier for some Multiracial American adolescents to choose a part of their ethnicity that they identify with most closely to avoid feeling as if they do not belong. In a study on the comparisons of identity development measures of mono- and biracial adolescents of various racial heritages (e.g., Asian, Latino) for instance, Herman (2004) found that more biracial adolescents chose their minority category rather than their White category, especially those of African American descent. Neighborhood and peer group were also found to play a role. For instance, Herman's study found multiracial adolescents who had a primarily ethnic minority peer group were more likely to identify with their minority race and those that were raised in affluent White neighborhoods, were more likely to identify as White (Herman, 2004).

Similar to differences within monoracial adolescents, it is important to explore within group differences in the racial/ethnic identity development of multiracial adolescents. Rockquemore and Brunsma (2002) found that multiracial individuals with darker physiognomy reported experiencing more ethnic discrimination than monoracial individuals and were more likely to identify with their ethnic minority heritage. Multiracial American racial/ethnic identity theorists also contend that gender alignment between Multiracial American youth and their monoracial parents may have significant implications for adolescent racial/ethnic identity development (Khanna, 2004). While some researchers posit that mothers often play more significant roles in ethnic socialization, others argue that the father more heavily influences the cultural practices of the family. Herman (2004) found that sharing gender with a parent significantly increased the likelihood of the adolescent identifying with the heritage of the same-sex parent over the heritage of the opposite-sex parent.

Miville, Constantine, Baysden, and So-Lloyd (2005) compared the efficacy of several developmental models of racial/ethnic identity to explain how Multiracial Americans make sense of ethnicity, including Poston's (1990) model, Kich's (1992) three-stage heuristic developmental model of biracial identity, Rockquemore's (1999) multidimensional model of biracial identity, and Maria P.P. Root's (2001) ecological meta-model of racial/ethnic identity development for multiracial Americans. Poston's model (1990) details a process by which multiracial adolescents move from excluding ethnicity from their reference group identity to appreciating and integrating all aspects of their ethnic heritage into their identity.

Kich (1992) posited that racial/ethnic identity development for multiracial adolescents begins with self-awareness of dissonance with the immediate environment, continues with a struggle for acceptance from self and others, and culminates with the affirmation of a multiracial identity. Other models approach racial/ethnic identity development for multiracial adolescents by examining the cultural knowledge, historical context, and the degree to which adolescents feel accepted or excluded by family and friends (Root, 2001; Suyemoto & Tawa, 2009).

In their study, Miville and associates (2005) found that parents, developmental period (i.e., elementary school years, high school years, college years) and certain places (e.g., school settings) were influential in the racial/ethnic identity development of participants during their adolescence. Miville et al. (2005) contended that these developmental periods heighten the multiracial adolescent's experience of being different from others in addition to influencing racial/ethnic identity development. For instance, if the multiracial adolescent's school is marked by tension surrounding ethnic issues, this tension may impinge upon one's self-acceptance (Miville et al., 2005).

Root (1996) proposed that youth with multiple racial heritages navigate this process by using four strategies, or border crossings. These border crossings include the ability to shift one's racial/ethnic identity to meet the needs of the environment, establish a multiracial reference status around family members, the ability to view life through more than one ethnic lens and the maintenance of a monoracial identity when the adolescent interprets this is warranted by the situation. Because multiracial youth have the genotype of more than two ethnic groups, it may be more difficult for this population to maintain a monoracial identity to meet the needs of their environment. Biracial racial/ethnic identity models propose that biracial youth can choose an identity somewhere on a spectrum with two points, but they do not account for the additional dimension of ethnicity for adolescents with three or more ethnic backgrounds.

It has been suggested that the Multiracial American racial/ethnic identity development literature is limited by the idea that Multiracial Americans are searching for a fully integrated racial/ethnic identity (Root, 1998, 1999, 2003b). On the contrary, it seems as if the process of identity development among this population is dynamic and continues throughout the person's childhood and young adulthood. Those Multiracial American young adults who achieve meaningful, balanced social identities demonstrate techniques such as shifting their ethnic identities when it is context-appropriate and the ability to access numerous cultural perspectives when communicating with others (Root, 1996, 2003b).

Implications for working with multiracial adolescents in school settings. Rather than being forced to choose those parts of themselves that are most salient or meaningful, Herman (2004) discussed how "multiracial youth are simply at greater liberty to embrace all their racial identity, when given a chance" (p. 746). Mental health professionals working in school settings can help to facilitate the process of racial/ethnic identity development of multiracial adolescents by identifying and supporting these strengths. School counselors can work with multiracial adolescents to explore all aspects of racial/ethnic identity and help further define what their various identities mean to them.

White American Adolescents

The term White American assumes membership to one or more sub-ethnic groups with European origins. At close to 64%, non-Hispanic White Americans comprise the largest portion of the U.S. total population, although this number has decreased more than 5% since the year 2000 (Hixson, Hepler, & Kim, 2011). It is projected that what is described as today's minority population will increase to the point at which it will represent the majority of people residing in the U.S. between 2040 and 2050, while the non-Hispanic White population is expected to decrease during this time (Ortman & Guarneri, 2009). These projections show rapid changes in the U.S. demographic landscape.

A group of British and other northwestern European settlers came to what is now called the United States of America during the years 1607 and 1634 (Tehranian, 2000). After this early settlement, waves of other European immigrants including Irish, Greek, and Jewish peoples joined the White American ethnic group. Intermarriage among this set of diverse sub-ethnicities was common (Warren & Twine, 1997).

When many of the German, Sicilian, and Irish immigrant groups first arrived to U.S. shores, they were immediately relegated to the bottom of the social pecking order and worked alongside Black people in building the country (Fussel, 2007). Gradually, these immigrant groups worked their way up the ethnic social hierarchy to transcend stereotypes. This process often involved distancing themselves from Black Americans (Warren & Twine, 1997).

Today, some White Americans may have little association with their race and dissociate from its meaning. McDermott and Samson (2005) propose three major characteristics of White American racial/ethnic identity: it is invisible and often taken for granted; it is rooted in social and economic privilege; and its meaning is highly situational. In their review of recent developments in White American racial/ethnic identity research, these researchers found privilege, social status, and invisibility of White racial/ethnic identity to be highly mutable (McDermott & Samson). For example, if a White American adolescent has a marginalized status, his/her racial/ethnic identity is more likely to be less privileged than other White American adolescents. White American youth from low income families may not enjoy the same social privilege as White American adolescents with no such socioeconomic limitations (Buck, 2001; Rasmussen, Klinenberg, Nexica, & Wray, 2001).

White racial identity development (WRID) is one framework to understand the experience of one's race as a White individual. Originally created by Helms (1990), this developmental model is comprised of six statuses of racial identity development, defined as constantly changing behavioral, cognitive, and emotional processes that determine how racial environments are interpreted within one's interpersonal environment (Helms, 1995).

The first racial identity status of the WRID model is *Contact*, where the White adolescent denies or avoids racial information perceived as sensitive. Once White adolescents experience a racial event they cannot ignore, the WRID model suggests they progress toward the *Disintegration* status, where they begin to question stereotypes and other misguided racial beliefs. White adolescents experience *Reintegration* when the growing dissonance between their previously held racially insensitive beliefs and invalid racial stereotypes causes them to regress to attitudes of White racial superiority. The fourth stage of Helms' (1990) WRID model suggests that White adolescents will begin to reject those superior attitudes when they reach *Pseudo-Independence* by beginning to consider how racism is maintained by White Americans. An understanding of race and racism during this status is primarily on an intellectual level.

At the fifth status, *Immersion-Emersion*, White adolescents commit to exploring one's Whiteness and its meaning. The final status of White American racial identity development, *Autonomy*, involves a rejection of racial oppression and being engaged in seeking out relationships across racial/ethnic groups (Clauss-Ehlers & Carter, 2005, 2006; Cross, 1991; Hardiman, 2001; Helms, 1995).

There are several positive implications of racial/ethnic identity development for White American adolescents, including the ability to recognize and understand racism, to avoid internalizing negative external perceptions of White racial/ethnic identity, and the freedom to enjoy cultural values and practices (Frankenberg, 2001; Grossman & Charmaraman, 2009; McIntosh, 2003; Phinney, 1990). These are all productive, constructive ways to internalize WRID.

It has been suggested that White American identity is shaped in part from social exposure to non-Whites and that this exposure shapes how White Americans think and feel about themselves and their ethnic group (Knowles & Peng, 2005). White American adolescents who gain exposure to other White Americans with more developed White racial identity are likely to have examples for developing their own healthy racial/ethnic identity (Clauss-Ehlers & Carter, 2005, 2006). Thus, White American adolescents with diverse social networks and White Americans at more developed White racial identity statuses may gain insight into differing cultural values and ways of being, and, in turn, be privy to engage in a process of understanding and awareness.

Implications for working with White American adolescents in school settings. Mental health professionals can engage White American youth in a dialogue about their perceptions of their own and other racial/ethnic groups in a safe environment. White adolescents can begin to construct their own racial/ethnic identities using positive messages and traits as building blocks. School administrators can aid in healthy development of racial/ethnic identity for White adolescents by creating multicultural opportunities and diverse social networks. It is hoped that this kind of outreach can initiate a process whereby White adolescents learn what it means to be White while also learning about cultural diversity, having diverse social networks, and have greater understanding of the ethnic minority experience in the U.S. (Mercer & Cunningham, 2003).

Conclusion

Our changing demographic landscape provides the context for diverse youth in the process of establishing their social and racial/ethnic identities. Adolescents at the crossroads of their racial/ethnic identity development face the challenge of how to merge individual values, traditional cultural/familial values, and societal values. Examining the complexities of present day adolescent identity development helps to shed light on some of the unforeseen challenges that tomorrow's adolescent may endure. Exploring racial/ethnic identity development among diverse racial/ethnic adolescents underscores the extent to which one must be cognizant of within-group differences (i.e., the vast array of differences within a racial/ethnic group) rather than merely focusing on between-group differences (i.e., differences between racial/ethnic groups). The amount of time required for *exploration* is shorter for some, longer for others; parents may wield explicit influence in the components of ethnicity their children will *commit* to, while some adolescents are more likely to rely upon peers in their decision making. For each ethnic group, an *achieved* racial/ethnic identity is certainly possible. When surveying the patterns of racial/ethnic identity development among diverse groups, it becomes clear that adolescents benefit from agents who are willing to facilitate, not control this process.

Mental health providers and school personnel are at the forefront of adults who work with adolescents on a day-to-day basis. Given this access, these professionals are encouraged to create safe environments that respect differences and guard against bias. Youth-serving professionals can be active advocates for adolescents, helping them navigate the complexities, not only of adolescence itself, but also those associated with acculturation and racial/ethnic identity development. The adaptive racial/ethnic identity development of tomorrow's adolescent may incorporate a complex network of community, family influences, and the adolescent him- or herself. By granting each component the respect it deserves, practitioners can help tomorrow's adolescent integrate multiple social/reference group identities.

References

Agbayani-Siewart, P. (2002). Filipino American culture and family values. In N. V. Benokratis (Ed.), *Contemporary ethnic families in the United States: Characteristics, variations, and dynamics* (pp. 36–42). Englewood Cliffs, NJ: Prentice Hall.

Ajrouch, K. J. (2000). Place, age, and culture: Community living and ethnic identity among Lebanese American adolescents. *Small Group Research, 31*, 447–469.

Ajrouch, K. J. (2004). Gender, race, and symbolic boundaries: Contested spaces of identity among Arab American adolescents. *Sociological Perspectives, 47*(4), 371–391.

Ali, S. R., Liu, W. M., & Humedian, M. (2004). Islam 101: Understanding the religion and therapy implications. *Professional Psychology, Research and Practice, 35*, 635–642.

Al-Krenawi, A., & Graham, J. (2000). Islamic theology and prayer: Relevance for psychology practice. *International Psychology, 43*(3), 289–304.

Altschul, I., Oyserman, D., & Bybee, D. (2006). Racial-ethnic identity in mid-adolescence: Content and change as predictors of academic achievement. *Child Development, 77*(5), 1155–1169.

American Psychological Association, Task Force on Resilience and Strength in Black Children and Adolescents. (2008). *Resilience in African American children and adolescents: A vision for optimal development*. Washington, DC: Author.

Bankston, C. L. (2006). Filipino Americans. In P. G. Min (Ed.), *Asian Americans: Current trends and issues* (pp. 180–203). Thousand Oaks, CA: Pine Forge Press.

Barringer, H. R., Gardner, R. W., & Levin, M. J. (1993). *Asian and Pacific islanders in the United States*. New York: Russell Sage Foundation.

Beauvais, F. (2000). Indian adolescence: Opportunity and challenge. In R. Montmeyer, G. Adams, & T. Gullotta (Eds.), *Adolescent diversity in ethnic, economic, and cultural contexts* (pp. 110–140). Thousand Oaks, CA: Sage.

Berry, J. W., Poortinga, Y., Segall, M. H., & Dasen, P. R. (2002). *Cross-cultural psychology: Research and applications* (2nd ed.). New York: Cambridge University Press.

Bowles, D. D. (1993). Biracial identity: Children born to African American and White couples. *Clinical Social Work Journal, 21*(4), 417–428.

Breland, A., Coleman, H., Coard, S., & Steward, R. (2002). Differences among African American junior high students: The effects of skin tone on ethnic identity, self-esteem, and cross-cultural behavior. *Dimensions of Counseling: Research, Theory and Practice, 30*, 15–21.

Buck, P. D. (2001). *Worked to the bone: Race, class, power, and privilege in Kentucky*. New York: Monthly Review.

Caldwell, C. H., Sellers, R. M., Bernat, D. H., & Zimmerman, M. A. (2004). Racial identity, parental support, and alcohol use in a sample of academically at-risk African American high school students. *American Journal of Community Psychology, 34*(1–2), 71–82.

Cauce, A. M., & Domenech-Rodriguez, M. (2002). Latino families: Myths and realities. In J. M. Contreras, K. A. Kerns, & A. M. Neal-Barnett (Eds.), *Latino children and families in the United States: Current research and future directions* (pp. 3–26). Westport, CT: Praeger.

Chan, C. S. (1991). *Asian Americans: An interpretive history*. Boston: Twayne.

Chang, T., & Kwan, K. L. K. (2009). Asian American racial and ethnic identity. In N. Tewari & A. N. Alvarez (Eds.), *Asian American psychology: Current perspectives* (pp. 113–133). New York: Erlbaum.

Cheung, M., & Nguyen, S. M. H. (2001). Parent-child relationships in Vietnamese American families. In N. B. Webb (Ed.), *Culturally diverse parent-child and family relationships* (pp. 261–281). New York: Columbia University Press.

Chirkov, V. I. (2009). A cross-cultural analysis of autonomy in education: A self-determination theory perspective. *Theory and Research in Education, 7*(2), 253–262.

Clauss, C. S. (1998). Language: The unspoken variable in psychotherapy practice. *Psychotherapy: Theory, Research, Practice, Training, 35*, 188–196.

Clauss-Ehlers, C. S., & Carter, R. T. (2005). Current manifestations of racism: An exploratory study of social distance and White racial identity. *Journal of Social Distress and the Homeless, XIV*(3 and 4), 261–285.

Clauss-Ehlers, C. S., & Carter, R. T. (2006). White American attitudes in interracial situations: An empirical examination of perceived behavioral options and White racial identity. *Journal of Social Distress and the Homeless, 15*, 117–139.

Clauss-Ehlers, C. S., Yang, Y. T., & Chen, W. J. (2006). Resilience from childhood stressors: The role of cultural resilience, ethnic identity, and gender identity. *Journal of Infant, Child, and Adolescent Psychotherapy, 5*, 124–138.

Cokley, K. (2005). Racial(ized) identity, ethnic identity, and Afrocentric values: Conceptual and methodological challenges in understanding African American identity. *Journal of Counseling Psychology, 52*, 517–526.

Cooper, S. M., McLoyd, V. C., Wood, D., & Hardaway, C. (2008). Racial discrimination and the mental health of African American adolescents. In S. M. Quintana & C. McKown (Eds.), *Handbook of race, racism, and the developing child* (pp. 287–312). Hoboken, NJ: Wiley.

Cordeiro, P. A. (1990). *Growing away from the barrio: An ethnography of high achieving at risk Hispanic youths at two urban high schools.* Unpublished doctoral dissertation, University of Houston, Houston, TX.

Cross, W. E. (1991). *Shades of Black.* Philadelphia, PA: Temple University Press.

Cross, W. E., & Vandiver, B. J. (2001). Nigrescence theory and measurement: Introducing the Cross Racial Identity Scale (CRIS). In J. G. Ponterotto, J. M. Casas, L. A. Suzuki, & C. M. Alexander (Eds.), *Handbook of multicultural counseling* (2nd ed., pp. 371–393). Thousand Oaks, CA: Sage.

Day-Vines, N. L., Patton, J. M., & Baytops, J. L. (2003). Counseling African American adolescents: The impact of race, culture, and middle class status. *Professional School Counseling, 7*, 40–51.

DeGarmo, D. S., & Martinez, C. R. (2006). A culturally informed model of academic well-being for Latino youth: The importance of discriminatory experiences and social support. *Family Relations, 55*(3), 267–278.

Erickson, C. D., & Al-Timimi, N. R. (2001). Providing mental health services to Arab Americans: Recommendations and considerations. *Cultural Diversity and Ethnic Minority Psychology, 7*, 308–327.

Erikson, E. H. (1968). *Identity: Youth and crisis.* New York: Norton.

Fang, S. S., McDowell, T., Goldfarb, K. P., Perumbilly, S., & Gonzalez-Kruger, G. E. (2008). Viewing the Asian American experience through a culturally centered research lens: Do scholarship in family science and related disciplines fall short. *Marriage & Family Review, 44*(1), 33–51.

Flanagan, C. A., Syvertsen, A. K., Gill, S., Gallay, L. S., & Cumsille, P. (2009). Ethnic awareness, prejudice, and civic commitments in four ethnic groups of American adolescents. *Journal of Youth and Adolescence, 38*, 500–518.

Flores, E., Cicchetti, D., & Rogosch, F. A. (2005). Predictors of resilience in maltreated and nonmaltreated Latino children. *Developmental Psychology, 41*(2), 338–351.

Frankenberg, R. (2001). The mirage of an unmarked Whiteness. In B. B. Rasmussen, M. Klinenberg, I. J. Nexica, & M. Wray (Eds.), *The making and unmaking of Whiteness* (pp. 72–96). Durham, NC: Duke University Press.

Fuligni, A. J., Tseng, V., & Lam, M. (1999). Attitudes toward family obligations with Asian, Latin American, and European backgrounds. *Child Development, 70*(4), 1030–1044.

Fussel, E. (2007). Constructing New Orleans, constructing race: A population history of New Orleans. *The Journal of American History, 94*(3), 846–855.

Garcia Coll, C. T., Meyer, E. C., & Brillon, L. (1995). Ethnic and minority parenting. In M. Bornstein (Ed.), *Handbook of parenting* (Biology and ecology of parenting, Vol. 2, pp. 189–209). Hillsdale, NJ: Erlbaum.

Goodstein, L. (2001, September 12). In U.S., echoes of rift of Muslims and Jews. *The New York Times*, p. A12.

Grossman, J. M., & Charmaraman, L. (2009). Race, context, and privilege: White adolescents' explanations of racial-ethnic centrality. *Journal of Youth and Adolescence, 38*(2), 139–152.

Haboush, K. L. (2007). Working with Arab American families: Culturally competent practice for school psychologists. *Psychology in the Schools, 44*(2), 183–198.

Hall, R. E., & Livingston, J. N. (2006). Mental health practice with Arab families: The implications of spirituality vis-à-vis Islam. *American Journal of Family Therapy, 34*, 139–150.

Hardiman, R. (2001). Reflections on White identity development theory. In C. L. Wijeyesinghe & B. W. Jackson III (Eds.), *New perspectives on racial identity development* (pp. 108–128). New York: New York University Press.

Harris-Britt, A., Valrie, C. R., Kurtz-Costes, B., & Rowley, S. J. (2007). Perceived racial discrimination and self-esteem in African American youth: Racial socialization as a protective factor. *Journal of Research on Adolescence, 17*(4), 669–682.

Hayashino, D. S., & Chopra, S. B. (2009). Parenting and raising families. In N. Tewari & A. N. Alvarez (Eds.), *Asian American psychology: Current perspectives* (pp. 317–336). New York: Erlbaum.

Hébert, T. P. (1996). Portraits of resilience: The urban life experience of gifted Latino young men. *Roeper Review, 19*, 82–90.

Helms, J. E. (Ed.). (1990). *Black and White racial identity: Theory, research, and practice.* Westport, CT: Greenwood Press.

Helms, J. E. (1995). An update of Helms' White and People of Color racial identity models. In J. G. Ponterotto, J. M. Casas, L. A. Suzuki, & C. M. Alexander (Eds.), *Handbook of multicultural counseling* (pp. 181–198). Thousand Oaks, CA: Sage.

Herman, M. (2004). Forced to choose: Some determinants of racial identification in multiracial adolescents. *Child Development, 75*(3), 730–748.

Hesse-Biber, S. N., Howling, S. A., Leavy, P., & Lovejoy, M. (2004). Racial identity and the development of body image issues among African American adolescent girls. *Qualitative Report, 9*(1), 49–79.

Hixson, L., Hepler, B. B., & Kim, M. O. (2011). *The White population: 2010* (Report No. C2010BR-05). Retrieved from http://www.census.gov/prod/cen2010/briefs/c2010br-05.pdf on Dec 8, 2011.

Hughes, D., Rodriguez, J., Smith, E. P., Johnson, D. J., Stevenson, H. C., & Spicer, P. (2006). Parents' ethnic-racial socialization practices: A review of research and directions for future study. *Developmental Psychology, 42*(5), 747–770.

Humes, K. R., Jones, N. A., & Ramirez, R. R. (2011). *Overview of race and Hispanic origin: 2010* (Report No. C2010BR-05). Retrieved from http://www.census.gov/prod/cen2010/briefs/c2010br-02.pdf on Dec 8, 2011.

Inayat, Q. (2002). The meaning of being a Muslim: An aftermath of the Twin Towers episode. *Counselling Psychology Quarterly, 15*, 351–359.

Ishii-Kuntz, M. (2000). Diversity within Asian American families. In D. H. Demo, K. R. Allen, & M. A. Fine (Eds.), *Handbook of family diversity* (pp. 274–292). New York: Oxford University Press.

Javier, R. A., & Camacho-Gingerich, A. (2004). Risk and resilience in Latino youth. In C. S. Clauss-Ehlers & M. E. Weist (Eds.), *Community planning to foster resilience in children* (pp. 65–81). New York: Kluwer Academic.

Johnson, D. J. (1992). Developmental pathways: Toward an ecological theoretical formulation of race identity in Black-White biracial children. In M. P. P. Root (Ed.), *Racially mixed people in America* (pp. 37–49). New York: Sage.

Jones, C. P. (2000). Levels of racism: A theoretic framework and a gardener's tale. *American Journal of Public Health, 90*, 1212–1215.

Keith, V. M., & Herring, C. (1991). Skin tone and stratification in the Black community. *The American Journal of Sociology, 97*(3), 760–778.

Khanna, N. (2004). The role of reflected appraisals in racial identity: The case of multiracial Asians. *Social Psychology Quarterly, 67*(2), 115–131.

Kich, G. K. (1992). The developmental process of asserting a biracial, bicultural identity. In M. P. P. Root (Ed.), *Racially mixed people in America* (pp. 250–264). Newbury Park, CA: Sage.

Knowles, E. D., & Peng, K. (2005). White selves: Conceptualizing and measuring a dominant-group identity. *Journal of Personality and Social Psychology, 89*(2), 223–241.

Kohler, A. D., & Lazarín, M. (2007). Hispanic education in the United States. *National Council of La Raza Statistical Brief, 8*, 1–16.

Kulczycki, A., & Lobo, A. P. (2002). Patterns, determinants, and implications of intermarriage among Arab Americans. *Journal of Marriage and the Family, 64*, 202–210.

LaFromboise, T. D., Hoyt, D. R., Oliver, L., & Whitbeck, L. B. (2006). Family, community, and school influences on resilience among American Indian adolescents in the upper Midwest. *Journal of Community Psychology, 34*(2), 193–209.

LaFromboise, T. D., & Medoff, L. (2004). Sacred spaces: The role of context in American Indian youth development. In C. S. Clauss-Ehlers & M. D. Weist (Eds.), *Community planning to foster resilience in children* (pp. 45–63). New York: Kluwer Academic.

Lee, R. (1999). *Orientals: Asian Americans in popular culture*. Philadelphia: Temple University Press.

Lee, J., & Cynn, V. (1991). Issues in counseling 1.5 generation Korean Americans. In C. C. Lee & B. Richardson (Eds.), *Multicultural issues in counseling: New approaches to diversity* (pp. 127–140). Alexandria, VA: American Association for Counseling and Development.

Lee, S. J., Wong, N. A., & Alvarez, A. N. (2009). The model minority and the perpetual foreigner: Stereotypes of Asian Americans. In N. Tewari & A. N. Alvarez (Eds.), *Asian American psychology: Current perspectives* (pp. 69–84). New York: Erlbaum.

Lu, X. (2001). Bicultural identity development and Chinese community formation: An ethno-graphic study of Chinese schools in Chicago. *Howard Journal of Communications, 12*, 203–220.

Luyckx, K., Schwartz, S. J., Berzonsky, M. D., Soenens, B., Vansteenkiste, M., Smits, I., et al. (2008). Capturing ruminative exploration: Extending the four-dimensional model of identity formation in late adolescence. *Journal of Research in Personality, 42*, 58–82.

Marcia, J. E. (1993). The ego identity status approach to ego identity. In J. E. Marcia, A. S. Waterman, D. R. Matteson, S. L. Archer, & J. L. Orlofsky (Eds.), *Ego identity: A handbook for psychosocial research* (pp. 1–21). New York: Springer.

Markus, H. R., & Kitayama, S. (2003). Models of agency: Sociocultural diversity in the construction of action. In V. M. Berman & J. J. Berman (Eds.), *Nebraska symposium on motivation: Cross-cultural differences in perspectives on the self* (Vol. 49, pp. 1–58). Lincoln: University of Nebraska Press.

Marotta, S. A., & Garcia, J. G. (2003). Latinos in the United States in 2000. *Hispanic Journal of Behavioral Sciences, 25*(1), 13–34.

Martinez, C. R., DeGarmo, D. S., & Eddy, J. M. (2004). Promoting academic success among Latino youth. *Hispanic Journal of Behavioral Sciences, 26*(2), 128–151.

McDermott, M., & Samson, F. L. (2005). White racial identity and ethnic identity in the United States. *Annual Review of Sociology, 31*, 245–261.

McGruder, A., Barnes, R., Brooks, A., Taylor, Y., & Veen, J. V. (Writers), & Kim, S. E., & Hathcock, R. (Directors). (2008). The Uncle Ruckus reality show [Television series episode]. In A. McGruder & R. Hudlin (Executive producers), *The boondocks*. Atlanta, GA: TBS Broadcasting.

McIntosh, P. (2003). Unpacking the invisible knapsack. In S. Plous (Ed.), *Understanding prejudice and discrimination* (pp. 191–196). New York: McGraw-Hill.

McLoyd, V. C., Cauce, A. M., Takeuchi, D., & Wilson, L. (2000). Marital processes and parental socialization in families of color: A decade review of research. *Journal of Marriage and the Family, 62*, 1070–1093.

McNeil, D. W., Kee, M., & Zvolensky, M. J. (1999). Culturally related anxiety and ethnic identity in Navajo college students. *Cultural Diversity and Ethnic Minority Psychology, 5*(1), 56–64.

McNeil, D. W., Porter, C. A., Zvolensky, M. J., Chaney, J. M., & Kee, M. (2000). Assessment of culturally related anxiety in American Indians and Alaska Natives. *Behavior Therapy, 31*(2), 301–325.

Mercer, S. H., & Cunningham, M. (2003). Racial identity in White American college students: Issues of conceptualization and measurement. *Journal of College Student Development, 44*, 217–230.

Min, P. G. (2006). Asian immigration: History and contemporary trends. In P. G. Min (Ed.), *Asian Americans: Current trends and issues* (pp. 7–32). Thousand Oaks, CA: Pine Forge Press.

Miville, M. L., Constantine, M. G., Baysden, M. F., & So-Lloyd, G. (2005). Chameleon changes: An exploration of racial identity themes of multiracial people. *Journal of Counseling Psychology, 52*(4), 507–516.

Nagel, C. R., & Staeheli, L. (2005). "We're just like the Irish": Narratives of assimilation, belonging, and citizenship amongst Arab-American activists. *Citizenship Studies, 9*(5), 485–498.

Neblett, E. W., Philip, C. L., Cogburn, C. D., & Sellers, R. M. (2006). African American adolescents' discrimination experience and academic achievement: Racial socialization as a cultural compensatory and protective factor. *The Journal of Black Psychology, 32*(2), 199–218.

Newman, R. S. (1994). Adaptive help seeking: A strategy of self-regulated learning. In D. H. Schunk & B. J. Zimmerman (Eds.), *Self-regulation of learning and performance: Issues and educational applications* (pp. 283–301). Hillsdale, NJ: Lawrence Erlbaum Associates.

Newman, D. L. (2005). Ego development and ethnic identity formation in rural American Indian adolescents. *Child Development, 76*(3), 734–746.

Ortman, J. M., & Guarneri, C. E. (2009). *United States population projections: 2000 to 2050*. Retrieved from http://www.census.gov/population/www/projections/analytical-document09.pdf on Dec 8, 2011.

Padgett, T. (2010, March 29). Still Black or White: Why the Census misreads Hispanics. *Time*. Retrieved December 23, 2010, from http://www.time.com/time/nation/article/0,8599,1975883,00.html

Perreira, K. M., Harris, K. M., & Lee, D. (2006). Making it in America: High school completion by immigrant and native youth. *Demography, 43*(3), 511–536.

Petersen, W. (1966). Success story, Japanese-American style. *New York Times Magazine*, pp. 20–43.

Phelps, R. E., Taylor, J. D., & Gerard, P. A. (2001). Cultural mistrust, ethnic identity, racial identity, and self-esteem among ethnically diverse Black university students. *Journal of Counseling and Development, 79*(2), 209–216.

Phinney, J. S. (1989). Stages of ethnic identity development in minority group adolescents. *The Journal of Early Adolescence, 9*, 34–49.

Phinney, J. S. (1990). Ethnic identity in adolescents and adults: Review of research. *Psychological Bulletin, 108*(3), 499–514.

Phinney, J. S. (1992). The multigroup ethnic identity measure: A new scale for use with diverse groups. *Journal of Adolescent Research, 7*(2), 156–176.

Poston, W. S. C. (1990). The Biracial Identity Development Model: A needed addition. *Journal of Counseling and Development, 69*, 152–155.

Ramirez, R. (2004). *We the people: Hispanics in the United States. U.S.: Census Bureau*. Retrieved from http://www.census.gov/prod/2004pubs/censr-18.pdf on Dec 8, 2011

Rasmussen, B. B., Klinenberg, E., Nexica, I. J., & Wray, M. (Eds.). (2001). *The making and unmaking of Whiteness*. Durham, NC: Duke University Press.

Red Horse, J. (1997). Traditional American Indian family systems. *Families, Systems & Health, 15*(3), 243–250.

Renn, K. A. (2008). Research on biracial and multiracial identity development: Overview and synthesis. In K. A. Renn & P. Shang (Eds.), *Biracial and multiracial students* (New directions for student services no. 123, pp. 13–32). San Francisco: Jossey Bass.

Roberts, R. E., Phinney, J. S., Masse, L. C., Chen, Y. R., Roberts, C. R., & Romero, A. (1999). The structure of ethnic identity in young adolescents from diverse ethnocultural groups. *The Journal of Early Adolescence, 19*, 301–322.

Rockquemore, K. A. (1999). Between Black and White: Exploring the biracial experience. *Race & Society, 1*, 197–212.

Rockquemore, K. A., & Brunsma, D. L. (2002). *Beyond Black: Biracial identity in America*. Thousand Oaks, CA: Sage.

Root, M. P. P. (1995). The multiracial contribution of the psychological browning of America. In N. Zach (Ed.), *American mixed race: The culture of microdiversity* (pp. 231–236). Lanham, MD: Rowman & Littlefield.

Root, M. P. P. (Ed.). (1996). *The multiracial experience: Racial borders as the new frontier*. Thousand Oaks, CA: Sage.

Root, M. P. P. (1998). Experiences and processes affecting racial identity development: Preliminary results from the Biracial Sibling Project. *Cultural Diversity and Mental Health, 4*, 237–247.

Root, M. P. P. (1999). The biracial baby boom: Understanding ecological constructions of racial identity in the 21st century. In R. Hernandez-Sheets & E. R. Hollins (Eds.), *Racial and ethnic identity in school practices: Aspects of human development* (pp. 67–90). Mahwah, NJ: Erlbaum.

Root, M. P. P. (2001). *Love's revolution: Interracial marriage*. Philadelphia, PA: Temple University Press.

Root, M. P. P. (2003a). Multiracial families and children: Implications for educational research and practice. In J. A. Banks & C. A. McGee Banks (Eds.), *Handbook of research on multicultural education* (pp. 110–124). San Francisco: Jossey-Bass.

Root, M. P. P. (2003b). Five mixed-race identities: From relic to revolution. In L. I. Winters & H. L. Debose (Eds.), *New faces in a changing America* (pp. 3–20). Thousand Oaks, CA: Sage.

Rosenbloom, S. R., & Way, N. (2004). Experiences of discrimination among African American, Asian American, and Latino adolescents in an urban school. *Youth & Society, 35*(4), 420–451.

Ryckman, R. M. (2007). *Theories of personality*. Belmont, CA: Wadsworth.

Schwartz, S. J., Côté, J. E., & Arnett, J. J. (2005). Identity and agency in emerging adulthood: Two developmental routes in the individualization process. *Youth & Society, 37*, 201–229.

Schwartz, S. J., Zamboanga, B. L., Weisskirch, R. S., & Rodriguez, L. (2009). The relationships of personal and ethnic identity exploration to indices of adaptive and maladaptive psychosocial functioning. *International Journal of Behavioral Development, 33*(2), 131–144.

Scott, L. D. (2004). Correlates of coping with perceived discriminatory experiences among African American adolescents. *Journal of Adolescence, 27*(2), 123–137.

Seaton, E. K., Scottham, K. M., & Sellers, R. M. (2006). The status model of racial identity development in African American adolescents: Evidence of structure, trajectories, and well-being. *Child Development, 77*(5), 1416–1426.

Shaheen, J. G. (2001). *Reel bad Arabs: How Hollywood vilifies a people*. Northampton, MA: Olive Branch Press.

Simpkins, S. D., O'Donnell, M., Delgado, M. Y., & Becnel, J. N. (2011). Latino adolescents' participation in extracurricular activities: How important are family resources and cultural orientation? *Applied Developmental Science, 15*(1), 37–50.

Sirin, S. R., & Fine, M. (2007). Hyphenated selves: Muslim American youth negotiating identities on the fault lines of global conflict. *Applied Developmental Science, 11*(3), 151–163.

Smith, L. R., Burlew, A. K., & Lundgren, D. C. (1991). Black consciousness, self-esteem, and satisfaction with physical appearance among African-American female college students. *Journal of Black Studies, 22*(2), 269–283.

Spina, S. U. (2002). *Urban youth re-imagine trauma: Making meaning of experiences with chronic community violence through the arts*. PhD Dissertation, Department of Psychology, The Graduate Center for the City University of New York, New York, NY.

Stanton-Salazar, R. D. (2001). *Manufacturing hope and despair: The school and kin support networks of U.S. Mexican youth*. New York: Teachers College Press.

Stanton-Salazar, R. D., & Spina, S. U. (2003). Informal mentors and role models in the lives of urban Mexican-origin adolescents. *Anthropology & Education Quarterly, 34*(3), 231–254.

Stilling, G. E. S. (1996). *Lumbee voices: North Carolina's Lumbee Indians in literature, art and music*. Boone, NC: Appalachian State University.

Suyemoto, K. L., & Tawa, J. (2009). Multiracial Asian Americans. In N. Tewari & A. N. Alvarez (Eds.), *Asian American psychology: Current perspectives* (pp. 381–398). New York: Erlbaum.

Tatum, B. D. (1997). *"Why are all the Black kids sitting together in the cafeteria?" And other conversations about race*. New York: Basic Books.

Tatum, B. D. (2004). Family life and school experience: Factors in the racial identity development of Black youth in White communities. *Journal of Social Issues, 60*, 117–135.

Tehranian, J. (2000). Performing Whiteness: Naturalization litigation and the construction of racial identity in America. *The Yale Law Journal, 109*(4), 817–848.

U.S. Census Bureau. (2007). *2000 Summary file 1, U.S. Census Bureau*. Retrieved December 29, 2010, from http://www.census.gov/prod/cen2000/doc/sf1.pdf

U.S. Census Bureau. (2009). *American Community Survey 1-year estimates, race—universe: Total population*. Retrieved December 29, 2010, from http://factfinder.census.gov/servlet/DTTable?_bm=y&-geo_id=01000US&-ds_name=ACS_2009_1YR_G00_&-_lang=en&-redoLog=false&-mt_name=ACS_2009_1YR_G2000_C02003&-mt_name=ACS_2009_1YR_G2000_C02005&-format=&-CONTEXT=dt

Umana-Taylor, A. J., Bhanot, R., & Shin, S. (2006). Ethnic identity formation during adolescence: The critical role of families. *Journal of Family Issues, 27*(3), 390–414.

Valenzuela, A. (1999). *Subtractive schooling: U.S.-Mexican youth and the politics of caring*. New York: SUNY Press.

Vandiver, B. J., Cross, W. E., Worrell, F. C., & Fhagen-Smith, P. E. (2002). Validating the Cross Racial Identity Scale. *Journal of Counseling Psychology, 49*, 71–85.

Villalba, J. A., Jr. (2007). Culture-specific assets to consider when counseling Latina/o children and adolescents. *Journal of Multicultural Counseling and Development, 35*, 15–25.

Vo-Jutabha, E. D., Dinh, K. T., McHale, J. P., & Valsiner, J. (2009). A qualitative analysis of Vietnames adolescent identity exploration within and outside an ethnic enclave. *Journal of Youth and Adolescence, 38*(5), 672–690.

Wakeling, S., Jorgensen, M., Michaelson, S., & Begay, M. (2001). *Policing on American Indian reservations*. Washington, DC: National Institute of Justice, US Department of Justice.

Ward, J. V. (2000). Raising resisters: The role of truth telling in the psychological development of African American girls. In L. Weis & M. Fine (Eds.), *Construction sites: Excavating race, class, and gender among urban youth* (pp. 85–99). New York: Teachers College Press.

Warren, J. W., & Twine, F. W. (1997). White Americans, the new minority: Non-Blacks and the ever-expanding boundaries of Whiteness. *Journal of Black Studies, 28*(2), 200–218.

Watts, R. J., Abdul-Adil, J. K., & Pratt, T. (2002). Enhancing critical consciousness in young African American men: A psychoeducational approach. *Psychology of Men & Masculinity, 3*(1), 41–50.

West, A. E., & Newman, D. L. (2007). Childhood behavioral inhibition and the experience of social anxiety in American Indian adolescents. *Cultural Diversity and Ethnic Minority Psychology, 13*(3), 197–206.

Wing, J. Y. (2007). Beyond black and white: The model minority myth and the invisibility of Asian American students. *The Urban Review, 39*(4), 455–487.

Wong, C. A., Eccles, J. S., & Sameroff, A. (2003). The influence of ethnic discrimination and ethnic identification on African American adolescents' school and socio-emotional adjustment. *Journal of Personality, 71*(6), 1197–1232.

Yeh, C. J. (2001). An exploratory study of school counselors' experiences with and perceptions of Asian American students. *Professional School Counseling, 4*(5), 349–356.

Culturally Responsive Strategies to Address Youth Gangs in Schools

13

Nicole Evangelista Brandt, Emily Sidway, Melissa Dvorsky, and Mark D. Weist

Youth gangs are a significant problem in elementary and secondary schools across the United States (US) and are associated with violent crimes and serious delinquency (Chandler, Chapman, Rand, & Taylor, 1998). The presence of youth gangs in schools may negatively affect the school climate relating to an increased level of school violence (Laub & Lauritsen, 1998) and contributing to overall student victimization (Howell & Lynch, 2000). Youth in gangs are responsible for up to seven times more violent crime offenses than youth who are not involved in gangs (Howell, 2003). Although the characteristics of youth gangs are heterogeneous, both within and across different geographic locations (Egley, Howell, & Major, 2006), in general, youth gangs are an organized group with three or more members, between 12 and 24 years old, stable over time, share a sense of identity (e.g., name, symbols/colors, geographic location), and are involved in criminal activities (Howell, 2009). Additionally, the group must perceive themselves as a gang and others must identify them as a gang.

As the focus of this book is to advance culturally responsive school mental health (SMH) prevention and intervention, it is important to highlight the connection between culture and gangs. Culture is defined as "a common heritage or set of beliefs, norms, and values" and it "refers to the shared, and largely learned, attributes of a group of people" (U.S. Department of Health and Human Services, 2001, p. 9). Gangs have a shared set of worldviews, values, and behaviors that include three overarching components: (a) reputation (related to power and status), (b) respect (includes disrespecting other gangs), and (c) retaliation/revenge (confrontation with other gangs who are disrespectful). To show their gang affiliation, youth wear certain types of clothes and specific colors, walk in a distinct manner, and communicate with unique vocabulary and nonverbal gestures (e.g., hand signals) (Howell, 2010).

Although there are several local, state, and national initiatives (e.g., Baltimore City Criminal Justice Coordinating Council, 2006; Office of Juvenile Justice and Delinquency Prevention, 2009) focused on prevention and intervention for youth gangs, there are limited training and practical recommendations for mental health professionals in *schools* who work with youth involved in gangs. In a survey of 213 school psychology training programs, results indicated that preservice training related to gang issues is lacking and is a low priority for many programs (Larson & Busse, 1998). Although the most effective prevention and intervention activities for addressing

N.E. Brandt (✉) • E. Sidway
University of Maryland School of Medicine, Center for School Mental Health, Baltimore, MD, USA
e-mail: Nbrandt@psych.umaryland.edu;
esidway@psych.umaryland.edu

M. Dvorsky • M.D. Weist
University of South Carolina, Columbia, SC, USA
e-mail: dvorskymr@vcu.edu; weist@mailbox.sc.edu

gangs come from interdisciplinary collaborations between various professionals and organizations (Arciaga, 2007), in our experience, SMH clinicians are more likely to work with youth in gangs in one-on-one approaches (e.g., individual therapy). Irrespective of whether SMH clinicians are a part of a team or are working alone, it is critical that they are competent to work with this culturally diverse population. This chapter compiles current research on youth gangs in the US by providing an overview of the prevalence and demographic characteristics, risk and protective factors, the impact of popular culture, and associated problems. Practical strategies to enhance cultural competency in working with youth members of gangs in schools, a continuum of prevention and intervention strategies to address youth gangs in schools, and culturally responsive practical strategies for school personnel and SMH clinicians working with youth gang members in schools will also be presented.

Overview of Youth Gangs

Prevalence and Demographics

According to the 2009 National Youth Gang Survey (Egley & Howell, 2011), there has been a 20% increase in gang problems in the US from 2002 to 2009. Further, gang problems are widespread, with approximately 4–15% of youth in the US belonging to a gang (Esbensen, Peterson, Taylor, & Freng, 2010) not only in larger cities, but also across smaller cities, and rural and suburban counties (Egley & Howell 2011). An annual report of school crime and safety statistics for the 2007–2008 academic year indicated that 20% of public schools and 23% of students reported gang activities at school (Robers, Zhang, & Truman, 2010). As expected, the amount of gang activity reported increases with the age of students, with the lowest percentage of gang activity in primary school and the highest percentage of gang activity in high schools (Robers et al., 2010). A survey of nationally representative law enforcement agencies reported that 90% of gang members are male (National Youth Gang, 2009). Gangs represent a wide range of race and ethnicity; specifically, 49% of gang members are Hispanic/Latino, 35% are African-American/Black, 9% are Caucasian/White, and 7% are other races/ethnicities (Robers et al., 2010).

Risk Factors for Joining Gangs

Many youth choose to join a gang because they are attracted to the powerful social network they believe the gang provides (Howell, 2010), the money from drug dealing (Centers & Weist, 1998; Decker & Van Winkle, 1996), and the perception of gaining respect (Esbensen, Deschenes, & Winfree, 1999). Other researchers have found that the most common reason youth indicate for joining a gang is the perception that the gang will provide protection for them (e.g., Decker & Curry, 2000; Peterson, Taylor, & Esbensen, 2004; Thornberry, Krohn, Lizotte, Smith, & Tobin, 2003). Extensive research has been conducted to identify risk factors across a variety of domains (individual, family, peer, school, and community) that increase the probability that youth will be involved in a gang (Howell & Egley, 2005). The most prominent risk factor is a history of delinquency (Howell 2010). Similarly, association with peers who are delinquent, use drugs, or are aggressive also increases the likelihood of becoming involved in a gang (Huizinga & Lovegrove, 2009; Kupersmidt, Coie, & Howell, 2003). Other individual risk factors that predict gang membership are antisocial behavior, alcohol and drug use, mental health problems (e.g., conduct disorder, externalizing behaviors, depression), negative life events (e.g., break ups, death of a close friend), and peer rejection (Wasserman et al., 2003). Parents/caregivers who are gang members and/or are highly influential and may encourage their children to join gangs and/or may be accepting of their children's gang membership. Further, weak family structure (e.g., multiple caretaker transitions), parental attitudes favoring violence, poverty, sibling antisocial behavior, poor family management, ineffective parental supervision, poor attachment and bonding with parents, parental drug and alcohol use, and child abuse and neglect are all family factors that put a child at risk for gang involvement (Hill, Lui, & Hawkins, 2001; Howell & Egley 2005).

School factors, including low academic achievement, lack of school commitment and involvement, low academic aspirations, learning disabilities, negative school climate, lack of teacher role models, and school violence (Hill et al., 2001; Howell, 2010; Howell & Egley, 2005), are strong risk factors for gang membership. Additionally, community and neighborhood risk factors include the presence of criminal and gang activities, availability and use of drugs, low neighborhood attachment, and availability and use of firearms (Hill et al., 2001; Howell & Egley 2005). In some cities, immigrant youth are at risk for joining a gang due to acculturation issues, inadequate parenting, and difficulty in school (Vigil, 2002; 2008).

The number and type of risk factors experienced by youth also has an impact on their likelihood of joining a gang. In a longitudinal study, youth with seven or more risk factors were 13 times more likely to join a gang than youth with fewer risk factors (Hill et al., 2001). In addition, 61% of boys and 40% of girls who reported risk factors across all domains (i.e., individual, family, peer, school, community) were members of a gang. In sum, risk factors are cumulative such that more risk factors lead to a greater chance of gang membership.

In contrast to risk factors, protective factors decrease the probability of youth becoming involved in gangs. The literature on protective factors for youth gangs is limited, with the exception of early academic success, which has been identified as a protective factor and is targeted in some prevention programs (Arciaga, Sakamoto & Jones, 2010). Other protective factors include being female, demonstrating prosocial behaviors (e.g., empathy, helping, sharing, cooperating) especially in preschool, average or better cognitive abilities, and attachment to parents and societal institutions (e.g., school) (Wasserman et al., 2003).

Influence of the Media and Popular Culture

In addition to the well-documented risk factors presented above, the influence of the media and popular culture should be considered. Popular culture often portrays gangs in an attractive manner by glamorizing gangs through songs, music videos, movies, and television shows (Miller, 1992). For example, often through obscene lyrics and music videos, popular music can romanticize the lifestyle of gangs with violent themes of stealing, drug dealing, violence, or murder. Further, the artists who sing these songs are often popular, wealthy, and influential individuals (Miller, 2001). This gang culture is integrating into the general American culture (Howell, 2010) via social media networks (e.g., Facebook, Twitter, YouTube); thus, gangs can be easily and instantaneously promoted through photos, videos, and message boards (Howell, 2010). Taken together, all of the above may lead youth to desire this gangster lifestyle (Miller, 1992).

Associated Problems

As discussed in the previous section, youth involved in gangs often have a number of other problems and, in fact, gangs tend to attract antisocial youth (Thornberry, Huizinga, & Loeber, 2004). It is probable that these problems increase the likelihood that youth will affiliate with gangs; in turn, this affiliation directly causes more problems in the young person's life. For example, youth in gangs are more likely to drop out of school, have poor mental health, have significantly lower problem-solving skills, obtain lower grades, and demonstrate fewer future academic plans (Ellickson, Saner, & McGuigan, 1997; Li et al., 2002; Wood, Foy, Layne, Pynos, & James, 2002). Youth tend to have higher rates of delinquency during their time in a gang with other problems persisting even after they leave the gang (Thornberry et al., 2003; 2004). Compared to youth who are not in a gang, youth gang members are more likely to be involved in assault, robbery, breaking and entering, drug trafficking, and felony theft, as well as more likely to be arrested, binge drink, and use drugs (Hill et al., 2001, Li et al.). In a study of the juvenile justice system, gang members were more likely than other arrestees to have stolen a gun and used a gun while committing a crime, indicating that gang involvement can increase the severity of crimes committed (Sickmund, Snyder, & Poe-Yamagata, 1997). Further, gang members in the juvenile justice system are twice as likely as arrestees overall to have been shot at and are at greater risk for Post-Traumatic Stress Disorder (Sickmund et al., 1997; Wood et al., 2002).

Interdisciplinary Approaches to Gang Reduction

Given the complexity and severity of gang problems, an individual or single discipline cannot address gang problems in schools alone. To support this shared agenda (see Andis et al., 2002), it is necessary to form an interdisciplinary team composed of individuals representing education, mental health, law enforcement, juvenile probation, social services, family services, adult probation, grassroots organizations, community organizations, faith-based organizations, and youth and families (Allen, 1998; Arciaga, 2007; Howell, 2010). The role of the team is to inform, implement, and sustain gang reduction strategies and programs. Use of such a diverse team will increase the effectiveness of gang reduction efforts by sharing information and resources, collaborating to implement strategies and programs, and helping to ensure that gang reduction activities are culturally competent (Arciaga 2007). For example, law enforcement officers can provide reports on criminal activity for a specific child or neighborhood; community organizations can share their insights into neighborhood factors such as the level of support and attachment among neighbors; mental health professionals can discuss psychological factors related to violence, trauma, and drug use; and school personnel can provide a description of the school climate, policies, and teacher–student relationships.

The interdisciplinary team should conduct a gang problem assessment for the community in order to agree on a definition for a gang, identify risk factors for gang involvement, determine who is involved in gangs, understand the history of the gangs, identify crimes being committed by gangs, locate where the crimes are being committed, and understand the reasons for the criminal activity (Arciaga et al., 2010; Howell, 2010). The OJJDP developed two free online resources that can assist communities in conducting a gang problem assessment: the *Strategic Planning Tool* (Office of Juvenile Justice and Delinquency Prevention, 2010a) and *A Guide to Assessing Your Community's Youth Gang Problem* (Office of Juvenile Justice and Delinquency Prevention, 2009) (see www.nationalgangcenter.gov for both resources).

After a thorough gang problem assessment is complete, the interdisciplinary team should develop and implement prevention, intervention, and suppression strategies and programs to combat the gang problem. The OJJDP developed a Comprehensive Gang Model (2009) based on research that includes five strategies (i.e., community mobilization, provision of opportunities, social intervention, suppression, and organizational change), and a strong, long-term commitment from multiple community partners. Although comprehensive gang reduction activities are needed to address the escalating gang problem, the focus of the discussion here will be exclusive to gang prevention and reduction within schools and practical strategies that school staff and mental health clinicians can implement. For the purpose of this chapter, discussion of cultural competence and sensitivity will exclude racial/ethnic issues as these issues are presented elsewhere in this book.

Culturally Responsive Strategies for Working with Youth Gangs in Schools

Given the unique gang culture, school staff and SMH professionals need to be culturally competent to effectively work with youth in gangs. According to Sue and Sue's (2008) model of cultural competency, mental health professionals should work towards "an awareness of one's own assumptions, values, and biases, understanding the worldview of culturally diverse clients, and developing appropriate intervention strategies and techniques" (pp. 44–45). Sue and Sue state that "cultural competence is an active, developmental, and on-going process and that it is 'aspirational' rather than achieved" (p. 44). This aspirational approach is essential to reducing the serious gang problems in schools across the US. In this chapter, Sue and Sue's model is applied to school staff and SMH clinicians who work with youth gangs in schools by (a) presenting how school staff and SMH professionals can increase their awareness and knowledge of youth gangs, and (b) discussing a continuum of prevention and intervention programs and culturally responsive strategies for working with youth and gangs in schools.

Increase Awareness and Knowledge

Gaining an awareness of personal values, biases, and assumptions about gangs is a complicated task as gangs constitute a very heterogeneous population with members living in various geographical regions and coming from all racial and ethnic backgrounds, and other minority groups (e.g., women, minority sexual orientations). Further, gangs with the same affiliation and/or name may greatly vary from one another with regard to structure, group dynamics, membership rules, and criminal activity (Wyrick, 2006). Although challenging and complex, individuals who work in schools should think about how their biases and values interfere with their work with youth members of gangs. For example, a SMH clinician may feel uncomfortable working with a client in a gang who is engaged in violent acts, illegal activity, and drugs. Due to her personal values, she may be unable to provide empathy when her client discloses that he/she witnessed a fellow gang member get shot and killed during retaliation from a rival gang due to drug trafficking. In order to facilitate and encourage increased awareness and knowledge, comprehensive training on gang awareness for administrators, teachers and staff, families, and SMH professionals is necessary. The training would provide information on (a) the presence of gangs in that community and school, (b) how to identify gang activity or gang presence, (c) how to recognize signs that your child or student may be involved in a gang, (d) the common gang identifiers (e.g., symbols, hand signals, clothing, colors) and names of gangs, and (e) what to do if you suspect gang activity at school and/or a specific child or student is involved.

Youth Gang Prevention and Intervention

Similar to a public health model, Wyrick (2006) suggests a four-tiered triangular model that utilizes a strategic risk-based approach to address youth gangs (see Fig. 13.1). The bottom tier represents primary prevention and applies to all youth living in communities with high crime or

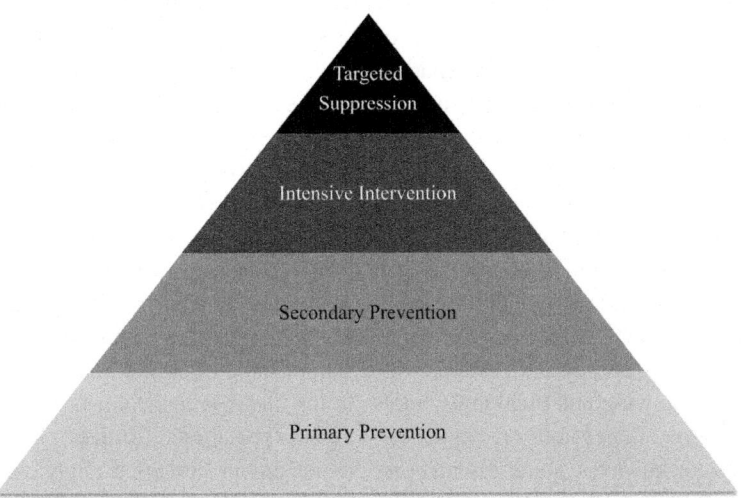

Fig. 13.1 *Youth Gang Prevention and Intervention Strategies. Note.* This figure provides a visual for Wyrick's (2006) model described in the section "Youth Gang Prevention and Intervention"

gang presence in order to reduce the number of youth who will join a gang. The next tier, secondary prevention, targets high-risk youth who have shown early signs of delinquency but are not yet in a gang, and need more intensive prevention, such as providing attractive alternatives, support systems, and holding the youth accountable for their actions. The third tier is for those youth already involved in gangs, thereby requiring intensive interventions, including group therapy, family therapy, mentoring, and individual therapy (e.g., cognitive-behavioral therapy). The top tier, is composed of youth members of gangs who are involved in chronic, serious, and violent crimes. At this level, it is necessary to involve law enforcement to help with suppression strategies to rehabilitate these youth. Because the focus of this chapter is on strategies for schools, particularly for SMH clinicians, a more detailed discussion of practical primary and secondary prevention and intervention activities that can be implemented in schools is provided.

Primary Prevention. Primary prevention activities involve participation from all school personnel to target the entire student population (Arciaga et al., 2010; Wyrick, 2006). First and foremost, schools must establish clear rules and consequences for all students, be dedicated to consistently and firmly enforcing all rules, and remain visible around the school. Further, school personnel must be willing to collaborate with school police or law enforcement, when appropriate, to ensure a safe school. For example, gang activities and problems often occur in hallways, lunchrooms, and bathrooms, so these areas should be closely monitored.

If the student violates the school policies or rules, there needs to be a consistent and appropriate consequence. It is imperative that the entire school staff present themselves as a unified staff with mutual respect. SMH clinicians can assist the school in developing appropriate rewards and consequences for following and breaking school rules. Out-of-school suspension or expulsion has been suggested; however, some researchers suggest that these disciplinary actions are ineffective and result in students being unsupervised and missing more academic instruction, and being sent out of school may actually be reinforcing negative behavior (Pesce & Wilczynski, 2005). Out-of-school suspension is most effective when paired with a prescriptive reentry program, such as parenting classes and mental health services for students. SMH clinicians can offer parent education (either individually or via group) and individual therapy for students who are re-entering school. Alternatively, in-school suspension may be utilized as a consequence that still allows for academic instruction and supervision (unlike out-of-school suspension and expulsion).

In order to prevent conflicts among rival gangs, schools should implement policies to help decrease gang members' ability to mark their territory or identify gang affiliation/membership. Schools may wish to adopt a dress code policy that would prevent gang members from wearing gang identifiers (e.g., colors) during school hours (Arciaga et al., 2010). Similarly, gang graffiti on school property should be documented, photographed, and removed as soon as possible. For these policies to be effective, schools need to have professional development trainings throughout the school year so that staff are aware and knowledgeable of gang identifiers, particularly because new trends are always emerging.

As previously discussed, a risk factor for joining a gang is poor teacher–student relationships and a poor sense of school belonging. Thus, all school personnel (e.g., bus driver, secretary, cafeteria worker, custodian, school nurse, teacher, principal, teacher's aide, etc.) are encouraged to build rapport and relationships with students to help them feel respected, supported, and engaged at school (Arciaga et al., 2010). In addition to building positive relationships with students, teachers should strive to build a positive classroom climate to help the students feel safe and connected to the school. To maintain a positive climate, teachers must consistently enforce school-wide rules and policies, provide structure in the classroom, establish clear classroom rules and expectations, utilize effective classroom management strategies, apply consistent rewards and consequences in the classroom, and provide interactive and cooperative lessons (Arciaga et al.). SMH clinicians can provide teacher consultation related to classroom management and behavior modification. If teachers need to discipline a student who is in a gang or suspected to be in a gang, teachers should calmly and quietly ask the student to remain after class to discuss the rule infraction and make sure that fellow gang members are not present during the conversation as youth members of gangs do not respond well if they are embarrassed in front of others.

Schools that implement after-school activities allow students to be involved in structured positive activities that can help them build a sense of belonging, obtain academic support, and build positive relationships with other peers and adult role models. Academic success was previously discussed as a protective factor; thus, academic intervention during after-school programs is an important prevention activity. It is important for schools to seek suggestions from youth to ensure that after-school activities fit their needs and interests.

Beyond school efforts, parents and caregivers should be involved in preventing youth from joining gangs. Parents and caregivers need to use effective parenting skills, strengthen family relationships, and be involved in their child's school (Arciaga et al., 2010). SMH clinicians can provide groups or classes on effective parenting strategies, organize parent events to increase awareness about gangs, or provide additional parent education or family therapy for specific families. In addition, it is important that schools collaborate with community organizations and leaders, as well as grassroots and faith-based organizations to provide after-school activities, community activities, and clubs to create violence-free areas. It is essential that all systems in the child's life are involved and committed to reducing gangs.

It is important to increase social–emotional skills and promote positive peer relationships in school-aged youth. A popular school-based prevention program taught by law enforcement officers is called the Gang Resistance Education and Training (G.R.E.A.T.) Program (Howell, 2010). This 13-week program teaches elementary and middle school students about the dangers of gang involvement and utilizes cognitive-behavioral training, social skills development, refusal skills, and conflict resolution. The overall goals are to reduce gang involvement and delinquency, gain knowledge of the consequences of gang involvement, and encourage positive relationships with law enforcement (Ashcroft, Daniels, & Hart, 2004). There is also a summer program and training for families.

In a national multisite evaluation of the G.R.E.A.T. Program, administrators, teachers, and counselors reported high acceptability and positive attitudes about the program (Peterson & Esbensen, 2004). Results indicated that 77% of school personnel reported that the program was appropriate for students, and 75% of school personnel indicated that the program taught students important skills to avoid gangs and improved their perceptions of law enforcement. In a different evaluation study of the G.R.E.A.T. Program, students were surveyed from 7th to 11th grade (Ashcroft et al., 2004). Results of this study revealed improved attitudes about law enforcement, more negative views about gangs, and increased prosocial peer activities 4 years after the program was delivered.

Secondary Prevention. For secondary prevention activities, schools need to identify high-risk youth and refer them to small groups such as anger management, conflict resolution, peer mediation, academic support, and/or self-esteem building (Arciaga et al., 2010; Wyrick, 2006). SMH clinicians are in an ideal position to lead these groups There are several secondary prevention programs and small prevention groups that are in the OJJDP Model Programs Guide (please visit http://www.ojjdp.gov/mpg/). One example of a secondary prevention program is Aggression Replacement Therapy (ART) that targets chronically aggressive, violent, and delinquent youth (Goldstein & Glick, 1994; Goldstein, Glick, & Gibbs, 1998). ART is an intensive 10-week (three one hour sessions per week) cognitive behavioral therapy group for youth that focuses on social skills training, anger control, and moral reasoning training with the goal of reducing aggression and violence in youth. The ART program is listed in the OJJDP Model Programs Guide as an effective program for aggressive and violent adolescents (2010).

Intervention. Intervention strategies focus on youth already involved in gangs and criminal activity, as well as the most frequently offending youth gang members who are involved in chronic, serious, and violent crimes (Wyrick, 2006). At this level, it is necessary to work intensely with youth on an individual and family level to help them get out of the gang by increasing their motivation to leave, and teaching them the knowledge and skills necessary to leave (Arciaga et al., 2010). SMH clinicians can provide cognitive behavioral therapy, substance abuse counseling, family therapy, and/or group therapy. When SMH clinicians work with youth in gangs, it is important that they show respect for the youth, listen to their stories, and be aware of their own biases. For youth who are frequent offenders, it will be essential to collaborate with law enforcement (given client's consent) for suppression strategies to rehabilitate these youth.

Safety Issues

As part of cultural competency training, school staff should be educated on safety issues related to gang violence (Arciaga et al., 2010). Gang members may respond with verbal exchanges, stare downs, nonverbal gestures, or physical aggression. Adults should avoid disrespecting anything related to the gang or gang member, embarrassing a gang member in public, or using their gang identifiers, hand signs, symbols, etc. Adults should be consistent and fair in enforcing rules across all students and groups. If rival gangs or gang members are in conflict or fighting at school, it is important to immediately separate the gang members and seek law enforcement assistance.

Importantly, there should be programs or meetings for students so they know what to do if they encounter problems with gangs. For example, there should be a confidential reporting system implemented for students to report possible gang violence and/or weapons at school. Students should be told that their reports will remain confidential and that they will receive support in order to prevent retaliation and being labeled a "snitch" (i.e., tattle-tail). Further, in the event of violence or crises, schools should assemble a crisis team and create a crisis plan in order to be prepared for emergencies. Similar to regular fire drills, "lock down" drills, or having students move to secured and locked areas, should be implemented in the event that there is an intruder in the school.

Conclusion

This chapter discussed the escalating youth gang problem and provided an overview of youth gangs. It is clear that multiple systems need to collaborate to successfully reduce youth gangs and related problems in schools. School staff and SMH clinicians can play an important role in helping to reduce gang problems in schools. Pre-service and in-service professional development trainings to gain competency in working with this population for SMH professionals are needed. Several practical culturally responsive strategies were presented that school staff and SMH clinicians can use to address gang problems in schools. Future research should examine the best mechanism for training mental health professionals to improve their cultural competency related to working with youth gangs, as well as studies investigating the effectiveness of strategies used by mental health professionals in their work with youth gangs.

References

Allen, M. P. (1998). The interdisciplinary movement. *Journal of Social Work Education, 34*(1), 2–5.

Andis, P., Cashman, J., Praschil, R., Oglesby, D., Adelman, H., Taylor, L., et al. (2002). A strategic and shared agenda to advance mental health in schools through family and system partnerships. *International Journal of Mental Health Promotion, 4,* 28–35.

Arciaga, M. (2007). Multidisciplinary gang intervention teams. *National Youth Gang Center Bulletin No. 3.* Tallahassee, FL: National Youth Gang Center.

Arciaga, M., Sakamoto, W., & Jones, E. F. (2010). Responding to gangs in the school setting. *National Gang Center Bulletin No. 5*. Tallahassee, FL: National Gang Center.

Ashcroft, J., Daniels, D. J., & Hart, S. V. (2004). *Evaluating G.R.E.A.T.: A school-based gang prevention program*. Washington, DC: U.S. Department of Justice Office of Justice Programs.

Baltimore City Criminal Justice Coordinating Council. (2006). *Baltimore city gang violence reduction plan*. Retrieved from http:www.jhsph.edu/research/centers-and-institutes/center-for-prevention-of-youth-violence/_pdfs/FINALGANGSTRATEGY.pdf. August 27, 2012.

Centers, N., & Weist, M. D. (1998). Inner city youth and drug dealing: A review of the problem. *Journal of Youth and Adolescence, 27*, 395–411.

Chandler, K. A., Chapman, C. D., Rand, M. R., & Taylor, B. M. (1998). *Students reports of school crime: 1989 and 1995*. Washington, D.C.: U.S. Department of Justice, Office of Justice Programs, Office of Juvenile Justice and Delinquency Prevention.

Decker, S. H., & Curry, G. D. (2000). Addressing key features of gang membership: Measuring the involvement of young members. *Journal of Criminal Justice, 28*, 473–482.

Decker, S. H., & Van Winkle, B. (1996). *Life in the gang: Family, friends, and violence*. New York, NY: Cambridge University Press.

Egley, A., & Howell, J. C. (2011). *Highlights of the 2009 National Youth Gang Survey. Fact Sheet*. Washington, D.C.: U.S. Department of Justice, Office of Justice Programs, Office of Juvenile Justice and Delinquency Prevention.

Egley, A., Howell, J. C., & Major, A. K. (2006). *National youth gang survey: 1999-2011*. Washington, D.C.: U.S. Department of Justice, Office of Justice Programs, Office of Juvenile Justice and Delinquency Prevention.

Ellickson, P., Saner, H., & McGuigan, K. A. (1997). Profiles of violent youth: Substance use and other concurrent problems. *American Journal of Public Health, 87*(6), 985–991.

Esbensen, F. A., Deschenes, E. P., & Winfree, L. T. (1999). Differences between gang girls and gang boys: Results from a multi-site survey. *Youth and Society, 31*, 27–53.

Esbensen, F. A., Peterson, D., Taylor, T. J., & Freng, A. (2010). Similarities and differences in risk factors for violent offending and gang membership. *The Australian and New Zealand Journal of Criminology, 42*, 1–26.

Goldstein, A. P., & Glick, B. (1994). Aggression replacement training: Curriculum and evaluation. *Simulation and Gaming, 25*(1), 9–26.

Goldstein, A. P., Glick, B., & Gibbs, J. (1998). *Aggression replacement training revision edition: A comprehensive intervention for aggressive youth*. Champaign, IL: Research Press.

Hill, K. G., Lui, C., & Hawkins, J. D. (2001). *Early precursors of gang membership: A study of Seattle youth. Bulletin*. Washington, D.C.: U.S. Department of Justice, Office of Justice Programs, Office of Juvenile Justice and Delinquency Prevention.

Howell, J. C. (2003). *Preventing and reducing juvenile delinquency: A comprehensive framework*. Thousand Oaks, CA: Sage Publications.

Howell, J. C. (2009). *Preventing and reducing juvenile delinquency: A comprehensive framework* (2nd ed.). Thousand Oaks, California: Sage Publications.

Howell, J. C. (2010). *Gang prevention: An overview of research and programs. Risk and protective factors of child delinquency*. Washington, D.C.: U.S. Department of Justice. Office of Justice Programs, Office of Juvenile Justice and Delinquency Prevention.

Howell, J. C., & Egley, A. (2005). Moving risk factors into development theories of gang membership. *Youth Violence and Juvenile Justice, 3*(4), 334–354.

Howell, J. C., & Lynch, J. (2000). Youth gangs in schools. *Juvenile Justice Bulletin: Youth gang series*. Washington, DC: U.S. Department of Justice, Office of Justice Programs, Office of Juvenile Justice and Delinquency Prevention.

Huizinga, D., & Lovegrove, P. (2009). *Summary of important risk factors for gang membership*. Boulder, CO: Institute for Behavioral Research.

Kupersmidt, J. B., Coie, J. D., & Howell, J. C. (2003). Building resilience in children exposed to negative peer influences. In K. I. Maton, C. J. Schellenbach, B. J. Leadbeater, & A. L. Solarz (Eds.), *Investing in children, youth, families, and communities: Strength-based research and policy* (pp. 251–268). Washington, DC: American Psychological Association.

Larson, J., & Busse, R. T. (1998). Specialist-level preparation in school violence and youth gang intervention. *Psychology in the Schools, 35*, 373–379.

Laub, J. H., & Lauritsen, J. L. (1998). The interdependence of school violence with neighborhood and family conditions. In D. S. Elliott, B. A. Hamburg, & K. R. Williams (Eds.), *Violence in American schools: A new perspective*. Cambridge, U.K. Cambridge University Press.

Li, X., Stanton, B., Pack, R., Harris, C., Cottrell, L., & Burns, J. (2002). Risk and protective factors associated with gang involvement among urban African American adolescents. *Youth and Society, 34*, 172–194.

Miller, W. B. (1992). *Crime by youth gangs and groups in the United States*. Washington, DC: U.S. Department of Justice, Office of Justice Programs, Office of Juvenile Justice and Delinquency Prevention.

Miller, W. B. (2001). *The growth of youth gang problems in the United States: 1970-1998*. Washington, DC: U.S. Department of Justice, Office of Justice Programs, Office of Juvenile Justice and Delinquency Prevention.

National Youth Gang Center (2009). *National Youth Gang Survey Analysis*. Retrieved from http://www.nationalgangcenter.gov/Survey-Analysis. August 27, 2012.

Office of Juvenile Justice and Delinquency Prevention. (2009). *OJJDP's comprehensive gang model: A guide to assessing your community's youth gang problem*.

Washington, DC: U.S. Department of Justice, Office of Justice Programs, Office of Juvenile Justice and Delinquency Prevention.

Office of Juvenile Justice and Delinquency Prevention. (2010). *OJJDP Strategic Planning Tool.* Retrieved from http:www.nationalgangcenter.gov/About/Strategic-Planning-Tool. August 27, 2012.

Office of Juvenile Justice and Delinquency Prevention. (2010). *OJJDP's Model Program Guide.* Retrieved from http://www.ojjdp.gov/mpg/

Pesce, R. C., & Wilczynski, J. D. (2005). Gang prevention. *Student Counseling 101.* Retrieved from http://www.nasponline.org/resources/principals/nassp_gang.pdf. August 27, 2012.

Peterson, D., & Esbensen, F. A. (2004). The outlook is G.R.E.A.T.: What educators say about school-based prevention and the gang resistance education and training (G.R.E.A.T.) program. *Evaluation Review, 28*(3), 218–245.

Peterson, D., Taylor, T. J., & Esbensen, F. A. (2004). Gang membership and violent victimization. *Justice Quarterly, 21*, 793–815.

Robers, S., Zhang, J., & Truman, J. (2010). Indicators of school crime and safety: 2010. National Center for Education Statistics, U.S. Department of Education, and Bureau of Justice Statistics, Office of Justice Programs. Washington, DC: U.S. Department of Justice.

Sickmund, M., Snyder, H. N., & Poe-Yamagata, E. (1997). *Juvenile offenders and victims: 1997 update on violence.* Washington, DC: Office of Juvenile Justice and Delinquency Prevention.

Sue, D. W., & Sue, D. (2008). *Counseling the culturally diverse: Theory and practice* (5th ed.). Hoboken, NJ: John Wiley and Sons, Inc.

Thornberry, T. P., Huizinga, D., & Loeber, R. (2004). Causes and correlates studies: Findings and policy implications. *Juvenile Justice, 10*(1), 3–19.

Thornberry, T. P., Krohn, M. D., Lizotte, A. J., Smith, C. A., & Tobin, K. (2003). *Gangs and delinquency in developmental perspective.* New York, NY: Cambridge University Press.

U.S. Department of Health and Human Services. (2001). *Mental health: Culture, race, and ethnicity—A supplement to Mental health: A report of the Surgeon General.* Rockville, MD: U.S. Department of Health and Human Services, Substance Abuse and Mental Health Services Administration, Center for Mental Health Services.

Vigil, J. D. (2002). *A rainbow of gangs: Street cultures in the mega-city.* Austin, TX: University of Texas Press.

Vigil, J. D. (2008). Mexican migrants in gangs: A second-generations history. In F. Van Gemert, D. Peterson, & I. L. Lien (Eds.), *Street gangs, migrations, and ethnicity* (p. 62). Portland, OR: Willan Publishing.

Wasserman, G. A., Keenan, K., Tremblay, R. E., Coie, J. D., Herrenkohl, T. I., Loeber, R., et al. (2003). *Risk and protective factors of child delinquency. Bulletin.* Washington, D.C.: U.S. Department of Justice, Office of Justice Programs, Office of Juvenile Justice and Delinquency Prevention.

Wood, J., Foy, D. W., Layne, C., Pynos, R., & James, C. B. (2002). An examination of the relationships between violence exposure, posttraumatic stress symptomatology, and delinquent activity: An "ecopathological" model of delinquent behavior among incarcerated adolescents. *Journal of Aggression, Maltreatment, & Trauma, 6*, 127–147.

Wyrick, P. A. (2006). Gang prevention: How to make the "front end" of your anti-gang effort work. *United States Attorneys' Bulletin, 54*, 52–60.

Part III

Specific Problems and Interventions

Training Transformed School Counselors

14

Marte Ostvik-de Wilde, Denise Park, and Courtland C. Lee

The last decade has seen a transformation in the role of the professional school counselor. National educational reform initiatives have influenced the nature of the theory and practice of school counseling (Trust, 2000). Like other educational professionals, school counselors are being called upon to contribute to a movement ensuring that all students achieve high academic standards, as measured by ever-increasing assessment initiatives. In an era of "No Child Left Behind" (U.S. Department of Education, 2001) and "Race to the Top" (U.S. Department of Education, 2009), educators are being held ever more accountable for students' academic achievement. As the field of education grapples with this call for accountability, the nature of educator preparation is coming under greater scrutiny.

This movement for accountability has compelled the profession of counseling to reflect on the role of school counselors and the nature of their preparation. Traditionally school counselors have been trained to facilitate student's academic, career, and personal–social development within a context that reflects the mental health traditions of the counseling profession (Herr, 2003). The mental health focus of many counselor preparation programs often overshadows aspects of educational theory and practice that should be emphasized in school counselor training. If not overshadowed, then training curriculum fails to emphasize a link between mental health and education. This often leads to role ambiguity when counselors enter schools. This ambiguity contributes to their role being considered ancillary to the main educational focus of schools (Erford, House and Martin, 2003). While many school counselors develop skills to address student problems, they often lack the ability to impact upon the overall educational program in ways that support the mission of schools—which is to promote academic achievement. Since academic achievement is the primary goal of schooling, it can be asserted that school mental health includes academic success for young people.

The purpose of this chapter is to provide a perspective on school counselor training which is based on a philosophy that there is a direct correlation between academic success and optimal mental health. This philosophy posits that if barriers to optimal mental health are effectively challenged and removed, then the likelihood of academic success increases. This chapter will explore the school counselor training experience at a major university, which is focused on ensuring that counselors are key participants in efforts to close the pervasive achievement gap in the American educational system.

M. Ostvik-de Wilde (✉) • D. Park • C.C. Lee
University of Maryland at College Park,
College Park, MD, USA
e-mail: mdewilde@umd.edu

Academic Success and the Link to Mental Health

It has been asserted that mentally healthy children enjoy a quality of life that includes success in school (Friedrich, Raffaele-Mendez, & Mihalas, 2010; Hoagwood, Jensen, Petti, & Burns, 1996). Academic success and mental health have been considered linked in an interdependent and cyclical fashion (Murray, Low, Hollis, Cross, & Davis, 2007). Lleras-Muney (2005) suggests that education has a causal relationship to health. As such, when students' social and psychological needs are appropriately addressed, the likelihood of succeeding in school increases (Anderson, Houser, & Howland, 2010). Further, Bradshaw, Buckley, & Ialongo (2008) suggest that addressing academic difficulties, as well detecting internalizing and externalizing problems in early school years, are key to preventing subsequent mental health and educational issues.

The University of Maryland at College Park Urban School Counseling Program

Since 2003, the school counseling program at the University of Maryland at College Park has been redesigned to align itself with major school counseling reform efforts. In particular, the program has used the conceptual framework developed by the Education Trust's Transforming School Counseling Initiative (Education Trust, 2000) as the basis for curriculum design. The Transforming School Counseling Initiative aims to place school counselors at the center of efforts to close the achievement gap that exists between children of color and poor children and their White middle class counterparts in American education (Haycock, 2001). Within this context, the faculty decided at that time that given the proximity of the University of Maryland to the major urban areas of Washington, DC and Baltimore, MD, it was logical for its school counselor preparation program to focus on arming counselors with skills to address urban educational challenges. The urban school districts surrounding the University of Maryland were characterized by a number of schools that were experiencing massive educational failure with achievement gaps based on race/ethnicity and social class. It was the faculty's firm belief that academic success was paramount to the school experience. Further, the faculty perceived school counselors as both mental health agents and educators tasked with the responsibility of ensuring that academic success was the foundation for school mental health.

In conceiving the program, the term *urban* was conceptualized to mean more than just *inner city*. Urban was defined as a metropolitan area that includes a large population nucleus, together with adjacent communities that have a high degree of economic and social interactions with that nucleus (U.S. Bureau of the Census, 2010). Schools in this environment often reflect many of the dynamics that characterize the urban experience such as population density, cultural diversity, and structural density (Lee, 2005). Schools in urban areas are characterized by significant variability when it comes to access to educational resources. While some schools prosper, others experience high levels of concentrated poverty and challenging school cultures. Measures of educational progress suggest that students in urban schools, particularly those with significant levels of poverty, experience greater challenges to academic, career, and social success than their peers in rural and suburban schools (Lippman, Burns, & McArthur, 1996). The combination of these variables associated with the urban educational context, often threatens educational achievement and the mental health of scores of children.

Program Mission. The mission of the Maryland program is to prepare counselors to work professionally with children in urban settings from kindergarten through high school.

The faculty's focus on preparing professional school counselors who can promote student growth and development in urban educational settings is the hallmark of this program. The faculty considers the promotion of student growth and development as the essence of optimal mental health in educational contexts.

The program emphasizes the development of school counselor competencies for work with culturally diverse urban student populations. It also promotes the development of competencies for working with stakeholders (e.g., parents, teachers, administrators, community leaders, etc.) who are crucial to students' academic success. A major theme in the program is the commitment to access, equity, and social justice in the delivery of counseling services to close the achievement gap in culturally diverse urban school settings. The program aims to develop professional school counselors who are educational leaders and advocates for systemic change.

The Admissions Process

Given the mission of the program, there are important qualities that are sought in applicants. The faculty considers the following qualities to be crucial for success in the program and, as a professional school counselor working in an urban environment: (1) a commitment to urban school counseling, (2) a commitment to social justice and closing the achievement gap, and (3) a commitment to multiculturalism and diversity. In addition to these aspects of commitment, the faculty also wants students who have passion, exhibit leadership qualities, and have the ability to "think outside the box" when it comes to conceptualizing and implementing a school counseling program.

In order to find individuals with these qualities, the program engages in a comprehensive admissions process inspired by the work of Stone and Hanson (2002). This process begins with an initial screening of applicant files. Applicants are required to complete a graduate school application and submit scores from the Graduate Record Exam. In addition, they must submit an undergraduate transcript, a statement of professional goals, and three letters of recommendation.

Applicants must also submit a program-specific application in which they must complete a brief response to a school equity scenario. This scenario is designed to assess an applicant's rudimentary understanding of issues related to cultural diversity and social justice in school counseling. After an initial screening of applications, selected candidates are invited to campus for an in-depth interview with a selection team consisting of program faculty and students.

The daylong interview process involves a number of evaluative experiences. First, each applicant is interviewed individually by a program faculty member and by current students. Second, the applicants take part in a group interview where they are observed interacting with other candidates as they work on a case study to jointly develop a counseling intervention. The presenting issue in the case study is that a talented African-American female student shows an interest in college, but her mother comes to the school counselor and expresses her concern that the family does not have the money for a college education and that she needs her daughter to get a job after graduation. Given this scenario, the group must brainstorm ideas for addressing the challenges presented in the case and agree on action steps. This group interview is structured to evaluate each applicant's ability to function in a small group. This activity is designed to assess how applicants assume roles as both collaborative participants and leaders while working to accomplish a task. The faculty and students who observe the group process evaluate each applicant on the following criteria: (1) the ability to focus on the task, (2) the ability to function as a team member and leader by inviting comments and listening to other group members, (3) the ability to offer useful information to accomplish the task, (4) the ability to comprehend the cultural dimension in the case study, and (5) the ability to summarize the group process and suggest a course of action.

Third, the applicants must participate in a writing exercise. They are given a journal article related to issues of access, equity, and social justice in education to which they must write a reaction. The writing sample is designed to assess the applicant's ability to think critically about social and educational issues. In addition, this writing assignment gives the faculty an assessment of the applicants' writing ability.

Finally, each candidate must give an extemporaneous 5-min speech to an audience composed of program faculty and students. Each applicant is shown data that graphically illustrate the achievement gap in American education. The candidate must then speak for five minutes to the question. "How will these data influence your work as a school counselor?"

Each applicant is then evaluated by the faculty and students in the audience on the following criteria: (1) the ability to think on one's feet, (2) degree of confidence in speaking to a group, (3) the extent to which the applicant grasps the magnitude of the achievement gap, and (4) the ability to discuss the relevance of such data to school counseling.

At the conclusion of the interview process, the admissions committee discusses each applicant and reviews the candidate's evaluations on each of the day's tasks. Those applicants who receive the highest evaluations and by group consensus are considered to have the greatest potential to experience success in the program and ultimately as professional school counselors are recommended to the Graduate School for admission.

While this process is extremely labor intensive for the program faculty, it tends to yield a cohort of students who have not only the ability, but also the commitment to succeed in the program. Those applicants who successfully complete the interview process are then admitted, and ultimately enroll in the program relate that this process is intense, but also gives them a realistic picture of the program and its expectations. They report that after going through the interview process they appreciate the selective nature of the program.

Curricular Experiences

The program curriculum is designed to assist students in developing the skills to promote academic, career, and personal/social development among K-12 students in urban educational contexts. A set of competencies proposed by Lee (2005) is the center of the training experience, including cultural competence, skills for promoting empowerment, adopting a systemic perspective on student issues, advocacy, collaboration, and leadership. The didactic and experiential components of the coursework in the program include an exploration of some aspect of these competencies. It is anticipated that graduates of the program will be urban school counselors who demonstrate:

1. Skills in assessing the influence of the urban social context on the psychosocial development of children and adolescents.
2. Increased sensitivity and clinical skills that represent awareness of the diversity of race, gender, religion, ethnicity, ability status, nationality, and sexual orientation within the student population.
3. Knowledge of the role and function of the professional counselor and how it relates to the mission of schools.
4. Leadership ability and advocacy skills in schools and communities to remove barriers to student learning.
5. The ability to build collaborative partnerships with all educational stakeholders to promote access, equity, and social justice in school settings.
6. Expertise in working individually and in groups with culturally diverse students on issues that impact upon student achievement.
7. Skills in developing a data-driven counseling program.
8. The ability to conduct research in school settings.
9. Comprehension of ethical and legal issues related to school counseling.

The nature of the coursework is rooted in the curricular areas delineated by the Council for the Accreditation of Counseling and Related Educational Programs (CACREP). CACREP is an independent agency recognized by the Council for Higher Education Accreditation (CHEA) to accredit masters degree programs in counseling. There is a set of core counseling curricular standards that forms the basis of a CACREP accredited counseling program. In addition, there are specialty standards that CACREP has developed for school counseling programs.

The program faculty has designed the coursework to comply with CACREP standards. While courses contain content that reflects traditional counseling theory and practice, students are also exposed to issues and concepts that reflect school counseling in contemporary urban environments. There are several pervasive themes that are infused throughout the training curriculum. These include: multicultural competency, social justice, and exploring the issues and dynamics of the achievement gap and the social injustices that surround them. As an example, in the Introduction to School Counseling class, which is the first course in the masters training sequence, students are exposed to the history and foundations of school counseling. Additionally, however, they read *Can We Talk About Race?* by Beverly Tatum (2007) and *School Counseling to Close the Achievement Gap: A Social Justice Framework for Success* by Cheryl Holcomb-McCoy (2007). These books underscore the issues of social justice and multicultural competence that serve as the framework for the rest of the students' experience in the program.

Field Experiences

In order to underscore the development of these competencies, the program emphasizes field experiences within urban educational settings. These experiences begin with a community volunteer experience in the introductory course. In order to better understand the role of the urban school counselor as advocate and leader, students are required to do volunteer work in an urban community agency, preferably one that focuses on youth issues. Students are expected to volunteer at least five hours per week at the agency. They must keep a log of their volunteer activities and turn it in at the end of the semester. In addition to the log, students complete a five-page reaction paper about their volunteer experience and how they perceive it contributing to their role as a professional school counselor.

As with most counselor training programs, the students are required to complete both a practicum and internship experience. However, these experiences are completed in urban schools and differ significantly from what is normally required in a field-based course. For example, a major feature of the internship experience is the Advocacy Project. All interns must complete a data-driven advocacy project as a part of their field experience. At the beginning of their internship, students must consult with their supervisor and identify data that is indicative of student needs, concerns, challenges, or issues. In examining the data, they must identify possible systemic contributions to the problem or issue. This includes any access or equity barriers that may be contributing to the problem. The students must also detail possible consequences of not addressing the problem or issue.

After an issue has been identified, students must then develop an action plan to address the concern. This plan must identify possible educational stakeholders who could be enlisted as allies in addressing the issue and plans for collaboration with these individuals. The next step in the process is to implement the action plan and measure its success. In reviewing the implementation of the project, interns must identify policies and practices that may need to change and then they must develop change strategies. They must assess which system policies and practices interfere with the project strategies and action steps and develop methods for addressing or challenging these systemic impediments.

Advocacy Project: An Example

One intern was assigned to an urban high school with a history of low academic performance. Her advocacy project began with an examination of the school's suspension data. She discovered that a large percentage of the student body was being suspended (often multiple times) for a wide variety of offenses. The typical length of any suspension was 10 days and the decisions to suspend were often arbitrary and capricious. During the time students were suspended, they could not come to school and were not given academic work to complete during their period away from school. In many instances, students who were suspended were left home alone and became involved in questionable and often dangerous street activities.

The intern identified a strong positive correlation between the suspension rate and the pervasive academic failure at the school. She also surmised that multiple suspensions were having a negative impact on the mental health of many students, as it appeared that they became more isolated from the school experience as their suspensions mounted.

Enlisting the support of parents and community representatives, the intern developed a plan for an alternative in-school suspension program. Rather than have students miss 10 days of school, they would be suspended, but remain in school and during this time they would receive academic help in the form of tutoring and personal counseling as needed. The intern then presented this suspension alternative to the school's principal.

The Culminating Experience

The culminating experience in the program takes place in a capstone course entitled *Program Planning: Principles and Practices of Urban School Counseling K-12*. This course focuses on the planning, implementation, and evaluation of a systemic data-driven and developmental urban school counseling program, in particular, school counseling programs that promote access and equity for all students. Specific emphasis is placed upon the integration of the school counseling program with a standards-based educational program. This course is competency based and is designed to have students develop a systemic data-driven school counseling program that is:
1. An integral component of the overall educational program.
2. Designed to promote the achievement of all students and assist in closing the achievement gap.
3. Aligned with state and national initiatives such as the ACSA National Model as well as *Maryland State Content Standards*.
4. Consistent with legislation such as *No Child Left Behind* and *Race to the Top*.
5. Sensitive to contemporary issues of family, society, and culture and their influence on students' psychosocial development.
6. Designed to foster a positive school climate and culture and enhance the teaching and learning process for all students.
7. Based on an understanding of the application of district policies, and state and federal laws.
8. Based on the application of developmental counseling strategies and interventions useful in the school setting.
9. Based on the understanding of the development, implementation, and evaluation of school counseling programs from a systemic change model.

In order to develop these competencies, students must create a systemic school counseling program. The program must be divided into four phases: Phase I must include an introduction and needs assessment; Phase II must include professional foundations and theory; Phase III must include the development of a year-long calendar of school counseling activities; Phase IV must include activities and policies for each component of the counseling program as well as a program evaluation. Each student organizes his or her program by section areas in a three-ring binder. In preparing their programs, students must select the content standards from one subject area in the *Maryland State Content Standards*. One section of those standards must be incorporated into one of the counseling interventions that are developed in their program. The program that students develop in this course becomes a reference source that as a professional school counselor they use, add to, and continue to develop to meet the diverse needs of students in a pluralistic society.

The Training Program Outcomes

The following is an example of how this training program impacts the school counseling practice of its graduates:

Ann (not her real name) is a recent graduate of the School Counseling Program. Her first job was as a counselor at a charter school in an urban, inner city area. The population of the school was predominantly Latino. In addition, the overwhelming majority of the students came from poor families. The school did not have much of a college-going culture and a large percentage of the students dropped out before graduation. Those who did graduate usually ended up in low-paying jobs or unemployed.

Armed with data that showed that Latinos are approximately 10% less likely than non-Hispanic Whites and 5% percent less likely than African-Americans to attend college (U.S. Department of Education, 2002), Ann decided to take action at her school. She committed herself to motivating and supporting students and their parents in a college access process. In addition to her intervention with students and parents, she used these data to challenge long-standing school and school system policies and procedures that blocked college access for Latino students. Against the advice of her colleagues and despite their skepticism, Ann had every senior fill out a college application. She also provided the students and their families with information about college and the college-going process. In addition, she worked with teachers at a nearby university to provide the students with supplemental academic support. As a result of her action, at the end of the academic year 70% of the senior class was accepted into a 2 or 4-year college or university.

Conclusion

Graduates of the School Counseling Program at the University of Maryland at College Park are in high demand, both in the Washington, DC metropolitan area and other urban school systems throughout the country. A principal who hires a graduate of this program can be assured of getting a professional school counselor with the awareness, knowledge, and skills to truly make a difference in the lives of young people in urban areas. In particular, program graduates have unique competencies to challenge the status quo that often prevents students of color and those who are economically disadvantaged from achieving their fullest academic and social potential. The graduates understand that the role of the school counselor has been transformed and they are committed to ensuring that all students achieve to high academic standards. Part of this commitment involves impacting the overall educational program in ways that support the mission of schools—which is to promote academic achievement. Program graduates work from a perspective that they are both educators and mental health professionals who are able to equate school mental health with academic success for all young people.

References

Anderson, J. A, Houser, J. H, & Howland, A. (2010). The full partnership model for promoting academic and socio-emotional success in schools. *The School Community Journal 20* (1).

Bradshaw, C. P., Buckley, J. A., & Ialongo, N. S. (2008). School based service utilization among urban children with early onset educational and mental health problems: The squeaky wheel phenomenon. *School Psychology Quarterly, 23*, 169–186.

Erford, B. T., House, R., & Martin, P. (2003). Transforming the school counseling profession. In B. T. Erford (Ed.), *Transforming the school counseling profession* (pp. 1–20). Upper Saddle River, NJ: Merrill Prentice-Hall.

Friedrich, A. A., Raffaele-Mendez, L. M., & Mihalas, S. T. (2010). Gender as a factor in school-based mental health service delivery. *School Psychology Review, 39*, 122–136.

Haycock, K. (2001, March 6–11). Closing the achievement gap. *Educational Leadership*.

Herr, E. L. (2003). Historical roots and future issues. In B. T. Erford (Ed.), *Transforming the school counseling profession* (pp. 21–38). Upper Saddle River, NJ: Merrill Prentice-Hall.

Hoagwood, K., Jensen, P. S., Petti, T., & Burns, B. J. (1996). Outcomes of mental health care for children and adolescents: A comprehensive conceptual model. *Journal of the American Academy of Child and Adolescent Psychiatry, 35*, 1055–1063.

Holcomb-McCoy, C. C. (2007). *School counseling to close the achievement gap: A social justice framework for success*. Thousand Oaks, CA: Corwin.

Lee, C. C. (2005). Urban school counseling: Context, characteristics, and competencies. *Professional School Counseling, 8*, 184–188.

Lippman, L., Burns, S., & McArthur, E. (1996). *Urban Schools: The challenge of location and poverty (NCES 96-184)*. Washington, DC: U.S. Department of Education, National Center for Education Statistics.

Lleras-Muney, A. (2005). The Relationship between education and adult mortality in the United States. *Review of Economic Studies, 72*, 189–221.

Murray, N. G., Low, B. J., Hollis, C., Cross, A. W., & Davis, S. M. (2007). Coordinated school mental health programs and academic achievement: A systematic review of the literature. *Journal of School Health, 77*(9), 589–600.

Stone, C. B., & Hanson, C. (2002). Selection of school counselor candidates: Future directions at two universities. *Counselor Education and Supervision, 41,* 175–192.

Tatum, B. D. (2007). *Can we talk about race?* Boston, MA: Beacon.

Education Trust. (2000). *National initiative for transforming school counseling summer academy for counselor educators proceedings.* Washington, DC: Author.

U.S. Bureau of the Census. (2010). Census 2010 urban and rural classification. Retrieved November 9, 2010, from http://www.census.gov/geo/www/ua/2010urbanruralclass.html.

U.S. Department of Education. (2001). *No Child Left Behind Act of 2001 (H.R. 1).* Washington, DC: Author.

U.S. Department of Education. (2002). *Profile of undergraduates in U.S. postsecondary institutions: 1999-2000 (NCES 2002-168).* Washington, DC: National Center for Education Statistics.

U.S. Department of Education. (2009). *Race to the top fund.* Washington, DC: Author.

Culturally Integrated Substance Abuse and Sex Education Prevention

Programming for Middle School Students

Desi S. Hacker, Faye Z. Belgrave, Jamie Grisham, Jasmine Abrams, and Darlene G. Colson

Co-occurring problems of early and unprotected sex and drug use can lead to several adverse social, health, and academic outcomes for youth, especially those who reside within low-resource communities. Early adolescence (age 11–14) can be an especially vulnerable period for the initiation of substance abuse and risky sexual activity. Two significant changes occur during this developmental period: puberty and the transition to middle school. With puberty comes movement away from family toward peers for affiliation and social needs. Affiliation with delinquent peers may contribute to early and/or risky sexual behavior and substance use. The transition from the more protective environment of elementary school to middle school brings greater independence and increased responsibilities. Consequently, this is a developmental crossroads at which children may embark upon a high-risk path. Accordingly, programming that is aimed at preventing substance abuse and early and/or risky sexual behavior among middle school students is critical. Such programming is necessary to prevent the onset of behaviors that would otherwise likely continue into adulthood with devastating consequences for the individual and society.

D.S. Hacker (✉) • J. Grisham • D.G. Colson
700 Park Ave, Norfolk State University, Norfolk, VA 23504, USA
e-mail: dshacker@nsu.edu

F.Z. Belgrave • J. Abrams
Virginia Commonwealth University, Richmond, VA 23284, USA

This chapter will (1) provide an overview of risk and protective factors related to substance use and early sexual behavior, (2) discuss the role of culture in addressing these behaviors, (3) describe existing school-based prevention programs targeting culturally diverse youth, and (4) present an example of a culturally-based, combined substance use prevention and sex education program for African American middle school girls.

Risk and Protective Factors

A risk factor increases the likelihood of a behavior that usually has negative consequences (Hawkins, Catalano, & Miller, 1992). A protective factor moderates or reduces the impact of a risk behavior, helps individuals not to engage in potentially harmful behavior, and/or promotes an alternative pathway. Risk and protective factors can exist in different contexts such as individual, family, peer, school, and community.

Substance use, early sexual activity, and other problem behaviors tend to co-occur among adolescents (Brookmeyer & Henrick, 2009; Wu, Witkiewitz, McMahon, Dodge, & Conduct Problems Research Group, 2010) and share similar risk factors. Some risk factors may be due to a constellation of underlying problems such as conduct disorder, family dysfunction, and neighborhood risk (Jessor & Jessor, 1977; Doherty, Green, & Ensiminger, 2008). In the Adverse

Childhood Experiences Study (ACE), child abuse and household dysfunction risk factors were correlated with delinquent behaviors in childhood and adolescence, including sexual activity, pregnancies, and early initiation of substance abuse (Middlebrooks & Audage, 2008). However, these risk factors may be difficult for prevention programs to address. Other risk factors, on the other hand, may be more amenable to change, for example students' attitudes, behaviors, and peer/institution affiliations. Research indicates that youth who associate with peers who have positive attitudes about drugs, alcohol, and deviant behavior, or youth who have problems academically, are at greater risk for both substance use and risky sexual behaviors. Alternatively, protective processes are at work for youth who associate with peers who have anti-drug attitudes, perceive negative consequences for drug use or sexual activity, and/or are connected to social institutions such as school or religious agencies (Kirby & Lepore, 2007; see Hogan, Gabrielsen, Luna, & Grothaus, 2002 for a more comprehensive review of risks and protective factors).

Culture, Substance Use, and Sexual Activity

While many factors may affect the risk for substance abuse and sexual behavior, the role of culture is particularly important. Culture is defined as "integrated patterns of human behavior that include the language, thoughts, communications, actions, customs, beliefs, values, and institutions of racial, ethnic, religious, or social groups" (U.S. Department of Health and Human Services, Office of Minority Health, 2005). Four culturally determined attributes important to consider for substance use and risky sexual behavior for ethnic minority students attending middle school are (1) age, (2) ethnicity, (3) gender, and (4) the middle school context.

The period of early adolescence is a risk factor for the initiation of substance use and sexual activity. Alcohol and tobacco are gateway substances that are initiated during early adolescence. For example, 7th and 8th grades, when most youth are 13–14 years old, are peak years for the initiation of drinking with forty percent of youth having consumed alcohol by 8th grade (Faden, 2006; Wu et al., 2010). In terms of sexual activity, a milestone during this developmental period is puberty which is accompanied by an awareness of self as a sexual being. Early puberty is a risk factor for problem behaviors, especially when youth reside in low resource communities (Obeidallah, Brennan, Brooks-Gunn, & Earls, 2004).

The initiation of substance use and sexual behavior varies across ethnic groups. The initial use of gateway substances such as alcohol and tobacco occurs earlier for White and Native American youth than it does for African American and Asian youth (Faden, 2006; Wu et al., 2010). However, the 2009 Centers for Disease Control and Prevention (CDC) National Youth Risk Behavior Survey (2010) found that early sexual initiation, sex prior to the age of 13, occurs at greater rates for African American and Hispanic youth than for White youth. Approximately 15% of Black students nationwide have had sexual intercourse before the age of 13, compared to 6.7% for Hispanics and 3.4% for White students.

Gender is also an important consideration as the motivation for engaging or not engaging in substance use and sexual behavior may differ for boys and girls. For example, there is a higher incidence of alcohol abuse among boys than among girls (Biglan, Brennan, Foster, & Holder, 2004; National Research Council and Institute of Medicine, 2009) and substance abuse develops more rapidly in boys (National Research Council and Institute of Medicine, 2009). However, a history of early victimization has a particularly negative impact on girls, resulting in increased substance use in middle school, increased alcohol use in high school (Biglan et al., 2004; Wright, Friedrich, Clinq-Mars, Cyr, & McDuff, 2004), and risky sexual practices (Wright et al., 2004).

A final cultural attribute to be considered is the school context. With the move to middle school come additional stressors and exposure to negative as well as positive peer influences. Peers have substantial influence on youth substance use and sexual behavior during this period and youth who affiliate with substance using and sexually active peers will use more substances and engage in more sexual risk than those who do not (Farrell & White, 1998; Reinherz, Giaconia, Hauf, Wasserman, & Paradis, 2000).

The school environment, including policies, can also influence risk and protective factors for youth. Schools with clearly articulated guidelines that enforce substance use infractions and that address substance and sex education as components of regular curricula provide a protective school environment. These schools would also have mechanisms to support positive academic and social development of youth, especially those with family, individual, and community risk. Biglan et al. (2004) argue for strengthening the protective power associated with a supportive school environment.

Prevention Programming in Schools

The school can be a good context in which to intervene because prevention interventions can take advantage of a captive audience. Additionally, the school environment provides a context in which peer norms can be changed, and peers can be used to promote prosocial and responsible behaviors. Prevention interventions must provide youth with the necessary knowledge base and skills with which to resist risky and unhealthy behavior along with the skills necessary to engage in safe, healthy, and prosocial behaviors. Interventions that simultaneously target risk factors and promote protective factors should be more effective than those that target a singular risk factor or problem behavior. In addition, preventive interventions that support positive youth development must address risks for both substance use and early sexual involvement before these problems surface and/or before they become serious problems.

Key Components of Effective Prevention Programs. Effective intervention programs share several common components: they are theory driven, of sufficient duration, responsive to the targeted population's needs, and address specific risk and protective factors while targeting specific behaviors (CDC, 2008; Nation et al., 2003; Wagner, Tubman, & Gil, 2004). Bukoski (2006) reported that good substance abuse prevention strategies, in addition to encompassing the above components, also focus on all forms of substance use, provide skill development on resistance, support commitment to avoid substance use, develop social competency, and foster negative attitudes toward substance use. Whereas, effective sex education programs should also address issues of contraceptive use, especially the use of condoms for youth who choose to become sexually active (Kirby, Laris, & Rolleri, 2006).

Examples of Universally Effective Substance Abuse Prevention Programs

There are some effective school-based prevention programs that do not include culturally specific adaptations but have been found to be effective with ethnically diverse middle school students. The following are examples of programs that have empirical support for their effectiveness with ethnically diverse youth. This list is not exhaustive, and a more complete list of substance abuse prevention programs is available in the Substance Abuse and Mental Health Services Administration's (SAMHSA) National Registry of Evidence-based Programs and Practices website.

- *Life Skills Training*, developed by Botvin and colleagues, has over 30 published studies on its effectiveness. It has been shown to work effectively with African American, Hispanic, and White youth. This program provides education on personal self-management, general social skills, and social resistance skills, along with substance refusal skills. The 35 core lessons in the curriculum are implemented throughout the 6–8th grade years (Botvin & Griffin, 2004).
- *Across Ages* is a generational mentorship program that pairs at-risk youth with an elder mentor (ages 55 years old and older) from the community to provide support. Mentors are matched to specific students and are expected to spend at least 2-hours per week with their mentee.

The youth must also participate in weekly community service, attend problem-solving skills classes, and engage in positive weekend activities with their family and their mentor.

- *Lion's Quest Skills for Adolescence* is designed to enhance youth's relationships within their families, school, and communities by becoming good citizens. It targets youth ages 10–14 years and engages them in community service, social skills training, as well as provides lessons designed to increase attitudes consistent with a substance-free lifestyle. In addition to addressing risk factors related to attitudes and behaviors, these programs also tend to focus on positive youth development and provide opportunities for youth to engage in activities that strengthen positive peer interactions as well as establish relationships with their communities and/or families which are protective factors against risky behavior.

Cultural Considerations in Prevention Programming

Cultural components that may be important for prevention programming include attending to ethnic identity and specific gender issues and needs. Kirby and colleagues (2006), in their review of effective sex education programs, found that programs that were responsive to youth's culture, age, and sexual experience were more effective interventions than those that did not attend to these elements.

Gender Issues. Programming for girls is likely to be effective if it considers their relational needs and the fact that substance use and risky sex usually occur within the context of close and intimate relationships (Belgrave, 2009). Prevention programming for all girls should consider their social and supportive networks and provide opportunities for positive relationships to develop and strengthen. These relationships might occur among girls or between girls and female adult staff. Prevention programming for boys should pay particular attention to whether or not they have a history of childhood behavioral problems.

For example, boys with a history of poor behavior control and disruptive behaviors are more likely to initiate and use substances during adolescence (Fallu et al., 2010). These boys are also more likely to affiliate with delinquent peers, another risk factor for substance use and other problem behaviors.

Ethnic Identity. Ethnic identity is a self-identification with a specific ethnic group and a sense of belonging and attachment to this group; it includes perceptions, behaviors, and feelings one has due to such membership; and involvement in the cultural and social practices of the group (Phinney & Kohatsu, 1997). The findings from several studies have shown that ethnic identity is directly and indirectly associated with lowered substance use and antisubstance attitudes, and less early and risky sexual attitudes and behavior among ethnic minority youth (e.g., Belgrave et al., 1994; Belgrave, Brome, & Hampton, 2002; Belgrave, Marín, & Chambers, 2000; Burlew et al., 2000; Corneille & Belgrave, 2007; Marsiglia, Kulis, & Hecht, 2001; Townsend & Belgrave, 2000). Ethnic identity may indirectly impact substance use and sex behaviors by enhancing prosocial adaptive behaviors and attitudes. For example, ethnic identity has been associated with higher academic achievement (Smith, Walker, Fields, Brookins, & Seay, 1999; Wong, Eccles, & Sameroff, 2003), more adaptive coping skills (Greig, 2003; Roberts et al., 1999), and higher psychosocial competence (Carter, DeSole, Sicalides, & Glass, 1997). Therefore, prevention interventions for ethnically diverse youth should consider using strategies that increase ethnic identity.

Cultural Competence in Service Provision. To deliver effective culturally sensitive programs, particular attention should be paid to cultural competence. Cultural competence consists of congruent behaviors, attitudes, practices, and policies that come together in a system, agency, or among professionals and enables that system, agency, or those professionals to work effectively in cross-cultural situations. Cultural competence facilitates culturally appropriate prevention and treatment strategies that are (1) based on the cultural values of the targeted group, (2) reflect the subjective cultural characteristics of members of the targeted group, and (3) reflect the behavioral preferences and expectations of members of the group (Marín, 2003). Terms that have been used to describe culturally competent programs are culturally sensitive, culturally tailored, culturally specific, culturally integrated, and culturally adapted.

Kumpfer, Alvarado, Smith, and Bellamy (2002) distinguish between intervention programs that are culturally sensitive and those that are culturally integrated. Culturally sensitive programs may make minor modifications to universal programs. These programs, for example, may ethnically match staff and program participants, and use videos and materials that reflect the ethnicity of participants. On the other hand, culturally tailored and culturally integrated programs consider core values and experiences that affect how individuals respond to and participate in the program. These programs would consider not only the content or what is presented, but the format and the ways in which information is presented and learned.

Culturally Specific Substance Abuse Prevention Programs

Several culturally sensitive programs for youth in middle school exist. Below are examples of programs that have published empirical evidence that they have a positive impact on youth's knowledge, intent to use, and use of a variety of substances, and reduce risky sexual behavior.

- *Hip Hop 2 Prevent Substance Abuse and HIV* (H2P; Turner-Musa, Rhodes, Harper, & Quinton, 2008). H2P has been used primarily with African American youth and targets youth ages 12–16. The program is designed to teach students to avoid substance use and risky sexual behavior, increase positive parent–child interactions, and increase constructive use of extracurricular time. It utilizes the hip hop culture to teach youth about substance use and HIV risk and has as its foundation the cultural competence model proposed by Resnicow, Soler, Braithwaite, Ahluwailia, and Butler (2000). This model highlights the importance of cultural sensitivity of program staff. Staff members are trained to understand the unique culture and needs of adolescents who are more inclined to respond to both the positive and negative messages in hip hop culture. The program provides information about substance use, HIV/AIDS, life skills training and counseling, and helps students become more involved in their communities. The program is delivered in ten 2-hour modules. School staff members are actively involved in providing the first four modules of the program. The remaining module includes a H2P camp that involves a three-day retreat where youth are engaged in interactive activities. This program is an example of a culturally tailored intervention that targets both substance use and sexual activity.
- *Project Venture* (Carter, Straits, & Hall, 2007). This program was developed for Native American youth in grades 5–8. It combines classroom instruction with outdoor experiential learning and community service. Project Venture utilizes Native American values that emphasize family, nature, spirituality, and service to others. Venture uses stories as metaphors for life skills development that is congruent with Native American culture and has a rites of passage component which builds on traditional ceremonial coming of age activities. While the program does not specifically focus on substance use, it encourages youth to develop a positive self-concept, effective social and communication skills, positive peer relationships, a community service ethic, self-efficacy, and sound decision-making and problem-solving skills. These skills can translate into a generalized resilience which can then be applied to resist the use of alcohol, tobacco, and other substances and promote related positive youth development outcomes (Carter et al., 2007). This program is highlighted because it targets risk and protective factors that should have spillover effects for increasing resiliency and decreasing risk.
- *Storytelling for Empowerment*. This program was developed for economically disadvantaged

Latino/Latina youth, ages 13–17 years old, at risk for substance abuse, HIV, and other negative behaviors. It has also been used with Native American youth. The program focuses on increasing the resiliency of youth to decrease the likelihood of substance use. It addresses the risk factors related to the presence of negative role models in the lives of the youth and the lack of positive cultural role models. It does this through the use of a Storytelling PowerBook that has 27 lessons which focus on Knowledge Power—understanding the brain and the physiological impact of substances, Skill Power—developing skills to make better decisions, Personal Power—multicultural lessons including symbol making that is more significant in Native American and Hispanic cultures, Character Power—historical figures and characteristics from the youth's culture, Culture Power—understanding their culture and subcultures, and Future Power—identification of positive role models in their community as well as development of goals for the future. The lessons are designed to be implemented over a 3-month period (Nelson & Arthur, 2003). This program is highlighted because it targets substance abuse reduction while simultaneously strengthening cultural pride, identity and attributes, as well as overall resiliency.

Promising and Empirically Supported Sex Education Programs

Sex Education programs typically focus on reducing risk through avoidance, increasing use of condoms and contraceptives, monogamy, and decreasing the number of sexual partners. Several governmental agencies have identified effective and promising programs for sex education (Advocates for Youth as cited by McKeon, 2006; U.S. Department of Health and Human Services, Office of Adolescent Health, The National Campaign to Prevent Teen and Unplanned Pregnancy, 2007) based on evaluation data demonstrating positive outcomes. Described below are three culturally responsive programs shown to be effective with ethnic minority middle school students.

Making Proud Choices. This program was originally developed for African American youth, ages 11–13, living in the inner city and from low-income families, to decrease their risk for pregnancy, HIV, and other STDs. However, it has also been found to be effective with Hispanic and Caucasian youth. The eight one-hour modules focus on teaching youth to abstain from sex or to engage in safe sex, specifically through the use of condoms. The program utilizes culturally sensitive videos, role plays, and games to help youth relate to program content. Youth participate in group discussions, practice problem solving and negotiation skills, as well as observe condom use demonstrations. There are four main goals of the program: (1) increasing youth's focus on their future and the impact unsafe sex could have on their choices; (2) increasing knowledge of STDs, HIV, and pregnancy; (3) changing attitudes and beliefs; and (4) developing refusal skills. This program is provided as an example of a culturally responsive program that can be implemented with diverse ethnic groups.

Reach For Health Community Youth Service (RFH CYS). This program combines health education with community service to prevent youth from engaging in high-risk sexual behavior (O'Donnell et al., 2002). It targets urban, African American, Hispanic, and socioeconomically disadvantaged at-risk seventh and eighth-grade students and is delivered in health education classes over 30 weeks. The curriculum is based on research that highlights gender- and cultural-based reasons for unhealthy sexual behavior. The curriculum has four classroom interactive lessons that are delivered during health education classes. The lessons revolve around four themes: protection of self and community well-being, responsibility for self and others, interdependence, and affirmation of positive behaviors. The program also includes a field placement where students spend two to three hours each week of the academic year in a service learning project. Youth who participate in this program are more likely to delay sexual initiation, increase condom and contraception use, and reduce the frequency of sexual activity (O'Donnell et al., 2002). This program is highlighted because it provides a good illustration of a comprehensive sex education program implemented within a classroom setting with a community component.

¡Cuídate! "Cuidate" translates to "taking care of yourself" and is a program developed for Latino/a youth ages 13–18. It utilizes the values of familialism (importance of family) and gender role expectations that are important in the Latino/a culture and uses these values to promote safe sex and thereby decrease youth risk for HIV. It is typically presented in an afterschool setting and uses six one-hour modules that can be delivered over two days. The program uses interactive, age appropriate activities that focus on education about safe sex, development of positive attitudes supporting safe sex behaviors, development of refusal and negotiation skills, and effective condom use. The program emphasizes cultural values that support safe sex (e.g., familialism: importance of family and taking care self for the family) and reinterprets values that may be perceived as barriers to safe sex (e.g., machismo or male dominance is reinterpreted to indicate that the male should protect and take care of his loved ones by engaging in safe sex). This program is a good example of a program that targets one cultural group by attending to the core values of this group and pays specific attention to gender issues that affect risky sexual behavior.

In Sum

Overall, we found few substance abuse prevention programs are specifically tailored for girls regardless of ethnicity. While girls may have lower risks for substance abuse problems, when these problems occur, they may have more severe negative outcomes (U.S. Department of Health and Human Services, 2001, 1998). Additionally, risk and protective factors are different for girls and boys and programs that target both are not always effective. In the review of effective programs provided by the National Campaign for Preventing Teen Pregnancy (1999), there were significantly more culturally sensitive sex education programs that were effective for boys than for girls in the middle school years.

Also worthy of note is that existing effective substance abuse prevention programs appear to target those populations that are more at risk for substance use during adolescence. Yet, it is important to address these issues for youth populations who might be at greater risk later in life. Of particular note is the paucity of empirically supported substance abuse programs in the literature specifically tailored to African American youth in middle school. This may be related to the lower incidence of substance use and abuse among African American youth (SAMHSA, 2010). However, given the increased risk of negative outcomes later in life (U.S. Department of Health and Human Services, 2001), early prevention is certainly warranted. In contrast to the absence of culturally specific substance abuse prevention for African American youth, there appear to be a plethora of sex education programs for this population. This, again, may reflect the higher prevalence of sexual activity, pregnancy, and HIV in this population (CDC, 2010). Given that African American and Hispanic girls have higher rates of teen pregnancy than their Caucasian counterparts, more programs need to address their unique sex education needs. In the section following, the *Sisters of Nia* program is described as an example of a program that specifically addresses the needs of African American girls and integrates a cultural curriculum with substance abuse and sex education curricula.

A Culturally Integrated Sex Education and Substance Prevention Program

With funding from the SAMHSA, Belgrave and colleagues developed and implemented a culturally integrated sex and substance abuse education program for African American middle school girls (Belgrave, Cherry, Butler, & Townsend, 2008). The program includes cultural features and components of two evidence-based curricula that address sex and substance use risk. The overall goal of the integrated program was to increase substance and sexual refusal efficacy and to increase positive cultural attributes, such as ethnic identity, body image, and specific gender role beliefs. The program encompasses: (1) a cultural curriculum—Sisters of Nia (Belgrave et al., 2008) to strengthen ethnic pride, gender role beliefs, and positive relationships; (2) an HIV prevention curriculum—Be Proud! Be Responsible (Jemmott, Jemmott, & McCaffree, 1995) to reduce sex and HIV risk; and (3) a substance prevention curriculum—Botvin's Life Skills Training (Botvin & Griffin, 2004) to increase substance refusal efficacy and to prevent and/or delay substance use. The program includes 17 sessions, approximately 90 minutes long that are held after school in both school and non-school settings.

Three hundred and eleven girls, 186 in the intervention group and 125 in the comparison group, participated in a grant-funded project. Participants at each intervention site were organized in small groups of six to ten participants. These small groups were facilitated by two young adult African American women. These women were referred to as 'mzees' which is a Swahili term for respected adult. Sessions began with a group ritual (i.e., giving thanks, acknowledging ancestors) where all girls and staff formed a unity circle. This was followed by participants going to their respective smaller groups to discuss the topic of the day. Session topics included: (1) orientation; (2) self-image; (3) self-image - media influence; (4) self-image: healing the hurt; (5) introduction to Africa and African culture; (6) Africa and African culture; (7) self-improvement: personal hygiene; (8) healthy relationships; (9) dating: deciding who to date; (10) healthy decisions; (11) negotiation and assertiveness in relationships; (12) sexual myths and responsibility; (13) introduction to HIV/AIDS; (14) vulnerability to HIV/AIDS; (15) smoking/marijuana/alcohol; (16) alcohol; and (17) ceremony and wrap-up. Guest speakers, team building and experiential activities, and videos were frequently used to provide variety and to enhance session topics. The last session of the program was a recognition ceremony during which girls were recognized for their achievement in becoming a "Sister of Nia." Parents, teachers, and others from the school and community were invited to this ceremony.

In both format and content, this program was culturally responsive to the age, gender, ethnicity, and life context of African American girls. For example, a relational and interdependent method of instruction was used whereby girls learn from each other and from an adult female role model in small group contexts. Activities were also interactive, engaging, and age appropriate. For example, in the personal hygiene session, girls discussed and experimented with hair and makeup, and for some sessions, natural care professionals and cosmetologists were invited speakers. Session topics focused on issues relevant particularly to girls (e.g., self-image) and being African Americans (e.g., Africa). Preliminary results indicate that girls who participated in the intervention reported higher ethnic pride, a higher satisfaction with their body shape and facial features, more instrumental gender role beliefs, and more positive relational and prosocial behavior, as well as more positive interpersonal relationships. Participants also reported having higher levels of efficacy regarding safer sexual communication. There were no improvements in substance use in part because the students reported very low levels of substance use at both pre- and post-test.

Implications and Conclusions

Culturally-specific and developmentally appropriate substance abuse and risky sexual behavior prevention programs are important for ensuring and promoting school mental health. The culturally sensitive programs described in our review all have the necessary components of an effective prevention program identified by the CDC (2008) earlier in the chapter (theory based, skill development, specific goals, etc.). The majority of the programs also identify specific cultural issues that are salient for the targeted population and integrate them into program content. However, Resnicow and colleagues, in a review of issues relevant to increasing cultural sensitivity in prevention programs for substance use, indicate that despite the fact that there are differences in initiation and risk factors for subgroups of youth, there is little research investigating how different racial/ethnic groups respond to different aspects of prevention programs. For example, do culturally sensitive programs that emphasize core values of specific populations work equally well with acculturated youth? Will these programs work as effectively with multiracial youth? These are questions with few available answers. It is also important to note that some universal programs are not as effective with all cultural groups. What distinguishes these programs from others that are less effective? While the field has clearly made progress, much more research is needed.

Our review of culturally responsive substance abuse and sex education programs for middle school students suggests key implications for future efforts to develop and implement such programs. Firstly, culturally responsive programs should move beyond surface level changes, such as changing the demographics of program staff and having program materials that reflect the culture of the participants, toward more culturally integrated programming where cultural matters are embedded in the context, values and unique issues pertinent to culturally diverse youth. For example, many of the cultural issues targeted by the programs, described in previous sections of this chapter, revolve around individual and cultural identity and the importance of both self and community. Four of the six identified programs have a strong community involvement element emphasizing the interconnectedness of youth to their social environments. As such, future programs for ethnic minority youth might emphasize communal and relational values by using interdependent instructional methods.

Secondly, culturally responsive programs must also address the social and environmental context in which students live. Students from urban communities may have different risk and protective factors than those from rural communities. Effective programs would also recognize the interdependence of relationships within families and communities and include these systems in prevention programming. A community service project would be one such example (e.g., students could paint an anti-drug mural on a building in the community). These programs would also strengthen cultural identity and include lessons relevant to their cultural group and the ways in which drug use and risky sexual practices negatively impact not only the youth but their families and communities.

At the policy level, substance abuse and sex education targeting the middle school years appears to be ideal to prevent the initiation of substance use and risky sexual behavior. Yet, school districts vary considerably from state to state and also within states in the degree to which programs are implemented as well as in the quality of the programs they offer. It would be optimal if each school district had a committee charged with recommending programs that were responsive to the cultural make-up of students and the socio-environmental context in which students and their families live.

For culturally tailored programs, a significant issue is the lack of research and an evidence base demonstrating their effectiveness. Even in a review of the programs listed by the National Registry of Evidence-based Programs and Practices by SAMHSA, there are limitations in the methodological quality of some of these programs. For example, some programs lack valid and reliable measurements and/or appropriate control conditions. As such, promising programs need additional data from multiple school settings with different youth groups to further strengthen our knowledge of the impact of these efforts.

In conclusion, several evidence-based programs are available that target substance use and sexual activity among middle school students. However, more are needed that promote overall positive youth development that will address both substance use and sexual risk and even more that target both in culturally responsive ways. We need to understand culturally diverse youth needs and to further develop appropriate methods to integrate cultural components into effective programming to address their unique needs.

References

Belgrave, F. Z. (2009). African American Girls: Reframing Perceptions and Changing Experiences London/New York: Springer.

Belgrave, F. Z., Brome, D. R., & Hampton, C. (2000). The contribution of afrocentric values and racial identity to the prediction of drug knowledge, attitudes, and use among African American youth. *Journal of Black Psychology, 26*(4), 386–401.

Belgrave, F. Z., Cherry, V., Butler, D., & Townsend, T. (2008). *Sisters of Nia: An Empowerment Cultural Curriculum for African American Girls.* Champaign, IL: Research Press.

Belgrave, F. Z., Cherry, V. R., Cunningham, D., Walwyn, S., Letdaka-Rennert, K., & Phillips, F. (1994). The influence of Africentric values, self-esteem, and black identity on drug attitudes among African American fifth graders: A preliminary study. *Journal of Black Psychology, 20*(2), 143–156.

Belgrave, F. Z., Marín, B. V., & Chambers, D. B. (2000). Culture, contextual, and intrapersonal predictors of risky sexual attitudes among urban African American girls in early adolescence. *Cultural Diversity and Ethnic Minority Psychology, 6*(3), 309–322.

Biglan, A., Brennan, P. A., Foster, S. L., & Holder, H. D. (2004). *Helping adolescents at risk: prevention of multiple problem behaviors.* New York: The Guildford Press.

Botvin, G. J., & Griffin, K. W. (2004). Life Skills Training: Empirical findings and future directions. *Journal of Primary Prevention, 25*(2), 211–232.

Brookmeyer, K. A., & Henrich, C. C. (2009). Disentangling adolescent pathways of sexual risk taking. *Journal of Primary Prevention, 30*(6), 677–696.

Bukoski, W. J. (2006). *Handbook of drug abuse prevention.* New York: Springer US.

Burlew, K., Neely, D., Johnson, C., Hucks, T. C., Purnell, B., Butler, J., Lovett, M., & Burlew, R. (2000). Drug attitudes, racial identity, and alcohol use among African American adolescents. *Journal of Black Psychology, 26*(4), 402–420.

Carter, R. T., DeSole, L., Sicalides, E. I., & Glass, K. (1997). Black racial identity and psychosocial competence: A preliminary study. *Journal of Black Psychology, 23*(1), 58–73.

Carter, S. L., Straits, J. E., & Hall, M. (2007). Project Venture: Evaluation of a positive, culture-based approach to substance abuse prevention with American Indian youth. Technical Report. The National Indian Youth Leadership Project. Gallup, NM.

Centers for Disease Control and Prevention. (2010). Youth Risk Behavior Surveillance-United States, 2009. Surveillance Summaries, SS-5. Morbidity and Mortality Weekly Report, 59.

Centers for Disease Control and Prevention, National Center for Chronic Disease Prevention and Health Promotion (2008). *Characteristics of an effective health education curriculum.* Retrieved from http://www.cdc.gov/HealthyYouth/SHER/characteristics/index.htm

Corneille, M. A., & Belgrave, F. Z. (2007). Ethnic identity, neighborhood risk, and adolescent drug and sex attitudes and refusal efficacy: The urban African American girls' experience. *Journal of Drug Education, 37*(2), 177–190.

Doherty, E. E., Green, K. M., & Ensminger, M. E. (2008). Investigating the long-term influence of adolescent delinquency on drug use initiation. *Drug and Alcohol Dependence, 93*(1-2), 72–84.

Faden, V. B. (2006). Trends in initiation of alcohol use in the United States 1975-2003. *Alcoholism: Clinical and Experimental Research, 30*(6), 1011–1022.

Fallu, J. S., Janosz, M., Brière, F. N., Descheneaux, A., Vitaro, F., Tremblay, R. E. (2010). Preventing disruptive boys from becoming heavy substance users during adolescence: A longitudinal study of familial and peer-related protective factors. *Addictive Behaviors, 35*(12), 1074–1082.

Farrell, A. D., & White, K. S. (1998). Peer influences and drug use among urban adolescents: Family structure and parent-adolescent relationships as protective factors. *Journal of Consulting and Clinical Psychology, 66*, 248–258.

Greig, R. (2003). Ethnic identity development: Implications for mental health in African-American and Hispanic adolescents. *Issues in Mental Health Nursing, 24*(3), 317–331.

Hawkins, J. D., Catalano, R. F., & Miller, J. Y. (1992). Risk and protective factors for alcohol and other drug problems in adolescence and early adulthood: Implications for substance abuse prevention. *Psychological Bulletin, 112*(1), 64–105.

Hogan, J., Gabrielsen, K., Luna, N., & Grothaus, D. (2002). *Substance abuse prevention: the intersection of science and practice.* Boston: Allyn & Bacon.

Jemmott L. S., Jemmott J. B. III, & McCaffree, K. (1995). *Be Proud! Be Responsible! Strategies to empower youth to reduce their risk for AIDS.* New York: Select Media Publications.

Jessor, R., & Jessor, S. L. (1977). *Problem behavior and psychosocial development: a longitudinal study of youth.* New York: Academic Press.

Kirby, D., Laris, B. A., & Rolleri, L. (2006). *Sex and HIV education programs for youth: Their impact and important characteristics.* Research Park, NC: ETR Associates.

Kirby, D. & Lepore, G. (2007). Sexual risk and protective factors: Factors affecting teen sexual behavior, pregnancy, childbearing and sexually transmitted disease: Which are important? Which can you change? ETR Associates. Retrieved on July 1, 2011 from http://www.teenpregnancy.ncdhhs.gov/docs/rfa/RiskProtectiveFactors-FullReport.pdf

Kumpfer, K. L., Alvarado, R., Smith, P., & Bellamy, N. (2002). Cultural sensitivity and adaptation in family-based prevention interventions. *Prevention Science, 3*(3), 241–246.

Marín, B. V. (2003). HIV prevention in the Hispanic community: Sex, culture, and empowerment. *Journal of Transcultural Nursing, 14*(3), 186–192.

Marsiglia, F. F., Kulis, S., & Hecht, M. L. (2001). Ethnic labels and ethnic identity as predictors of drug use among middle school students in the Southwest. *Journal of Research on Adolescence, 11*(1), 21–48.

McKeon, B. (2006). Advocates for Youth: Effective sex education. Retrieved from http://www.advocatesforyouth.org/storage/advfy/documents/fssexcur.pdf

Middlebrooks, J. S., & Audage, N. C. (2008). The Effects of Childhood Stress on Health Across the Lifespan. Atlanta (GA): Centers for Disease Control and Prevention, National Center for Injury Prevention and Control.

Nation, M., Crusto, C., Wandersman, A., Kumpfer, K. L., Seybolt, D., Morrissey-Kane, E., & Davino, K. (2003). What works in prevention: Principles of effective prevention programs. *American Psychologist, 5*(6-7), 449–456.

National Registry of Evidence-based Programs and Practices. (2011). Retrieved from http://nrepp.samhsa.gov/

National Research Council and Institute of Medicine. (2009). *Preventing mental, emotional, and behavioral disorders among young people: progress and possibilities.* Committee on the Prevention of Mental Disorders and Substance Abuse Among Children, Youth, and Young Adults: Research Advances and Promising Interventions. M.E. O'Connell, T. Boat, and K.E. Warner, Editors. Board on Children, Youth, and Families, Division of Behavioral and Social Sciences and Education. Washington, DC: The National Academies Press.

Nelson, A. & Arthur, B. (2003). Storytelling for empowerment: Decreasing at-risk youth's alcohol and marijuana use. *Journal of Primary Prevention, 24*(2), 169–180.

Obeidallah, D., Brennan, R. T., Brooks-Gunn, J., & Earls, F. (2004). Links between pubertal timing and neighborhood contexts: Implications for girls' violent behavior. *Journal of the American Academy of Child & Adolescent Psychiatry, 43*(12), 1460–1468.

O'Donnell, L., Stueve, A., O'Donnell, C., Duran, R., San Doval, A., Wilson, R. F., Haber, D., Perry, E., & Pleck, J. H. (2002). Long-term reductions in sexual initiation and sexual activity among urban middle schoolers in the Reach for Health service learning program. *Journal of Adolescent Health, 31*(1), 93–100.

Office of Adolescent Health. (n.d.) Retrieved from http://www.hhs.gov/ash/oah/

Phinney, J., & Kohatsu, E. (1997). Ethnic and racial identity development and mental health. In J. Schulenberg, J. Maggs, & K. Hurrelman (Eds.), *Health risks and developmental transitions in adolescence* (pp. 420-443). New York: Cambridge University Press.

Reinherz, H. Z., Giaconia, R. M., Hauf, A. C., Wasserman, M. S., & Paradis, A. D. (2000). General and specific childhood risk factors for depression and drug disorders by early adulthood. *Journal of the American Academy of Child & Adolescent Psychiatry, 39*(2), 223–231.

Resnicow, K., Soler, R., Braithwaite, R. L., Ahluwalia, J. S., & Butler, J. (2000). Cultural sensitivity in substance use prevention. *Journal of Community Psychology, 28*(3), 271–290.

Roberts, R.E., Phinney, J.S., Masse, L.C., Chen, Y.R., Roberts, C.R., & Romero, A. (1999). The structure of ethnic identity of young adolescents from diverse ethnocultural groups. *The Journal of Early Adolescence, 19*(3), 301–322.

Smith E. P., Walker, K., Fields, L., Brookins, C. C., & Seay, R. C. (1999). Ethnic identity and its relationship to self-esteem, perceived efficacy and prosocial attitudes in early adolescence. *Journal of Adolescence, 22*(6), 867–880.

Substance Abuse and Mental Health Services Administration. (2010). *Results from the 2009 National Survey on Drug Use and Health: Volume I. Summary of National Findings* (Office of Applied Studies, NSDUH Series H-38A, HHS Publication No. SMA 10-4586Findings). Retrieved from http://oas.samhsa.gov/NSDUH/2k9NSDUH/2k9ResultsP.pdf

The National Campaign to Prevent Teen Pregnancy. (1999). *Get Organized: A Guide to Preventing Teen Pregnancy.* Washington, DC: Author.

The National Campaign to Prevent Teen and Unplanned Pregnancy. (2007). Emerging Answers. Retrieved from http://www.thenationalcampaign.org/ea2007/postitive_impact.pdf

Townsend, T. G., & Belgrave, F. Z. (2000). The impact of personal identity and racial identity on drug outcomes among African American children. *Journal of Black Psychology, 26*, 424–436.

Turner-Musa, J. O., Rhodes, W. A., Harper, P. T. H., & Quinton, S. L. (2008). Hip-hop to prevent substance use and HIV among African American youth: A preliminary investigation. *Journal of Drug Education, 38*(4), 351–365.

U.S. Department of Health and Human Services, Office of Minority Health. (2005). *What is cultural competency?* Retrieved July 10, 2011, from http://minorityhealth.hhs.gov/templates/browse.aspx?lvl=2&lvlID=11

U.S. Department of Health and Human Services. (2001). *Women and Smoking: A Report of the Surgeon General, 2001.* Atlanta, Georgia: U.S. Department of Health and Human Services, Centers for Disease Control and Prevention, National Center for Chronic Disease Prevention and Health Promotion, Office on Smoking and Health, 1998.

U.S. Department of Health and Human Services. *Tobacco Use Among U.S. Racial/Ethnic Minority Groups—African Americans, American Indians and Alaska Natives, Asian Americans and Pacific Islanders, and Hispanics: A Report of the Surgeon General.* Atlanta, Georgia: U.S. Department of Health and Human Services, Centers for Disease Control and Prevention, National

Center for Chronic Disease Prevention and Health Promotion, Office on Smoking and Health, 1998.

Wagner, E. F., Tubman, J. G., & Gil, A. G. (2004). Implementing school-based substance abuse interventions: Methodological dilemmas and recommended solutions. *Addiction, 99*(2), 106–119.

Wong, C. A., Eccles, J. S., & Sameroff, A. (2003). The influence of ethnic discrimination and ethnic identification on African American adolescents' school and socioemotional adjustment. *Journal of Personality, 71*(6), 1197–1232.

Wright, J., Friedrich, W., Clinq-Mars, C., Cyr, M., & McDuff, P. (2004). Self-destructive and delinquent behaviors of adolescent female victims of child sexual abuse: Rates and covariates in clinical and nonclinical samples. *Violence and Victims, 19*(6), 627–643.

Wu, J., Witkiewitz, K., McMahon, R. J., Dodge, K. A., & Conduct Problems Research Group. (2010). A parallel process growth mixture model of conduct problems and substance use with risky sexual behavior. *Drug and Alcohol Dependence, 111*(3), 207–214.

Promoting Culturally Competent Assessment in Schools

Toni Harris, Scott Graves, Zewelanji N. Serpell, and Brittney Pearson

Assessment as an informal and formal process has and continues to play a critical role in the school mental health of culturally diverse students. Performance evaluation, referral, and placement for needed mental health services all depend on the outcomes of an assessment process. Given the increasing number of students from diverse cultural backgrounds entering public school settings, less than 20% of public school teachers identifying as nonwhite (U.S. Department of Education 2006), and the fact that standard assessment tools continue to be based primarily on white middle class norms (Nisbett, 2009), cultural competence in assessment requires concerted effort. For assessment to effectively serve the needs of culturally diverse youth it must entail nonbiased tools and instruments, culturally responsive processes and policies, and implementation by culturally-competent people (Skiba, Knesting, & Bush, 2002). This chapter: (1) reviews work that suggests that a lack of culturally competent assessment practices threatens the mental health status of culturally diverse youth in schools; (2) examines how assessment is situated in the general discussion about increasing cultural competence in schools; and (3) describes existing models for promoting culturally competent assessment and, the benefits and challenges associated with their application.

Evidence of a Persistent Cultural Bias in School-Based Assessment

Assessment—particularly as it relates to school mental health—has a troublesome history and entails significant challenges in educational contexts. Assessment sits at the center of an ongoing debate about inequities in school settings, particularly the over- and under-representation and placement of racial and ethnic minority students in special education. Noted disparities in access to appropriate referral and services also suggest bias in school assessment (Fierros & Conroy, 2002; Zito, Safer, DosReis, & Riddle, 1998), including the overuse of suspension and expulsion with racial/ethnic minorities (Skiba et al., 2003, 2011).

Disproportional Rates of Placement in Special Education. The disproportionate representation of ethnic minorities, males, and children from low-income backgrounds in special education has been a problem since the inception of special education (Donovan & Cross, 2002). A comprehensive study of disproportionality conducted by a group of scholars under the auspices of the Harvard Civil Rights Project documented pervasive disproportionality in referral and placement,

T. Harris (✉) • Z.N. Serpell • B. Pearson
Virginia State University, Petersburg, VA, USA
e-mail: tsharris@vsu.edu

S. Graves
Duquesne University, Pittsburgh, PA, USA

and showed African American children to be almost three times as likely as Caucasian children to be labeled mentally retarded and almost twice as likely to be labeled emotionally disturbed (Parrish, 2002). According to a more recent report—the *Twenty-Eighth Annual Report to Congress on the Implementation of IDEIA* (2006)—African American and Latino students were, respectively, 1.42 and 1.15 times more likely to be placed in the Specific Learning Disability category. Furthermore, African Americans were 2.83 and 2.24 times more likely to be placed in Mental Retardation (MR) and Emotional Disturbance (ED) categories, respectively. African Americans had the highest risk for placement in MR and ED of all racial groups (U.S. Dept. of Education, 2006; Serpell, Hayling, Stevenson, & Kern, 2009).

Although it receives far less attention, underrepresentation in special education is also a serious problem. Underrepresentation across disability categories is evident for Latino children (Pérez, Skiba, & Chung, 2008). It is also well documented that African American and Latino children are underrepresented in Gifted and Talented programs (Ford, Grantham, & Whiting, 2008).

There is a strong sentiment among researchers that the issue of disproportional representation of particular groups in disability labels and placement is associated less with the instruments used to determine eligibility and more to do with the people administering them (Skiba et al., 2002). It is noteworthy that referrals of racial/ethnic minorities to special education classes targeted for students with emotional and behavioral problems have been shown to decrease when the number of African American teachers rises (Serwatka, Deering, & Grant, 1995).

Bias in Social–Emotional and Behavior Ratings. There is substantial evidence to indicate pervasive bias in social–emotional and behavior ratings (Skiba et al., 2002). Several studies document elevations in teacher ratings of impulsivity and hyperactivity among African American students (DuPaul et al., 1997; Epstein, March, Conners, & Jackson, 1998; Reid et al., 1998). However, many researchers have rejected the notion that African Americans have higher rates of behavioral issues and argue that the key factor is bias in assessment practices (Lambert et al., 2005; Muroff, Edelsohn, Joe, & Ford, 2008).

Researchers examining bias consistently document a relationship between the ethnicity of the informant and their perception of children's behavior (De Los Reyes & Kazdin, 2005). In general, African American students rated by same-race informants are rated significantly lower in terms of behavior problems than when rated by European American informants. European American teachers are more likely to rate the behaviors of African American children as evidence of externalizing disorders (Lau et al., 2004). They are also more likely to describe the behaviors as more serious and indicating a worse prognosis than are African American raters (Nguyen, Huang, Arganza, & Liao, 2007). This type of bias has been found in studies that use direct observation measures (Harvey et al., 2009), diagnostic interviews of parents (Hillemeier et al., 2007), and behavior rating scales completed by multiple informants (Achenbach, 2006). Discrepancies between teacher and parent ratings may reflect actual observed differences in behavior (e.g., disruptive behaviors exhibited at school but not at home), but much of the evidence suggests discrepancies are better explained by specific biases teacher raters have towards specific ethnic groups (Lambert, Puig, Lyubansky, Rowan, & Winfrey, 2001; Youngstrom, Loeber, & Stouthamer-Loeber, 2000).

Bias in Referral and Disciplinary Action. Skiba and colleagues have been documenting a long-standing discrepancy between ethnic minority youth and their Caucasian counterparts in the receipt of disciplinary action, nature of infractions that yield disciplinary action, as well as the severity of disciplinary measures for comparable behaviors. Their work shows that African American and Latino students are punished at higher rates, for more subjective and less serious behavioral infractions, and experience higher rates of expulsion and suspension than Caucasian students (Skiba et al., 2002, 2011). Minority youth within special education are also more likely than their Caucasian counterparts to experience more severe disciplinary action, such as corporal punishment, placement in restrictive settings, school suspension and expulsion (Osher, Woodruff, & Sims, 2002; Raffaelle Mendez, 2003; Skiba, Poloni-Staudinger, Gallini, Simmons, & Feggins-Azziz, 2006; Zito et al., 1998). Noteworthy is the fact that while African American students experience more severe punishments, their infractions are less serious (Skiba, Michael, Nardo, & Peterson, 2002, 2011). In sum, research in this area suggests that culturally diverse youth are more likely to be routed to a disciplinary track (office referral, suspension, and expulsion) than they are to be referred for evaluation and receipt of school-based services (Skiba et al., 2002).

Test Bias. The evidence for standardized tests being biased and contributing to overrepresentation and underrepresentation in special education is not especially strong (Skiba et al., 2002). However, there is a long-standing criticism leveled against behavioral scientists' indiscriminant use of diagnostic measures across ethnic groups without regard to measurement equivalence (Jones, 1996). According to Knight, Roosa, & Umana-Taylor (2009), measurement equivalence is important in making scientific inferences regarding developmental changes, developmental differences, as well as group differences. However, these inferences are subject to random measurement error because of the additional influence of a number of cultural factors, including ethnicity, socioeconomic status, urbanicity, and religiosity.

Evaluation of measure equivalence entails harnessing theory on the basic nature of the underlying construct in the population being studied. It is important to consider the possibility that the basic nature of the construct may be influenced by the developmental stage and other key characteristics of research participants. The scientific credibility of the inferences regarding assessment processes is seriously compromised by the absence of measurement equivalence among different demographic groups (see Knight, Roosa, & Umana-Taylor, 2009, for more detail). Underestimation/overestimation of the underlying construct (i.e., behavior problems), or differences in the accuracy with which the construct is assessed because of differences in the validity of the measure, may yield results that do not reflect the same degree, magnitude, or intensity of the assessed behavior across different groups.

A joint report by the American Educational Research Association, American Psychological Association, and National Council on Measurement in Education (1999) delineates standards for educational and psychological testing that includes a fairness code. This "code of fairness" applies to all uses of tests (admission, educational assessment, diagnosis, and placement) in educational contexts, and while not intended for teachers per se, includes guidelines they can use in their assessment practices. Test users are encouraged to examine existing evidence on the test's use among diverse groups. Users are encouraged to use this knowledge to assess whether performance differences may be attributed to factors not related to the skills being tested (Lane, Plake, Herman, Cook, & Worrell, 2010). Specific guidelines are as follows:

1. Use test design, development administration, and scoring procedures that minimize barriers to valid test interpretations for all individuals.
2. Conduct studies to examine the validity of test score inferences for the intended examinee population.
3. Provide appropriate accommodations to remove barriers to the accessibility of the construct measured by the assessment and to the valid interpretation of the assessment scores.
4. Guard against inappropriate interpretations, use, and/or unintended consequences of test results for individuals or subgroups.

Culturally Competent Practitioners

The President's New Freedom Commission report (2003) identifies cultural competence as the most promising vehicle for eliminating mental health care disparities. Teachers are in a unique position to facilitate access to evaluation, treatment through referral, and school-based services (Snider, Busch, & Arrowood, 2003). They are critical to the identification and amelioration of problems that can inhibit learning (Lambert et al., 2001), and improving their cultural competence has been identified as a critical mechanism through which to address achievement gaps and disproportionate rates of special education placement (Klotz & Canter, 2006). Skiba, Knesting, & Bush (2002) also contend that racial disparities in school discipline are most effectively addressed through the training of teachers in culturally competent classroom management practices.

Significant advances have been made to define and guide efforts toward cultural competence among practitioners serving culturally diverse youth. Cultural competence is now widely accepted as not just important, but as a critical component of all service provision in education and health contexts. As such, it is no longer considered an add-on, but an integral part of the work that psychologists, social workers, educators, and others involved with school mental health.

Policy. The National Association of School Psychology (NASP) and the American Psychological Association (APA) have published policy documents that specifically address cultural competence in assessment. NASP has a website (http://www.nasponline.org/resources/cultural-competence/index.aspx) that includes a wealth of regularly updated reading materials, slide presentations, references, and resources for understanding and implementing culturally competent assessment. APA's *Guidelines on Multicultural Education, Training, Research, Practice and Organization Change for Psychologists* (1992) is a comprehensive guide aimed at providing psychologists with the rational and need for addressing multiculturalism. Standard 2.04 of this code of ethics prompts practitioners to be diligent in their knowledge and awareness of the limitations of typical assessment methods, diagnostic and other standardized instruments, including the populations on which instruments are normed, issues of validity, and applicability across cultural groups. This document further recommends the use of this knowledge to exercise critical judgment when interpreting data derived from culturally diverse individuals.

Theoretical and Conceptual Frameworks. A number of frameworks and models have been developed to guide efforts toward culturally competent assessment. Ponterotto, Gretchen, and Chauhan (2001) propose that multicultural assessment entails a detailed consideration and assessment of client's cultural identity, along with clinicians' use of the multicultural counseling competencies framework which includes self-exploration and scrutiny for bias. The Center for School Mental Health (Cunningham et al., 2006) recommends an ethnocultural assessment approach that incorporates information about acculturation level, migration history of the family, and the salience of ethnicity with family and peers. Ortiz's (2004) Stage Model of Nondiscriminatory Assessment provides the most comprehensive set of guidelines about how to effectively assess children whose first language is not English. A major premise of the model is that if the learning ecology is not carefully examined, the likelihood that children will be identified as deficient and disabled increases. As such, this model prioritizes consideration of the child's learning ecology prior to seeking an internal explanation when children do not perform to their optimal potential.

Other models emphasize the implementation of a culturally responsive assessment process. For example, the Multicultural Assessment Procedure (MAP; Ridley, Li, & Hill, 1998) includes a four-phase process, beginning with an interview to collect data pertinent to establishing the client's cultural background and ending with a more "typical" assessment process that includes psychological testing and the use of the DSM. The authors note that to minimize bias, it is critical for clinicians to recognize how they and the tools they use contribute to bias, as well as how client's characteristics may impact their clinical judgment. Similarly, the Hierarchical Assessment Procedures described by Roysircar-Sodowsky and Kuo (2001) highlight the importance of rapport building, explaining the assessment process to clients, consulting professionals from the client's cultural group, and asking clients for feedback on results. It also advocates for multiple sources of information—including record reviews and family interviews.

On the whole, experts in the field of multicultural assessment agree that the following are key characteristics of culturally competent practitioners:

1. Recognize the limits of their skills, training and expertise when working with culturally diverse children and seek help to fill gaps or defer to others
2. Understand limits of the assessment instruments and procedures (validity and reliability) with diverse groups
3. Recognize linguistic barriers when client is bilingual and should interact in client's primary language
4. Understand and document in the client's records evidence of cultural and sociopolitical factors

(Quoted from Gopaul-McNicol & Armour-Thomas, 2002, p. 24)

Challenges to Implementing Culturally Competent Assessment

Case Example

Sean Jackson a 10-year-old 4th grader was referred to the school psychologist for an Emotional and Behavior Disorder (EBD) evaluation. According to Sean's teacher: he is constantly out of his seat, frequently aggressive in the classroom and on the playground (pushes other children), and often challenges his teachers during class.

Sean's mother was extremely surprised by the letter she received that stated Sean's teacher wanted him to be assessed and potentially placed into an EBD classroom. She indicated that Sean goes to Sunday school, he is a member of the youth choir, and he plays football for the neighborhood team. However, she agrees to have him evaluated by the school psychologist.

The school psychologist began Sean's evaluation by administering teacher and parent adaptive rating scales, a Wechsler Intelligence Scale for Children (WISC) IQ test, completing a review of his academic achievement records, and conducting teacher and parent interviews. Each of his teachers rating scales and interviews indicated he had adaptive behavior issues, while his IQ test score was in the average range. During the evaluation team meeting, there was not a consensus on whether Sean would qualify for EBD with the teachers and school psychologist being in favor, while the parent and school social worker were not. Consequently, the team recommended the school social worker gather additional information by conducting community interviews and thorough interview with Sean.

During the course of the social workers interview, Sean was asked about pushing other children, he stated, "Sometimes I get into it with my friends because they *test me*. In my neighborhood people will tease you, if you let them think you're *soft*." Sean also indicated that he questions his teachers sometimes because that's how his mother talks to him, "She tells me to always question things people tell you, that way you can find out the truth." After gathering this additional information, the team agreed that Sean should not be placed in EBD, but rather he should be given supports to facilitate a medium between his behavior and vocalizations that are protective in his home environment, but inhibitive during some portions of his school day.

From a cultural competence framework, it is important to recognize that assessment standards and preassessment considerations may be specific to particular cultural groups. While general frameworks are an excellent starting point for resources each ethnic group must be considered unique. Cultural competence has been defined as the integration and transformation of knowledge about individuals and groups of people into specific standards and policies used to increase the quality of services (Davis, 1997). This definition prioritizes translation of knowledge into practice.

It is very important to pay attention to the ways in which the experiences of racial/ethnic minorities are similar or distinct from those of majority youth (Johnson, Jaegar, Randolph et.al., 2003). Culturally diverse students bring skills and strengths into their learning environment that may differ from skills valued by European American middle class values, and these skills have developed within a context influenced by social position variables (e.g., race, social class, ethnicity, and gender), social stratification mechanisms (e.g., racism, discrimination, and prejudice), and segregation. A consideration of ecological contexts is therefore critical as the complex interactions of child, family, school, and neighborhood factors play a role in school mental health.

For ethnic minorities, racism and discrimination must be addressed, as these experiences are very closely tied to social functioning among these youth. Adolescents of color report experiencing at least one discriminatory act in the previous 12 months (Seaton, Caldwell, Sellers, & Jackson, 2008) and were more likely than their European American counterparts to experience discrimination from adults (Huynh & Fuligni, 2010). Perceived discrimination during adolescence has been shown to predict increased depressive symptoms, physical complaints, alienation, risky behaviors, and feelings of distress; and decreased self-esteem, life satisfaction, school engagement, and grades (Benner & Kim, 2009; Huynh & Fuligni, 2010; Seaton et al., 2008; Umana-Taylor, Updegraff, & Gonzales-Backen, 2011). In contrast, healthy adult/student relationships at school have been shown to contribute to positive self-esteem and lower rates of depression among students (Reddy, Rhodes, & Mulhall, 2003).

At the core of many racial/ethnic disparities in school mental health is cultural misunderstanding linked to experiences, beliefs, values, and related expectations. These misunderstandings lay the foundation for insipid biases that undermine the utility of assessment for culturally diverse youth. Differences in communication styles and racial/ethnic stereotypes may lead teachers to have different behavioral expectations for Latino and African American youth. Environments that are perceived by ethnic minority youth as hostile might yield negative/aggressive behavioral repertoires albeit adaptive ones (Stevenson, 2008). Further, adaptive behaviors in a child's neighborhood context may translate into a profound disconnect between culturally diverse students and their teachers (see Case Example above). It is essential that teachers are able to recognize when exhibited behaviors are indicative of an underlying dysfunction within an individual versus a reaction to the immediate social context.

Language Issues. Several factors should be considered when engaging culturally and linguistically diverse populations. It is critical that language and culture be considered inextricably linked. However, there is vast variation among Spanish speaking peoples and understanding that language is a mode of communication that extends beyond vocabulary is critical in the assessment process.

Meaningful Engagement of Families. In our work, we consistently find that one of the most critical parts of effective assessment is data gathering from families. In numerous circumstances, the integration of knowledge related to family circumstances and documentation of a student's strengths can reduce over-referrals and disproportional placement into special education maybe avoided. In the case example presented earlier, Sean's behaviors may have been indicative of a student who is generally placed in EBD classrooms, but an examination of his cultural background and ecological circumstances demonstrated that placement would have been inappropriate.

Teachers often believe that parents do not want to be involved (Kohl et al., 1994) — a belief shown to be particularly salient among teachers who are socioeconomically or culturally different from the parents of their students (Epstein & Dauber, 1991). Yet, it is paramount that teachers listen carefully to parents and children without judgment and, trust that parents often have the most insight and knowledge about the normality or abnormality of children's behaviors. Additionally, it is crucial that we know when to recommend assessments that will accurately reflect a child's cognitive abilities, even when that choice goes against what is standard practice. This requires cultural competence and is a type of training rarely provided to teachers, school counselors, and other school staff, although there are an increasing number of resources that help practitioners communicate with culturally diverse families (Chandler, A'Vant, & Graves, 2008; Clauss-Ehlers, 2006). There are also resources that guide practitioners to use culturally competent assessment methods to decrease disproportional identification and placement of different racial/ethnic groups

(Sullivan, A'Vant, Baker, Chandler, Graves, & McKinney et al., 2009).

Promising Assessment Approaches in School Mental Health

As the field moves forward, two approaches, School-Wide Positive Behavioral Interventions and Supports (SWPBIS) and Strength-Based Assessment, are emerging as strategies through which cultural competence in assessment can be achieved. School Wide Positive Behavioral Interventions and Supports (SWPBIS) is a proactive approach for addressing student behavior and is grounded in applied behavior analysis and empirically-based approaches to behavior management. This approach is a multitiered framework that offers a range of interventions that are systematically applied to students based on their demonstrated level of need (Cheney, Flower & Templeton, 2008). To be effective for all students, whole-school initiatives such as SWPBIS must be supported by culturally responsive practices when addressing learning and behavior (e.g., identifying specific interventions found to be effective for CLD groups). If this is done and SWPBIS is implemented comprehensively and with fidelity, SWPBIS could help reduce discipline problems in schools and the high number of emotionally disturbed certifications among African American students and improve the learning environment for all students. However, more research is needed to see the actual effect of these practices.

Strength-based assessment is the measurement of emotional and behavioral assets and characteristics that enhances an individual's sense of accomplishment and promotes their social and academic development (Epstein & Sharma, 1998). This type of assessment is in direct contrast to typical special education practices in which students' deficits are identified and are essential for determining special education eligibility. The exclusive focus on deficits is problematic for numerous reasons; it frequently results in less information being collected, which in turn, yields an incomplete view of children's ecological circumstances (Lambert et al., 2005). Consequently, researchers are beginning to focus on dual models of mental health that include strength-based measures as well as traditional measures (Suldo & Shaffer, 2008). This entails examining cultural constructs that are often left out of assessment processes, such as racial socialization, level of acculturation, and perception of racial climate (Serpell, Hayling, Stevenson, & Lee, 2010). Research that utilizes strength-based instruments such as the Behavioral Assessment for Children of African Heritage (BACAH) and the Behavior and Emotional Rating Scale-2 (BERS) is necessary to document the benefits of using a strength-based approach in comparison to traditional methodologies.

Conclusions

Assessment plays an important role in educational contexts, but more importantly, it has been identified as a critical point of intervention if racial/ethnic disparities in school mental health are to be adequately addressed. Research shows beliefs do not necessarily lead to particular practices; hence actualizing multicultural competence requires that practitioners move from knowledge, awareness, and sensitivity to actually implementing a different approach. Culturally competent assessment must include an explicit consideration of how worldview and family background might necessitate adjustments to the assessment process. Additionally, students' unique cultural values, experiences, and behavioral repertoires must be considered in tandem to beliefs and values inherent in the school system to help identify when behavioral issues are attributable to areas of disconnect. Culturally competent assessment is a delicate balance of identifying when cultural variables are operating: "when diversity is seen as extraneous to someone's personality, behavior is misidentified and mistakenly pathologized. Or if diversity becomes an exclusive focus, people of color are assumed to be similar, within-group differences are ignored, and behavior is misidentified and under pathologized" (Roysircar, 2005, p. 22). Culturally competent assessment begins and ends with an emphasis on the child—it embraces the perspective that the purpose of assessment is to ensure an appropriate match between the child's learning context and their learning needs—the focus being on finding ways to enable success, and not to label and sort children (Darling-Hammond, 2006).

References

Achenbach, T. M. (2006). As others see us: Clinical and research implications of cross-informant correlations for psychopathology. *Current Directions in Psychological Science, 15*, 94–98.

American Educational Research Association, American Psychological Association, & National Council on Measurement in Education. (1999). *Standards for educational and psychological testing*. Washington, DC: Author.

Benner, A. D., & Kim, S. Y. (2009). Experiences of discrimination among Chinese American Adolescent and the consequences for socioemotional and academic development. *Developmental Psychology, 45*, 1682–1694.

Chandler, D., A'Vant, E., & Graves, S. (2008). Effective communication with Black families and students. *Communiqué, 37*, Special Pull-out Section, 1–3. education. National Research Council. Committee on Minority Representation in Special Education. Washington, DC: National Academy Press.

Cheney, D., Flower, A., & Templeton, T. (2008). Applying response to intervention metrics in the social domain for students at risk of developing emotional or behavioral disorders. *The Journal of Special Education, 42*, 108–126.

Clauss-Ehlers (2006). *Diversity Training for Classroom Teaching: A Manual for Students and Educators*. New York City, NY: Springer Publishing.

Cunningham, D.L., Ozdemr, M., Summers, J., & Ghunney, A. (2006). Cultural Competence. Baltimore, MD: Center for School Mental Health Analysis and Action, Department of Psychiatry, University of Maryland School of Medicine. Retrieved from http://csmh.umaryland.edu/resources.html/Cultural CompetenceIB-CSMHA.pdf.

Darling-Hammond, L. (2006). Constructing 21st-century teacher education. *Journal of Teacher Education, 57*(3), 300–314.

De Los Reyes, A., & Kazdin, A. E. (2005). Informant discrepancies in the assessment of childhood psychopathology: A critical review, theoretical framework, and recommendations for further study. *Psychological Bulletin, 131*, 483–509.

Donovan, M. S., & Cross, C. T. (Eds). (2002). *Minority students in special and gifted education*. Washington, DC: National Academy Press.

Davis, K. (1997). *Exploring the intersection between cultural competency and managed behavioral health care policy: Implications for state and county mental health agencies*. Alexandria, VA: National Technical Assistance Center for State Mental Health Planning.

DuPaul, G. J., Anastopoulos, A. D., Power, T. J., Reid, R., Ikeda, M. J., & McGoey, K. E. (1997). Teacher ratings of attention-deficit/hyperactivity disorder symptoms: Factor structure and normative data. *Psychological Assessment, 9*, 436–444.

Epstein, J. L. & Dauber, S. L. (1991). School programs and teacher practices of parent involvement in inner-city elementary and middle schools. *Elementary School Journal, 91*, 289–305.

Epstein, M. H., & Sharma, H. M. (1998). Behavioral and Emotional Rating Scale: A strength based approach to assessment. Austin, TX: PRO-ED.

Epstein, J. N., March, J. S., Conners, K., & Jackson, D. L. (1998). Racial differences on the Conners teacher rating scale. *Journal of Abnormal Child Psychology, 26*, 109–118.

Fierros, E. G., & Conroy, J. W. (2002). Double jeopardy: An exploration of restrictiveness and race in special education. In D. J. Losen & G. Orfield. (Eds.), *Racial inequality in special education* (pp. 39–70). Cambridge, MA: Harvard Education Press.

Ford, D., Grantham, T., & Whiting, G. (2008). Culturally and linguistically diverse students in gifted education: Recruitment and retention issues. *Exceptional Children, 74*, 289–306.

Gopaul-McNicol, S., & Armour-Thomas, E. (2002). *Assessment and culture: Psychological tests with minority populations*. San Diego: Academic Press.

Harvey, E., Friedman-Weieneth, J., Miner, A., Bartolomei, R., Youngwirth, S., Hashim, R., & Arnold, D. (2009). The role of ethnicity in observers ratings of mother child behavior. *Developmental Psychology, 45*, 1497–1508.

Hillemeier, M. M., Foster, E. M., Heinrichs, B, & Heier, B. (2007). Racial differences in parental reports of attention-deficit/hyperactivity disorder behaviors. *Journal of Development and Behavioral Pediatrics, 28*, 353–361.

Huynh, V. W., & Fuligni, A. J. (2010). Discrimination hurts: The academic, psychological, and physical well-being of adolescents. *Journal of Research on Adolescence, 20*, 916–941.

Johnson, D., Jaeger, E., Randolph, S., Cauce, A., & Ward, J. (2003) Studying the effects of early child care experiences on the development of children of color in the United States: Toward a more inclusive research agenda, *Child Development, 74*, 1227–1244.

Jones, R. L. (Ed.). (1996). *Handbook of tests and measurements for Black populations* (1st ed.). Hampton, VA: Cobb & Henry.

Klotz, B., & Canter, A. (2006). Culturally competent assessment and consultation. Bethesda, MD: NASP Publications.

Knight, G. P., Roosa, M. W., & Umana-Taylor, A. J. (2009). *Studying ethnic minority and economically disadvantaged populations: Methodological challenges and best practices*. Washington, DC: American Psychological Association.

Knight, G. P., & Zerr, A. A. (2010). Informed theory and measurement equivalence in child development research. *Child Development Perspectives, 4*, 25–30.

Kohl, G. K., Weissberg, R.P., Reynolds, A.J., Kasprow, W. J. (1994). Teacher perceptions of parent involvement in urban elementary schools: Sociodemographic and school adjustment correlates. Paper presented at the annual meeting of the American Psychological Association, Los Angeles, C.A. Aug, 1994.

Lambert, M. C., Puig, M., Lyubansky, M., Rowan, G. T., & Winfrey, T. (2001). Adult perspectives on behavior and emotional problems in Black/African American children. *Journal of Black Psychology, 27*, 64–85.

Lambert, M. C., Rowan, G. T., Kim, S., Rowan, S. A., An, A. S., Kirsh, E. A., et al. (2005). Assessment of behavioral and emotional strengths in Black children: Development of the Behavioral Assessment for Children of African Heritage (BACAH). *Journal of Black Psychology, 31*, 321–351.

Lane, Plake, B., Herman, J., Cook, L. & Worrell, F. (2010). *Fairness in testing.* Paper presented at American Educational Research Association, Denver, CO.

Lau, A. S., Garland, A. F., Yeh, M., McCabe, K. M., Wood, P. A., & Hough, R. L. (2004). Race/ethnicity and inter-informant agreement in assessing adolescent psychopathology. *Journal of Emotional and Behavioral Disorders, 12*, 145–156.

Muroff, J., Edelsohn, G. A., Joe, S., & Ford, B. C. (2008). The role of race in diagnostic and disposition decision making in a pediatric psychiatric emergency service. *General Hospital Psychiatry, 30*, 269–276.

Nguyen, L., Huang, L. N., Arganza, G. F., & Liao, Q. (2007). The influence of race and ethnicity on psychiatric diagnosis and clinical characteristics of children and adolescents in children's services. *Cultural Diversity and Ethnic Minority Psychology, 13*, 18–25.

Nisbett, R. E. (2009). *Intelligence and how to get it: Why schools and cultures count.* New York, NY: W. W. Norton & Company.

Ortiz, S. (2004). *Comprehensive assessment of culturally and linguistically diverse students: a systematic, practical approach for nondiscriminatory assessment* Bethesda, MD: National Association of School Psychologists.

Osher, D., Woodruff, D., & Sims, A. E. (2002). Schools make a difference: The overrepresentation of African American youth in special education and the juvenile justice system. In D. Losen & G. Orfield (Eds.), *Racial inequity in special education* (pp. 93–116). Cambridge, MA: Harvard Education Publishing Group.

Parrish, T. (2002). Racial disparities in the identification, funding, and provision of special education. Schools make a difference: The overrepresentation of African American youth in special education and the Juvenile Justice System. In D. Losen & G. Orfield (Eds.), *Racial inequity in special education* (pp. 15–38). Cambridge, MA: Harvard Education Publishing.

Perez, B., Skiba, R. J., & Chung, C. (2008). Latino students and disproportionality in special education. Bloomington, IN: Center for Evaluation & Education Policy.

Ponterotto, J. G., Gretchen, D., & Chauhan, R. V. (2001). Cultural Identity and multicultural assessment: Quantitative and qualitative tools for the clinician. In L. A. Suzuki, J. G. Ponterotto, & P. J. Miller (Eds.), *Handbook of multicultural assessment: Clinical, psychological and educational practices* (2nd ed., pp. 67–99). San Francisco: Jossey-Bass.

Raffaele Mendez, L. M., & Knoff, H. M. (2003). Who gets suspended from school and why: Demographic analysis of schools and disciplinary infractions in a large school district. *Education and Treatment of Children, 26*, 30–51.

Reddy, R., Rhodes, J. E., & Mulhall, P. (2003). The influence of teacher support on student adjustment in the middle school years: A latent growth curve study. *Development & Psychopathology, 15*, 119–138.

Reid, R., DuPaul, G. J., Power, T. J., Anastopolous, A. D., Rogers-Adkinson, D., Noll, M. B., et al. (1998). Assessing cultural different students for attention deficit hyperactivity disorder using behavior rating scales. *Journal of Abnormal Child Psychology, 26*, 187–198.

Ridley, C. R., Li, L. C., & Hill, C. L. (1998). Multicultural assessment: Reexamination, reconceptualization, and practice application. *Counseling Psychologist, 26*, 810–827.

Roysircar-Sodowsky, G., & Kuo, P. Y. (2001). Determining cultural validity of personality assessment: Some guidelines. D. Pope-Davis & H. Coleman (Eds.), The intersection of race, class, & gender: Implications for multicultural counseling (pp. 213-239). Thousand Oaks, CA: SAGE.

Roysircar, G. (2005). Culturally sensitive assessment, diagnosis, and guidelines. In D. W. Sue (Ed.), *Strategies for building multicultural competence in mental health and educational settings* (pp. 19–38). Hoboken, NJ: Wiley.

The condition of education 2010. National Center for Education Statistics, Institute of Education Sciences, U.S. Department of Education, Washington, DC.

Seaton, E. K., Caldwell, C. H., Sellers, R. M., & Jackson, J. S. (2008). The prevalence of perceived discrimination among African American and Caribbean Black youth. *Developmental Psychology, 44*, 1288–1297.

Serpell, Z., Hayling, C., Stevenson, H., & Kern, L. (2009). Cultural considerations in the development of school-based interventions for African American adolescent boys with emotional and behavioral disorders. *Journal of Negro Education, 78*, 321–332.

Serwatka, T. S., Deering, S., & Grant, P. (1995). Disproportionate representation of African Americans in emotionally handicapped classes. *Journal of Black Studies, 25*, 492–506.

Skiba, R. J., Knesting, K., & Bush, L. D. (2002). Culturally competent assessment: More than non–biased tests. *Journal of Child and Family Studies, 11*(1), 61–78.

Skiba, R., Michael, R., Nardo, A., & Peterson, R. L. (2002). The color of discipline: Sources of racial and gender disproportionality in school punishment. *The Urban Review, 34*, 317–342.

Skiba, R. J., Poloni-Staudinger, L., Gallini, S., Simmons, A. B., & Feggins-Azziz, L. R. (2006). Disparate access: The disproportionality of African American students with disabilities across educational environments. *Exceptional Children, 72*, 411–424.

Skiba, R. J., Simmons, A. B., Staudinger, L. P., Rausch, M. K., Dow, G., & Feggins, L. R. (2003). Consistent removal: Contributions of school discipline to the school-prison pipeline. Paper presented at the Harvard Civil Rights Conference School-to-Prison Pipeline Conference, Cambridge, MA.

Skiba, R. J., Horner, R. H., Chung, C. G., Rausch, M. K., May, S. L., & Tobin, T. (2011). Race is not neutral: A national investigation of African American and Latino disproportionality in school discipline. *School Psychology Review, 40*, 85–107.

Snider, V. E., Busch, T., & Arrowood, L. (2003). Teacher knowledge of stimulant medication and ADHD. *Remedial and Special Education, 24*(1), 46–56.

Stevenson, H. C. (2008). Fluttering around the racial tension of trust: Proximal approaches to suspended Black student-teacher relationships. *School Psychology Review, 37*, 354–358.

Suldo, S. M., & Shaffer, E. J. (2008). Looking beyond psychopathology: The dual-factor model of mental health in youth. *School Psychology Review, 37*, 52–68.

Sullivan, A. L., A'Vant, E., Baker, J., Chandler, D., Graves, S., et al. (2009). Confronting inequity in special education: Understanding the problem of disproportionality: Part I. *NASP Communiqué, 38*(1), 1–16.

Umana-Taylor, A. J., Updegraff, K. A., & Gonzales-Backen, M. A. (2011). Mexican-origin adolescent mothers' stressors and psychosocial functioning: Examining ethnic identity affirmation and familism as moderators. *Journal of Youth and Adolescence, 40*, 140–157.

U.S. Department of Education, National Center for Education Statistics, (2006). *The Condition of Education* (NCES 2006-071). Washington, DC: U.S. Government Printing Office.

Youngstrom, E., Loeber, R., & Stouthamer-Loeber, M. (2000). Patterns and correlates of agreement between parent, teacher, and male adolescent ratings of externalizing and internalizing problems. *Journal of consulting and clinical psychology, 68*, 1038–1050.

Zito, J. M., Safer, D. J., DosReis, S., & Riddle, M. (1998). Racial disparity in psychotropic medications prescribed for youths with Medicaid insurance in Maryland. *Journal of the American Academy of Child and Adolescent Psychiatry, 37*, 179–184.

Work–Family Balance: Challenges and Advances for Families

17

Patricia M. Raskin

Introduction

The importance of understanding work–family issues for both public and private school personnel cannot be understated, as much of what goes on in and around schooling is mandated. Indeed, teachers and administrators do not have a lot of flexibility when it comes to the school day, and everyone who is involved with the school community as a whole is affected by these government regulations, whether they are at the local, state, or federal level.

The issues associated with work–family balance are not new; indeed, researchers and institutions have been thinking and writing about them since the mid-1960s (see, for example: Bailyn, 1978; Ginzerg, Ginsburg, Axelrad, & Herma, 1966). Since the mid-1980s, by which time more than 50% of mothers had entered the workforce, the issue of balance and work–family conflict had become considerably more salient; it has been studied by anthropologists, economists, demographers, sociologists, health, industrial-organizational, and developmental psychologists, to name a few, as well as by organizations seeking to reduce turnover, and those nonprofit institutions (such as Catalyst for Women) whose goal is to increase the number of women who reach higher managerial levels.

Further, demographers forecast an increasingly ethnically diverse population of men and women, who will have competing needs and responsibilities to care for their families. More than half of our workforce has to attend to family caregiving as well as work (Berkman & Glass, 2000). That is not to say that one has to be a parent to fit into the work–family paradigm. Everyone has a life outside of work, and there is no intent to suggest that only parents should be studied. Because the focus of this *Handbook* is on school mental health practitioners, however, this chapter is limited to a discussion of families with children and/or eldercare responsibility. It is also intended to inform school personnel, as everyone who works in education is also affected by work–family advantages and constraints.

Over the past three decades, women have experienced much success in the classroom as well as in industry, and nowhere is this progress more evident than in higher education. In the United States (U.S.) today, women now earn 62% of the associate's degrees, 57% of the bachelor's degrees, and 60% of the master's degrees awarded each year. In addition, approximately 50% of professional degrees and nearly 50% of PhDs are now given to women. This compares to 1970, when women earned fewer than 10% of professional degrees and PhDs in the United States (Mason, 2009). According to the Bureau of Labor Statistics, at age 22, 185 women have graduated

P.M. Raskin, Ph.D (✉)
Teachers College, Columbia University,
New York, NY, USA
e-mail: pmr12@columbia.edu

from college for every 100 men who have done so (Bureau of Labor Statistics, 2011).

Finally, according to the National Study of the Changing Workforce, for the first time since 1992, young women and young men do not differ in terms of their desire for jobs with greater responsibility (Galinsky, Aumann, & Bond, 2009). As a result, young women will likely be less prone to be the "accommodating" or "trailing" spouse in two-career couples, where they would place their career aspirations second to that of their husbands. Historically, young women, cognizant of both the professional obstacles they faced as well as needs and expectations related to childbearing and child rearing, were less likely to seek jobs with greater responsibility than their male counterparts. Today for the first time in recent history, it appears that this is no longer the case.

In part this is due to the highly unequal impact of the recession of 2008–2010 on men, who lost more than 70% of the 8 million total jobs lost in the United States. This disparity is also due in great measure to the industries that have been most affected by the recession—housing and construction, automotive, manufacturing, and financial services, which are typically male-dominated industries. By contrast, service industries and education, sectors where women have a stronger presence, were less adversely impacted by the recession. As we look to the future, of the 15 job categories projected to have the greatest growth rate in next decade, 12 are dominated by women (Boushey, 2009). We still do not know much, however, in part, because women's full-time participation in the workforce is so recent (Table 17.1).

As you can see, not much has changed in 30 years, but relative to the population as a whole, low-income women have less opportunity than they did. In part, these data reflect the upward trend in education. Fewer positions are available to individuals who have less than some posthigh school training. Manufacturing has decreased as well, so factory jobs have decreased significantly.

In Table 17.2, one can see that low- and middle-income families actually earn less than they did in the 1970s, both in actual dollars, and relative to their professional counterparts. Income increases are restricted to the professional class.

Table 17.1 Women in the Work Force

Stay-at-home married mothers, by family income, in the late 1970s and the late 2000s

	Low income (%)	Middle income (%)	Professional (%)
1977–1979	55	35	35
2006–2008	60	23	20

Source: Heather Boushey and Jeff Chapman's analysis of Miriam King, Steven Ruggles, Trent Alexander, Donna Leicach, and Matthew Sobek. Integrated Public Use Microdata Series, Current Population Survey: Version 2.0. (Machine-readable database). Minneapolis, MN: Minnesota Population Center (producer and distributor), 2009)

Table 17.2 Diverging Classes

Median family income by income, 1979 and 2008, 2008 dollars

	Low income ($)	Middle income ($)	Professional ($)
1979	26,709	74,244	137,547
2008	19,011	64,465	147,742

Source: Heather Boushey and Jeff Chapman's analysis of Miriam King, Steven Ruggles, Trent Alexander, Donna Leicach, and Matthew Sobek. Integrated Public Use Microdata Series, Current Population Survey: Version 2.0 Survey: Version 2.0. (Machine-readable database). Minneapolis, MN: Minnesota Population Center (producer and distributor), 2009

Differential Treatment at Work

Converging attitudes toward work do not result in undifferentiated treatment in the workplace. We know that employers see mothers and fathers as different from each other and from nonparents, to such a degree that we describe the effects as a "motherhood penalty" and "fatherhood bonus" (Blair-Loy, 2003; Harrington, Van Deusen, & Ladge, 2010). And yet, there is no evidence to suggest that mothers and fathers behave differently at work. Indeed, Kmec (2010) found that mothers and fathers were similar on 5 out of 7 pro-work dimensions and outperformed fathers on the other two. Nor does it mean that all working women are alike, despite the fact that they continue to hold most of the responsibility for their households (Bianchi, Robinson, & Milkie, 2006).

Although attitudes are changing in some quarters, gender has been a stable predictor of the division of labor when it comes to domestic and work responsibilities for many years. The system functions as a result of how we define our values about work, defining the ideal worker as one who takes no time for childbirth or childcare, whose commitment is first and foremost to the workplace. This view clashes with our equally held belief that children should be cared for by parents. Everyone in this system suffers: men, women, and children.

Williams (1999) documents that mothers remain economically marginalized, and points out that when mothers first marginalize and then divorce, their children often accompany them into poverty. Williams argues that designing workplaces around the bodies of men (who need no time off for childbearing) and men's life patterns (for women still do 80% of the child care) often constitutes discrimination against women. "Since women in the workforce aren't offered any special dispensation to raise their children or care for sick or elderly family members, they're forced to work part time, take pay cuts and sidetrack the progress of their work lives" (Harrington et al., 2010; Kornbluh & Homer, 2009, p. 2, Retrieved on 3/7/11). Gender is sometimes treated as a "one-size fits all" variable that describes biological, and therefore, parental differences.

Although in principle, work–family balance is not a gendered issue, in practice it is, as mores in the U.S. have not changed much since the Industrial Revolution. Indeed, Congress first passed the "living wage" law in 1938, based on the principle that men went to work and women stayed home to raise children and keep the household. In essence, this was the first legal acknowledgement that men should be wage earners, and women should engage solely in childcare. In a time of economic downturn, servants were no longer the norm, and it was in this same federal law that child labor was prohibited (Fair Labor Standards Act), meaning that children were at home after school. This principle still has force, despite evidence that for the most part, both American men and women are at work, work longer hours and more weeks/per year and that those women who are not at work are largely low-income part-time workers who would prefer to work more.

Low-wage workers. Nearly 1 in 5 rural Americans over the age of 25 were classified as low-wage workers in 2005. Typically what that means is not only do they earn less than higher paid workers, they also do not have access to benefits, nor control over their hours. When we generalize to all low-wage workers, we see that women are overrepresented (7 of the 11 million hourly workers who earned under $7.25/h are female), yet they account for a smaller share of all hourly workers. Minorities, particularly Hispanics, are also overrepresented in the low-wage group, as are nonnative workers. "Lack of meaningful input into work schedules and unpredictable and unstable work schedules can have a number of serious consequences for workers—including unstable child care, difficulty accessing job training and work supports, transportation problems, inability to hold down a second job, lost wages, and job loss" (Workplace Flexibility, 2010, Retrieved on 3/1/11). Low-income mothers, especially, suffer from role strain, irrespective of ethnicity (Morris & Coley, 2004).

Race and Ethnicity

Although there is little empirical research on the relationship between race and ethnicity in the U.S. and work–family balance, work–family issues are closely associated with class, which, in turn, overlap substantially with race. Culture also comes into play here in multiple ways, especially when it comes to childcare arrangements.

For example, sense of community and family (which varies widely among ethnic/racial groups in the U.S.) may be a differentiating factor. We have both quantitative and qualitative data to suggest that sense of community is considerably stronger in non-European Americans than in Americans of European descent. In a small study of 151 employees, 77 of whom were Nez Perce Indians, it was found that employees' sense of community and sense of control at work mediate the relationship among four personal/work factors (employees' ethnicity, family-sensitive supervision, the intrinsic value they place on their work, and work flexibility) and work–family role conflict (Clark, 2002). Clauss-Ehlers (2007) argues similarly, as do Pituc and Lee (2007) and Raskin (2006) who also found support for this data.

In a qualitative study of Asian women, there was some indirect corroboration for these findings: Researchers observed little work–family conflict as working was perceived as caring for the family in and of itself (Thein, Austen, Currie, & Lewin, 2010). The same conclusions were drawn for a Mexican sample of working women (Cavazos-Garza, 2011). The conclusion, however, has not been affirmed. There is little research directed particularly towards non-White families, and far more research is necessary to make the argument that social support accounts for a meaningful portion of the variance in either work or family circumstance variables (Zhang, 2011). Ethnic groups vary widely on other dimensions as well: length of time in the U.S., immigration status, the value placed on education, community safety, any and all of which can account for some variance in work–family balance.

Class

"The bottom 30% of American families try to get by on a median annual income of $19,000, earning less than $35,000 dollars a year. Their median income has fallen 29% since 1979 (in inflation adjusted dollars). These families get few benefits from their employers to help manage work-life conflict and often hold jobs with inconsistent or unpredictable schedules that exacerbate these conflicts. Government policies to help these families are too often inadequate and underfunded, and often critics of governmental support suggest that this is an individual rather than societal issue" (Williams & Boushey, 2010, p. ii). One of the biggest sources of work–family stress is either not knowing when you will have work during the week (e.g., unpredictable shift changes) or having to work during times that are at odds with the community as a whole.

Nonstandard work hours: "One in five employees in the United States works mostly at nonstandard times—during the evening, at night, or on rotating shifts and one in three works on the weekend. Despite their prevalence, nonstandard hour workers are remarkably invisible, remaining largely off the radar screen of policy-makers, unions, and other groups concerned with jobs, workers, and working conditions" (Gornick, Presser, & Batzdorf, 2009, p. 21). The nonstandard hour workforce is diverse, comprising white-, blue-, and pink-collar workers (semiskilled workers such as waitresses and construction workers), Whites and non-Whites, immigrants and nonimmigrants, and both part- and full-time workers. And, of course, the 24/7 work force includes both men and women—with men slightly more likely to work nonstandard hours (Kalil, Ziol-Guest, & Epstein, 2010).

Overall, women are not overrepresented among shift workers, full-time, full-week employment definitely has a greater effect on women. "Consumer demand for 24/7 access to services and retail has been driven in part by increases in women's—especially mothers'—employment". The increase in women's daytime employment has raised demand for services during evenings, nights, and weekends, because women are less able to shop or to purchase services during weekdays. In addition, the expansion of the United States' service economy has increased demand for employees to work during nonstandard hours, doing jobs such as waiting tables in restaurants—which are overwhelmingly held by women. Other factors contribute, too. The graying of the population has raised demand for around-the-clock medical and caregiving services, which are primarily staffed by women. Although not specific to women, technological and economic shifts have intensified globalized markets, pushing and pulling diverse commercial activities into 24-h schedules (Gornick et al., 2009, p. 21).

Increased mothers' employment is linked to rising nonstandard hour work in other ways as well. A substantial number of American workers with children organize their work lives so that two caregivers work different shifts. "This so-called "tag team" or "split shift" caregiving allows families to forgo out-of-home child care—which saves crucial dollars, especially during economic downturns.... Working atypical hours affects the temporal structure of family life, particularly among dual-earner couples and those with children, often compromising the quality and stability of marriages" (Gornick et al., 2009, p. 22). Further, nonstandard work hours reduce contact among family members, a factor associated with lower marital happiness, higher levels of conflict, and poorer family adjustment (Kalil et al., 2010). In addition, nonstandard work hours may have a negative impact on child development (Han & Waldfogel, 2007), even when they are predictable. Researchers have found unfavorable effects of increased maternal work hours on three of six outcomes: skipping school, performing above average, and parental contact about behavior problems. Adolescent-aged sons seem to be particularly sensitive to changes in mothers' hours of work (Crouter, Head, McHale, & Tucker, 2004; Gennetian, Lopoo, & London, 2008; Rapoport & Le Bourdais, 2008) and recent research suggests that when parents are not home in the evening, homework suffers, even when parental schedules are predictable.

Hall (2011) asks "Why are working mothers treated as one undifferentiated group? There are 16 million working mothers in the United States alone. What are the motivations, support networks and economic circumstances that drive their behaviors? Can segments be defined among these working mothers to create meaningful context for the choices that they make?" The founder and owner of "The Primary Dilemma, LLC," she identifies Working-Mother Methods: Each working mother has her own formula, but there are some shared approaches to the work–family juggle. This website was developed by the author based on her research on working mothers. *The Primary Dilemma.com* identifies 5 approaches and calls them Working-Mother Methods:

1. *Fully loaded*: She is a single parent, solely responsible for the balance of work and family. Among the more than 100 women who responded to the *Primary Dilemma* research, 10% were Fully Loaded. Of note, a higher percentage of respondents reported to be single mothers but acknowledged co-parenting with someone else.
2. *Workable*: She holds the primary career in her family. She spends more physical time working than she does in physical childcare. The Workable is enabled by someone else providing primary childcare. Of note, the Workable is highly engaged with her children emotionally. Among working mothers responding to the *Primary Dilemma* research, 22% identified themselves as a Workable.
3. *Equalizer*: She is actively engaged in work and parenting. She must carefully coordinate with an equally involved and accountable partner to share childcare and household responsibilities. Of women responding to *primary dilemma* research, 21% were Equalizers. This person has the opportunity to be a primary careerist and a primary parent, just not at the same time.
4. *Obliged*: She is the primary physical parent who also supplies a required second income. Of the women responding to the *Primary Dilemma* research, 24% identified as Obliged. This is a complicated method. Most of the childcare responsibility will fall on the shoulders of this person but there is also significant pressure on her job. The greatest dissatisfaction for work was expressed among survey respondents in this cohort. The dissatisfaction typically reflected inflexible work arrangements and an overall shortage of time.
5. *Parentess*: She is the primary physical parent, supplying a discretionary second income for her family. Among working mothers responding to the *Primary Dilemma* research, 22% identified themselves as Parentesses. Part-time or flexible work indexes are highest for this method. In addition, she acknowledges that her method may be transitional. She wants to keep her options open and does not want to opt out of work (Hall, 2011).

This nomenclature is one of many used to differentiate women in the labor force, capturing the kinds of circumstances, and in some case, choices, working women have. This recent research corroborates past scholarship, beginning in the late 1960s (Almquist & Angrist, 1970; Greenhaus, 1971) that catalogues how women manage work and home. One of the assumptions embedded in most of these taxonomies is that all women have choices. Coping strategies (Carver, Scheier, & Weintraub, 1989; Raskin, Kummel, & Bannister,

1998) are often seen as active decisions, but that is not necessarily the case. The correlation between income and choice has to be taken into account. Clearly, single mothers working nonstandard hours have far fewer options than married middle-class professionals.

For the most part, when we talk about work–family issues, we do so because of the huge shift of mothers' entry into the labor force, even when they have new babies. But fathers are changing too. Indeed, men are more likely than women to experience work–family conflict (Galinsky et al., 2009). In part, that may have to do with the fact that although some (not all) fathers are "ramping down" to have more time with their families, they tend to do so informally (Hewlett, 2007, p.137), and somewhat surreptitiously, in corporate cultures. During economic downturns, fathers are more likely to be actively involved at home, especially if moms are still at work. Nevertheless, more men are committed to actively parenting (Baird, 2010; Parker-Pope, 2010) and believe that it is a given that they will be present in their children's lives in a way that their fathers were not. There is little data on fathers' choices and almost none on single fathers, gay fathers, and non-White fathers (Roberts, 2010).

Childcare

The typical American middle-income family puts in an average of 11 more hours a week in 2006 than it did in 1979. Not only do American families work longer hours, but they do so with fewer laws to support working families.

One of our oldest legacies is our fierce attachment to "bootstrap" achievement—taking care of ourselves and our families, without assistance. Our debates between big and small government have an impact on childcare. We are the only developed country that does not subsidize parental leave for the care of newborns. More than178 countries guarantee paid parental leave, and 50 of those offer paid paternal as well as maternal leave (Human Rights Watch, 2011). Only the U.S. lacks paid maternity-leave laws among the 30 industrialized democracies in the Organization for Economic Cooperation and Development. Family leave available to Americans is unpaid, limited to 3 months, and covers about half the labor force. Discrimination against workers with family responsibilities, illegal throughout Europe, is forbidden only indirectly here, e.g., one has to sue to prove that discrimination. Americans also lack paid sick days, limits on mandatory overtime, the right to request work-time flexibility without retaliation, and proportional wages for part-time work. All of these supports exist elsewhere in the developed world (Williams & Boushey, 2010). The absence of societal support, the fact that Americans work more hours, and have fewer days off than any other developed countries, means that our attempts to balance work and family result in individual solutions rather than broad policy changes.

Work–family Crossover, Spillover, Overload, and Conflict

Although most married adults in the U.S. feel at least somewhat successful in balancing work and family (Milkie & Peltola, 1999), among parents, almost half report difficulty in balancing the two domains (Bellavia & Frone, 2005).

Crossover refers to "the process that occurs when the psychological well-being experienced by one person affects the level of well-being of another person" (Bakker, Westman, & Van Emmerik, 2009, p. 112). Researchers have found associations between anxiety, depression, and burnout when crossover is negative. But crossover may be positive as well: marital satisfaction, flow at work, and work engagement have been associated with positive crossover; some of these associations are related to the ability to take perspective (Bakker, Shimazu, Demerouti, Shimada, & Kawakami, 2011). In other words, the more we can take our family members' perspective on work and family, the less likely we are to experience work–family conflict.

Spillover can be positive or negative, and is defined as any aspect of work and family that extends into the other domain. When it is positive, the synergy can enhance beneficial effects for both the individual and the family (Beutell, 2010).

Work–family conflict is much higher in the United States than elsewhere in the developed world. One reason is that Americans work longer hours than workers in most other developed countries, including Japan, where there is a word, karoshi, for "death by overwork" (Keene & Quadagno, 2004; Milkie & Peltola, 1999; Moen, 2003). Other causes for conflict include lack of affordable childcare, inadequate family leave policies, inflexible work schedules, and feeling that one is not spending the "right" amount of time with children (Milkie, Kendig, Nomaguchi, & Denny, 2010).

Work–family conflict, however, is not defined only by the presence or absence thereof. It is bidirectional, i.e., conflict arising from work that interferes with family functioning, or conflict that arises from family that interferes with work functioning. There is a wealth of data to suggest that negative work–family associations are associated with stress, irrespective of the source of that conflict (Byron, 2005; Ford, Heinen, & Langkamer, 2007). Many of us make the assumption that work-to-family conflict is more prevalent. Yet prevalence is not a stand-in for importance.

Family-to-work conflict. The quintessential family-to-work conflict is one that arises when family members require more than usual care, as in the case of either child or adult disability (Jang & Appelbaum, 2010; Taylor et al., 2005). This kind of responsibility almost always falls on women (Baker & Drapela, 2010; Brandon, 2007; Crow & Florez, 2006; Leiter, Krauss, Anderson, & Wells, 2004, Parish, 2006) and tends to increase with time and age of dependent (Franklin, Ames, & King, 1994). Approximately 13% of children and adolescents in the United States have a special health care need (Van Dyck, Kohan, McPherson, Weissman, & Newacheck, 2004). Families with disabled children experience greater financial hardship (Kulthau, Smith Hill, Yucel, & Perrin, 2005), poorer mental health (Tliyen, Terres,Yazdgerdi, & Perrin, 1998), and increased stress (Sliver, Westbrook, & Stein, 1998).

Disability within the family is not, however, the only source of family-to-work conflict. Marital difficulties and domestic violence are other sources of work-to-family conflict, and they are much more likely to be unknown to others. Researchers have, however, investigated the quality of marital relationships (Byron, 2005), number and ages of children at home (Davis & Pirretti, 2008), and concluded that spousal support mitigates family-to-work conflict.

Work-to-family conflict (negative spillover) is the kind of conflict most workers think of when work–family conflict is described. Primarily, it is seen as a function of not enough time, or more specifically, not enough flexible time. For professionals, the expectation of 24/7 commitment to the job is increasing, and there is increasing work interference with family because of our global connectedness. Global employees are expected to be in touch, irrespective of time zone. Moreover, the willingness to put work ahead of family is essential to promotion in some occupations.

Interestingly, it is on this dimension that the highest paid professions and the lowest wage occupations are similar: low-wage nonstandard hour workers have little flexibility in their schedules, as do highly paid professionals whose commitment to the profession in one way organizations (accounting, financial services, and law firms for example) that make "up or out" promotion decisions. For someone who has invested more than a quarter of a million dollars in education, repaying debt plays a part in conforming to expectation. The antecedents of work–family conflict come from multiple sources and include individual differences such as demographic and personality variables, family issues, including marital quality, but any and/or all of these may play out at work, seeming to originate in the workplace.

Time, however, is not the only source of work-to-family conflict. There is some data to suggest that supervisor support is inversely related to the experience of work-to-family conflict (Major & Morganson, 2011; Raskin, 2006), and more specifically, that supervisors' interactions with low-income working mothers can spill over to mother–child interactions (Gassman-Pines, 2011).

Desrochers and Sargent (2003) have suggested that knowing that the boundaries between work and family are permeable permits us to articulate the following propositions:

- Keeping work and family separate makes it easier to manage work–family borders.
- Integrating work and family facilitates transitions between these domains.
- Either strategy can improve the well-being of employees, depending on the characteristics of employees (e.g., time management skills, being a "self starter," or social influence at home and work), the idiosyncratic meanings they attach to work and family (e.g., the extent to which they see these as similar roles), their preferences for integration versus segmentation, contextual factors (e.g., "family friendly" workplace norms and policies, long or irregular work hours, or social support from supervisors, coworkers, and family), and the fit between their preferences and the boundaries allowed by their social context. Positive spillover is defined as positive moods, skill sets, values, and behaviors that transfer from one role to another (Poelmans, Stepanova, & Masuda, 2008).

Work–Family Balance

The idea of balance is proving to be illusory. Rather, researchers and policy-makers are more likely to call the concept "juggling" or "coping" with the "time bind" (Hochschild, 1997) or "time famine" imposed by the demands of the separate domains of work and family. Although often defined as an individual's cognitive appraisal of the effects of the family domain on the work domain, or the effects of the work domain on the family domain (Voydanoff, 2005), the prevailing view on balance is that it is somewhat unlikely, especially in families with children. Nevertheless, feeling balanced is important across both work and family domains because that sense is associated with several well-being outcomes (Milkie et al., 2010), such as satisfaction with the amount of time parents feel they are spending with their children, and their subjective sense of how their children are doing psychologically.

Flexibility

By 1994, the Alfred P. Sloan Foundation had developed a program on Working Families, and since then, hundreds of grants have been awarded by that foundation. Over the course of the last 15 years, some consensus has emerged; as more and more women not only entered the workforce, but did so with the intent of remaining there and developing careers, it became clear that the model of "Three jobs, two people," i.e., each parent goes to work; the 3rd job is taking care of the family (Christensen & Schneider, 2010) does not work.

Among the consistent findings in recent research, it is evident that flexibility in all its forms (temporal, spatial, and project-based) can mitigate this dilemma somewhat (Hill, Hawkins, Ferris, & Weitzman, 2001), and that the more autonomy one has at work, the less work-to-family conflict there is. In the past decade, interest in work flexibility has become mainstream, and even the White House has called for the implementation of workplace flexibility policies (Workplace Flexibility, 2010).

But flexibility solutions do not seem particularly attractive to many men, nor to many career salient (Hall, 2011; Raskin, 2006) women. In some ways, this may be because of the premise that career-oriented men put work first, that they belong to their jobs and that responsibility for children and the household belongs to wives (the "ideal worker," (someone who works at least 40 h a week year-round) Williams, 1999). In the mid-1970s, in a study for Bell Labs identifying high potential managers, Bray, Campbell and Grant (1974) found that one of the differentiating characteristics between high-potential managers and nonhigh potential managers was their primary allegiance to work over family. In a follow-up study on Ginzberg, Ginsburg, Axelrad, and Herma's college-educated women, Yohalem (1978) obtained similar results (Fannin, 1981). Not much has changed. In a recent study of career-oriented women, young men and women did not differ substantially in their ambition: 47% of women 30 and younger describe themselves as "very ambitious," as compared to 62% of men (Hewlitt & Marshall, 2011). Child-bearing, however, can derail ambition in women. As Hewlitt and Marshall (2011) suggest, "Women are confronted with a choice that men simply don't have to make: to reach for the brass ring at great personal sacrifice, or to embrace marriage and parenthood at the expense of their dreams". There is a wealth of economic research to support that women's wages, relative to men's, have not increased since the early 1970s (Catalyst, 2011, Retrieved on 3/4/11 from www.Catalystwomen.org)—$.75/$1.00. That is, women continue to earn only $.75 for every $1.00 that men earn. This inequity compounds over time, and becomes part of the equation that sees women more likely than men to drift closer to poverty as they age.

Parental leave and flexibility are not gendered. Corporate policies put in place to assist with work–family balance are independent of gender and are in fact available not specifically to help families, but to increase productivity, attract and retain talented workers, reduce turnover and absenteeism, and increase profitability. Yet these policies are overwhelmingly used by women when they are used at all, not just to care for children, but also to give care to elders. When these corporate benefits are used, individual differences emerge. Employees who have fewer career ambitions or believe that they lack the skill sets to move up in an organization, and/or are unambivalently family oriented, and/or who earn lower wages who do not see opportunity in their organization, might see no reason to look like "the ideal worker." These data, however, hold only for large corporations. People who work in mid-size and smaller companies tend to negotiate flexibility considerably more informally. Raskin (2006) found that lower middle-class families were more likely to involve everyone in household responsibilities; as in many extended families, everybody worked and everybody contributed to domestic tasks and childcare. This finding has been corroborated in more recent research (Baird, 2010).

The definition of workplace flexibility varies; often researchers and policy-makers define it narrowly, in terms of hours at work. Workplace flexibility is one solution to actual "time binds," a phrase originated by Hochschild (1997). Hochschild (1997) was one of the first researchers to write about the scarcity of time and the need to allocate it among competing demands. According to some data, flextime policies are available to about 80% of working families. This 80% figure, however, is not universally accepted. According to the American Federation of Labor-Congress of Industrial Organizations (AFL-CIO), 75% of working adults say they have little or no control over their work schedules. Income accounts for much of the variance in this statistic: flextime is available to nearly 2/3 of those workers who earn more than $71,000 per year, but to less than 1/3 (31%) of working parents with annual incomes of less than $28,000. Flexibility is relative to other variables as well: industry, social class, age, career stage, and marital status.

For single, poor, underemployed women, flexibility is no solution, even when the institutions they work for offer that policy. In that a case, the absence of sufficient income takes precedence, and the dearth of childcare options complicate their lives to such a degree that flexibility does not usually come into play. Further, the current recession has had a huge effect on working families: job loss, unemployment, underemployment, the lack of healthcare and housing costs put the idea of balance on the back burner. According to Galinsky et al. (2009), workplace flexibility is not used to cut companies' costs; rather, employers are doing their best to show employees how important they are, even when profits have decreased. This finding is proving useful. As organizations become aware of the positive effect on the bottom line, more and more companies are putting options into place, and developing best practices for industry as a whole (Bond & Galinsky, 2008; Koblenz, 2003).

Due to technological advances and the availability of *telecommuting*, individuals are much more likely to work at home now than they have been since the beginning of the Industrial Revolution; many workers never meet their colleagues, especially those working in Information Technology (IT). In many managerial jobs at IBM, for instance, working means telecommuting, and, as virtual engagement becomes easier and of higher quality (see Cisco systems software, for example), meeting online means cost cutting for the company, and increased flexibility for the worker. There are costs, however, to virtual work, such as the loss of workplace camaraderie, and the drift toward work–family "bleed," i.e., the loss of clear boundaries between work and home, both in terms of time and physical space. According to a survey by the human resources group WorldatWork the number of Americans who work either from their homes or remotely at least 1 day a month rose by 74% between 2005 and 2008, to more than 17 million. If you add to that figure the so-called contract telecommuters—folks who are self-employed or run their own businesses—the number jumps to nearly 34 million people.

"Opting Out"

Even though the press has exaggerated the phenomenon of leaving careers to be stay-at-home mothers, some women do just that. Opting out is described as an upper middle-class choice for women with partners who earn a "living wage," i.e., enough of an income to take care of the family. Beneath the surface, however, is a less glamorous story. Some women leave the labor force because of the difficulty of combining paid and unpaid work (Kuperberg & Stone, 2008). It is a costly decision since returning to the labor market after childrearing years is precarious, even if a woman exits for as little as 2 years. It is unlikely that she will return to work in a similar capacity, that she will earn as much as she had been earning, or that she will advance in the career trajectory she was pursuing. Hewlett and Luce (2005) estimated that even a short break can result in a 30% decline in professional women's re-entry. But some women do leave their careers, in part because of economics.

Women who are married to men who work long hours and who also engage in more nonpaid work are more likely to exit the labor force than women who are married to men who work less than a 46 h/week. Further, women whose income is low in proportion to their husbands' may see their unpaid household work as contributing more to family well-being than the income they provide. Shafer (2011) points out that these findings reinforce gender stereotypes: since women earn less than men, they are more likely to earn less than their husbands, therefore are more like to leave the labor force, reinforcing the idea that women are not committed to their jobs. In addition, Shafer's findings reinforce the literature that suggests that wives make career sacrifices because of their husbands' career demands, even when their career ambitions are similar to their husbands.

Implications for School Mental Health Practitioners

The question now becomes: How do we as practitioners learn from the scholarship that has emerged in the last 15 years? What are the implications for those of us who work in schools with highly diverse populations? Once we get beyond the obvious, it is not so clear.

There are currently important *workplace effects on families and schooling.*

Rosen (2007) suggested that our inability to distribute work and family roles has resulted in a "care crisis." Parents who work may be dependent on others to drop off and pick up children, for instance, or to take care of them after school. As a result, this country's family policies lag far behind those of the rest of the world. A just-released study by researchers at Harvard and McGill found that of 173 countries studied, 168 guarantee paid maternal leave—with the United States joining Lesotho and Swaziland among the laggards. At least 145 countries mandate paid sick days for short- or long-term illnesses—but not the United States. "One hundred thirty-four countries legislate a maximum length for the workweek; not us" (Rosen, 2007, p.13).

After-school care is a genuine concern for many parents. More than 25% of America's schoolchildren are on their own after the school day ends and before parents get home from work. Despite our awareness that children are at particular risk at those times, the number of children who are left on their own has increased by more than a million in 5 years. Thirty percent of middle school children and 4% of elementary school students are unsupervised. These statistics vary somewhat by race/ethnicity. More Asian American, African American, Hispanic, and American Indian children are enrolled in after school programs, yet more than 20% of those ethnically diverse children have no adult presence after school. On average, children in self-care spend 8 h per week unsupervised and 45% of those children are from low-income households. Those who work nonstandard hours or have fluctuating schedules have an even harder time arranging affordable child care. It is estimated that over three million children between the ages of 6 and 12 are "latchkey kids" who are left to look after themselves after school while their parents are at work.

Parental after school stress results from aftercare concerns. There is some data to suggest that the worst time of the day for working parents is after school, when they are not sure of children's activities and/or whereabouts (Catalyst, 2006). Barnett, Gareis, Sabbatini, and Carter (2010) found that parents' long hours, lack of schedule control, and children's unsupervised time after school indeed predicted parental concerns and job disruptions, irrespective of gender.

Nutrition and exercise is influenced by work–family balance questions. The decrease in exercise and increase in obesity affects children all over the world. Conflicts between paid work and family life are likely to constitute some barriers for a physically active lifestyle and possibly also for healthy food habits. The U.S. culture has experienced profound changes over the last 40 years—the family structure and maternal employment has changed significantly since the 1960s. In 1960, only 9% of children lived in single-parent households. By 1998, that number rose to 27%. There has also been substantial growth in maternal employment, with 74% of mothers with children ages 6–17 being employed outside the household. This trend alone has implications on many areas of family life including fewer family meals, less time for meal preparation, and increased demand for convenience and prepared foods (Blake, Wethington, Farrell, Bisogni, & Devine, 2011).

In addition, longer work hours and distances to travel for work coupled with advances in technology can produce overall less physical activity for the entire family (Moag-Stahlberg, Miles, & Marcello, 2003). Blake et al. (2011) studied 50 Black, White, and Latino parents in upstate New York and found that having fewer family dinners was characterized by nonstandard work hours, having a working partner, single parenthood and with family meals away from home, grabbing quick food instead of a meal, using convenience entrées at home, and missing meals or individualized eating. Parents who cooked at home included considerably more married fathers with nonemployed spouses and more home-cooked family meals. Food-choice coping strategies affecting dietary quality reflect parents' work and family conditions.

It has been well documented that neither children nor adults get enough sleep in this 24/7 economy (Patlak, 2005). This is true worldwide. In theory, employed people spend about a third of their time at work and an equally long time asleep, but that seems to be less and less true (Lallukka, Rahkonen, Lahelma, & Arber, 2009). Too little sleep accounts for much of the variance in occupational accidents, especially in shift workers, in attention at school, on psychosocial job strain, marital quality, health-related issues, and in posttraumatic stress (e.g., Burgard & Ailshire, 2009; Frone, Russell, & Cooper, 1997; Knudsen, Ducharme, & Roman, 2007). Further, Maume, Sebastian, and Bardo (2010) found in a qualitative study that many women sacrifice sleep more than men do, defending the decision on the basis of husband as primary wage earner, even though these women are working as many hours as their husbands.

Military Families

"The work of war is very much a family affair" (Dao & Einhorn, 2010, p. A1). Approximately 43% of the Active Duty Force and 43% of the Selected Reserves have one or more children (DoD, 2006, p. 42, 96). More than a million U.S.

troops have been deployed to the Middle East since September 11, 2001, and the number of families with both parents in the military is up 35% from 2000 to 2007 (Nelson, 2010). Seventy-nine percent of all spouses say they and their soldier spouse have dependent children living with them and the soldier (U.S. Army Community and Family Support Center, 2005, p. 6.). Often, both parents deploy at the same time, and often not in the same place (Nelson, 2010). The active-duty military includes nearly 73,000 single parents, which equates to 5.3% of the total force, according to Defense Department statistics from 2008. The Army leads the way with more than 35,000 single parents, followed by the Navy with more than 16,000, and the Air Force with more.

The children of these families vary enormously in their capacity to adjust to parental deployment. They are more likely to report anxiety than children in civilian families, and the longer the deployment, the more difficulty children have in school and at home. In a qualitative study of adolescents from military families, Mmari, Bradshaw, Sudhinaraset, and Blum (2010) found that adolescents in military families were most worried about making frequent moves and having a parent deployed. The stronger the social support for both parents and teenagers, the more likely they were to make better adjustments. Bradshaw and her colleagues found that move-related stressors were associated with school adjustment (Bradshaw, Sudhinaraset, Mmari, & Blum, 2010).

The adjustment of the whole family to parental return from deployment is even more varied. It takes time to readjust, and often there are infants in the house that dad has never met. Children change, grow up, and even though they have missed their deployed parent, they can be reluctant to re-attach. Households change; the stay-at-home parent has taken charge, developed coping strategies that are not always easy to relinquish. Orthner and Rose (2005) reported that 47% of military spouses do not consider the adjustment easy. Of those who indicated difficulty, changes to soldier's personality/moods, restoring co-parenting, and communication with one another were considered most difficult.

Relevance to School Mental Health Professionals

Although there is little empirical data to support particular recommendations for school psychologists, we know enough from the work–family literature to draw some conclusions that most school personnel already know:

- More school children come from working families than from families who have one parent at home.
- Mothers may believe that teachers tend to connect children's academic achievements to their own involvement (Garey, 1999), i.e., in the United States, parents, especially mothers, tend to think that the more time they spend with parents, the better they are as parents.
- Finding the time and resources to communicate with these families is increasingly dependent on electronic access.
- Children who exhibit behavior problems are more likely to have parents whose careers are negatively affected by that family-to-work conflict.
- Negative work experiences reduce both quality of parenting and parent–child interaction, low parental self-efficacy, stress, burnout, and depressive symptoms in parents (Cinamon, Weisel, & Tzuk, 2007; Costigan, Cox, & Cauce, 2003; Franche et al., 2006; Grzywacz, Almeida, & McDonald, 2002; Innstrand, Langballe, Espnes, Falkum, & Aasland, 2008).
- In military families, both deployment and return from deployment can be stressful for children.
- Even with external support strategies in place, e.g., family-friendly policies at work, good childcare, challenges at work and at home can still occur.
- Working mothers may feel guilty for working, even when their income is necessary to the well-being of their families, despite the lack of evidence of poor child outcomes when both parents work.
- Stay-at-home mothers may be sacrificing their careers to be at home with their children, even though they feel it is the right decision.

Schools are often a stand-in for childcare, medical, and mental health care. Most of the time, we make the assumption, usually a good one, that parents want to be involved, and that they want to be in touch, that they believe that partnering with schools is a good thing. Further, the community the school provides can ease the burden on working parents by enabling social support—a key factor in work–family issues. As schools become technologically sophisticated, it becomes easier to be in touch with parents, even when they are at work. One of the keys to making the partnership successful is early communication: when teachers tell us that there may be a concern about a student, early intervention may sometimes be called for, and the sooner the parent is brought into the loop, the less stress the school places on the family. If parents are working long hours, it is sometimes difficult to schedule meetings with teachers and support staff. There is a fair amount of data to suggest that when children are having trouble in school, parents who do not have flexibility at work take sick days and vacation days to meet with school personnel—they risk their jobs for their families.

Conclusions

The more we know about the interactions between parents and their working worlds, the more equipped we are to provide school mental health practitioners the resources they need to engage in meaningful dialogue about students' needs and concerns, as well as those of the school. Ultimately, each family will have a unique set of circumstances, and these individual conditions affect and are affected by school policies and personnel. Of course, school mental health practitioners are members of families too and so constraints exist all around. Most parents want to do well by their children, and most schools want to do well by the families served by them. A willingness to be flexible, to respect individual circumstances and choices, creative use of available technology, and continued dialogue are more likely to result in good child outcomes than inflexible policies, procedures, and attitudes. To the extent that the school community can be a resource for the family as a whole, work–family issues need not be individual burdens, but rather situations and states of affairs that may be amenable to remediation. As Bass, Butler, Grzywacz, and Linney (2008) concluded, family life education programs can benefit families by identifying individual family resources and strengths. When schools and their personnel bring these resources together, they benefit the entire community.

References

Almquist, E. M., & Angrist, S. S. (1970). Career salience and atypicality of occupational choice among college women. *Journal of Marriage and the Family, 32,* 242–249.

Bailyn, L. (1978). Accommodation of work to family. In R. Rapoport & R. N. Rapoport (Eds.), *Working couples*. New York: Harper & Row.

Baird, J. (2010, April 8). Beyond the bad boys: A quiet revolution in male behavior. Retrieved March 11, 2011, from Newsweek.com.

Baker, D. L., & Drapela, L. A. (2010). Mostly the mother: Concentration of adverse employment effects on mothers of children with autism. *The Social Science Journal, 47,* 578–592.

Bakker, A. B., Shimazu, A., Demerouti, E., Shimada, K., & Kawakami, N. (2011). Crossover of work engagement among Japanese couples: Perspective taking by both partners. *Journal of Occupational Health Psychology, 16*(1), 112–125.

Bakker, A. B., Westman, M., & Van Emmerik, I. J. H. (2009). Advancements in crossover theory. *Journal of Managerial Psychology, 24,* 206–219.

Barnett, R. C., Gareis, K. C., Sabbatini, L., & Carter, N. M. (2010). Parental concerns about after-school time: Antecedents and correlates among dual-earner parents. *Journal of Family Issues, 31*(5), 606–625.

Bass, B. L., Butler, A. B., Grzywacz, J. G., & Linney, K. D. (2008). Work–family conflict and job satisfaction: Family resources as a buffer. *Journal of Family and Consumer Science, 100,* 24–30.

Bellavia, G. M., & Frone, M. R. (2005). Work –family conflict. In J. Barling, E. K. Kelloway, & M. R. Frone (Eds.), *Handbook of work stress* (pp. 113–148). Thousand Oaks, CA: Sage.

Berkman, L., & Glass, T. (2000). Social integration, social networks, social support, and health. In L. Berkman (Ed.), *Social epidemiology* (pp. 137–173). New York: Oxford University Press.

Beutell, N. (2010). The causes and consequences of work-family synergy: An empirical study in the United States. *International Journal of Management, 27*(3, Part 2), 650–664.

Bianchi, S. M., Robinson, J. P., & Milkie, M. A. (2006). *Changing rhythms of American family life.* New York: Russell Sage.

Blair-Loy, M. (2003). *Competing devotions: Career and family among women executives.* Cambridge, MA: Harvard University Press.

Blake, C. E., Wethington, E., Farrell, T. J., Bisogni, C. A., & Devine, C. M. (2011). Behavioral contexts, food-choice coping strategies, and dietary quality of a multi-ethnic sample of employed parents. *Journal of the American Dietetic Association, 111*, 401–407.

Bond, J., & Galinsky, E. (2008). *National study of the changing workforce.* New York: Families and Work Institute.

Boushey, H. (2009, October). The new breadwinners. In Maria Shriver and the Center for American Progress, *The Shriver report: A woman's nation changes everything* . Washington, DC: Center for American Progress.

Bradshaw, C. P., Sudhinaraset, M., Mmari, K., & Blum, R. W. (2010). School transitions among military adolescents: A qualitative study of stress and coping. *School Psychology Review, 19*(1), 84–105.

Brandon, P. (2007). Time away from "smelling the roses": Where do mothers raising children with disabilities find the time to work? *Social Science & Medicine, 65*, 667–679.

Bray, D. W., Campbell, R. J., & Grant, D. L. (1974). *Formative years in business: A long-term AT&T study of managerial lives.* Huntington, NY: R.E. Krieger.

Bureau of Labor Statistics (2011). *Women in the labor force,* 1970–2009, Washington, DC.

Burgard, S., & Ailshire, J. (2009). Putting work to bed: stressful experiences on the job and sleep quality. *Journal of Health and Social Behavior, 50*, 476–492.

Byron, K. (2005). A meta-analytic review of work-family conflict and its antecedents. *Journal of Vocational Behavior, 67*, 169–198.

Catalyst (2006). *After-school worries: Tough on parents, bad for business.* New York: Author.

Carver, C. S., Scheier, M. F., & Weintraub, J. K. (1989). Assessing coping strategies: A theoretically based approach. *Journal of Personality and Social Psychology, 56*, 267–283.

Cavazos-Garza, A. (2011). Work and family conflict: A comparison between American and Mexican women. *International Journal of Management and Marketing Research, 4*(1), 31–47.

Christensen, K., & Schneider, B. (2010). *Workplace flexibility: Realigning 20th-century jobs for a 21st-century workforce.* Ithaca, NY: ILR Press (an imprint of Cornell University Press).

Cinamon, G. R., Weisel, A., & Tzuk, K. (2007). Work family conflict within the family: Crossover effects, perceived parent child interaction quality, parental self-efficacy, and life role attributions. *Journal of Career Development, 34*, 79–100.

Clark, S. C. (2002). Employees' sense of community, sense of control, and work/family conflict in Native American Organizations. *Journal of Vocational Behavior, 61*(1), 92–108.

Clauss-Ehlers, C. S., (2007). Extending work-family concepts to the lives of Latinas. In Sweet, S., & Casey, J (Eds.), *Work and family encyclopedia.* Chestnut Hill, MA: Sloan Work and Family Research Network. Retrieved March 3, 2011, from http://wfnetwork.bc.edu/encyclopedia.

Costigan, C. L., Cox, M. J., & Cauce, A. M. (2003). Work–parenting linkages among dual-earner couples at the transition to parenthood. *Journal of Family Psychology, 17*, 397–408.

Crouter, A. C., Head, M. R., McHale, S. M., & Tucker, C. J. (2004). Family time and the psychosocial adjustment of adolescent siblings and their parents. *Journal of Marriage and the Family, 66*(1), 147–162.

Crow, T. K., & Florez, S. I. (2006). Time use of mothers with school-age children: A continuing impact of a child's disability. *American Journal of Occupational Therapy, 60*, 194–203.

Dao, J., & Einhorn, C. (2010, December 31). Families bear brunt of deployment strains. New York: *New York Times*, p. A1. SIRS Researcher.

Davis, K. D., Goodman, W. B., Pirretti, A. E., & Almeida, D. M. (2008). Nonstandard work schedules, perceived family well-being, and daily stressors. *Journal of Marriage and Family, 70*, 991–1003.

Desrochers, S., & Sargent, L. (2003) Boundary/border theory and work-family integration. In Raskin, P. M., & Pitt-Catsouphes, M. (Eds.), *Work and family encyclopedia.* Chestnut Hill, MA: Sloan Work and Family Research Network. Retrieved March 3, 2011, from http://wfnetwork.bc.edu/encyclopedia.

Ford, M. T., Heinen, B. A., & Langkamer, K. L. (2007). Work and family satisfaction and conflict: A meta-analysis of cross-domain relations. *Journal of Applied Psychology, 92*, 57–80.

Fannin, P. M. (1981, Summer). Essay review: The careers of professional women. *Teachers College Record, 82*(4), 689–693.

Franche, R.-L., Williams, A., Ibrahim, S., Grace, S. L., Mustard, C., Minore, B., et al. (2006). Path analysis of work conditions and work–family spillover as modifiable workplace factors associated with depressive symptomatology. *Stress and Health, 22*, 91–103.

Franklin, S. T., Ames, B. D., & King, S. (1994). Acquiring the family eldercare role: Influence on female employment adaptation. *Research on Aging, 16*(1), 27–42.

Frone, M. R., Russell, M., & Cooper, M. L. (1997). Relation of work-family conflict to health outcomes: A four-year longitudinal study of employed parents. *Journal of Occupational and Organizational Psychology, 70*, 235–335.

Galinsky, E., Aumann, K., & Bond, J. T. (2009). *NSCW 2008: Times are changing: Gender and generation at work and at home.* New York: Families and Work Institute.

Garey, A. (1999). *Weaving work and motherhood.* Philadelphia: Temple University Press.

Gassman-Pines, A. (2011). Associations of low-income working mothers' daily interactions with supervisors and mother-child interactions. *Journal of Marriage and the Family, 73*, 67–76.

Gennetian, L. A., Lopoo, L. M., & London, A. S. (2008). Maternal work hours and adolescents' school outcomes among low-income families in four urban counties. *Demography, 45*(1), 31–53.

Ginzerg, E., Ginsburg, S. W., Axelrad, S., & Herma, J. L. (1966). *Lifestyles of educated women*. New York: Columbia University Press.

Gornick, J. C., Presser, H. P., & Batzdorf, C. (2009). Outside the 9-to-5. *The American Prospect, 20*(5), 21–24.

Greenhaus, J. H. (1971). An investigation of the role of career salience in vocational behavior. *Journal of Vocational Behavior, 1*(3), 2009–2216.

Grzywacz, J. G., Almeida, D. M., & McDonald, D. A. (2002). Work–family spillover and daily reports of work and family stress in the adult labor force. *Family Relations, 51*, 28–36.

Hall, L. (2011) *The primary dilemma*. Retrieved February 16, 2011 from http://wfnetwork.bc.edu/blog/primary-dilemma-a-study-of-the-choices-working-mothers-make.

Han, W.-J., & Waldfogel, J. (2007). Parental work schedules, family process, and early adolescents' risky behavior. *Children and Youth Services Review, 29*, 1249–1266.

Harrington, B., Van Deusen, F., & Ladge, J. (2010). *The new dad: Exploring fatherhood within a career context*. Boston: Boston College Center for Work & Family.

Hewlett, S. A. (2007). *Off-ramps and on-ramps: Keeping talented women on the road to success*. Cambridge, MA: Harvard Business School Press.

Hewlett, S. A., & Luce, C. B. (2005, March). Off-ramps and on-ramps: Keeping talented women on the road to success. *Harvard Business Review*, pp. 43–54.

Hewlitt, S.A., & Marshall, M. (2011) Does female ambition require sacrifice? Retrieved February 28, 2011 from http://blogs.hbr.org/hbr/hewlett/2011/02/does_female_ambition_require_a.html.

Hill, E. J., Hawkins, A. J., Ferris, M., & Weitzman, M. (2001). Finding an extra day a week: The positive influence of perceived job flexibility on work and family life balance. *Family Relations, 50*(1), 49–58.

Hochschild, A. R. (1997). *The time bind: When work becomes home and home becomes work*. New York: Henry Holt.

Human Rights Watch (2011). *United States: Failing its families: Lack of paid leave and family supports in the US*. New York, NY.

Innstrand, S. T., Langballe, E. M., Espnes, G. A., Falkum, E., & Aasland, O. G. (2008). Positive and negative work–family interactions and burnout: A longitudinal study of reciprocal relations. *Work and Stress, 22*, 1–15.

Jang, S. J., & Appelbaum, E. (2010). Work-life balance in extraordinary circumstances. *Journal of Women, Politics & Policy, 31*, 313–333.

Kalil, A., Ziol-Guest, K. M., & Epstein, J. L. (2010). Nonstandard work and marital instability: Evidence from the National Longitudinal Survey of Youth. *Journal of Marriage and the Family, 72*, 1289–1300.

Keene, J. R., & Quadagno, J. (2004). Predictors of perceived work—Family balance: Gender difference or gender similarity? *Sociological Perspectives, 47*, 1–23.

Kmec, J. A. (2010). Are motherhood penalties and fatherhood bonuses warranted? Comparing pro-work behaviors and conditions of mothers, fathers, and non parents. *Social Science Research, 40*, 444–459.

Knudsen, H. K., Ducharme, L. J., & Roman, P. M. (2007). Job stress and poor sleep quality: Data from an American sample of full-time workers. *Social Science & Medicine, 64*, 1997–2007.

Koblenz, M. (2003). Ten best practices of companies that care. *Employment Relations Today, 30*(3), 1–7.

Kornbluh, K., Homer, R. (2009). Paycheck feminism: *Ms, 19*(4), 28. Retrieved March 7/SIRS.

Kulthau, K., Smith Hill, K., Yucel, R., & Perrin, J. (2005). Financial burden for families of children with special health care needs. *Maternal and Child Health Journal, 9*(2), 207–218.

Kuperberg, A., & Stone, P. (2008). The media depiction of women who opt out. *Gender and Society, 22*(4), 497–517.

Lallukka, T., Rahkonen, O., Lahelma, E., & Arber, S. (2009). Sleep complaints in middle-aged women and men: The contribution of working conditions and work-family conflicts. *Journal of Sleep Research, 19*, 466–477.

Leiter, V., Krauss, M. W., Anderson, B., & Wells, N. (2004). The consequences of caring: Effects of mothering a child with special needs. *Journal of Family Issues, 25*, 379–403.

Major, D. A., & Morganson, V. J. (2011). Coping with work-family conflict: A leader-member exchange perspective. *Journal of Occupational Health Psychology, 16*(1), 126–138.

Mason, M. A. (2009). Ask the expert: Patching America's leaky pipeline in the sciences. Center for American Progress. ret. 9/23/12.

Maume, D. J., Sebastian, R. A., & Bardo, A. R. (2010). Gender, work-family responsibilities, and sleep. *Gender and Society, 24*(6), 746–768.

Milkie, M. A., Kendig, S. M., Nomaguchi, K. M., & Denny, K. E. (2010). Time with children, children's well-being, and work-family balance among employed parents. *Journal of Marriage and the Family, 72*, 1329–1343.

Milkie, M. A., & Peltola, P. (1999). Playing all the roles: Gender and the work—Family balancing act. *Journal of Marriage and the Family, 61*, 476–490.

Mmari, K. N., Bradshaw, C. P., Sudhinaraset, M., & Blum, R. (2010). Exploring the role of social connectedness among military youth: Perceptions from youth, parents, and school personnel. *Child Youth Care Forum, 39*, 351–366.

Moag-Stahlberg, A., Miles, A., & Marcello, M. (2003). What kids say they do and what parents think kids are doing: The ADAF/Knowledge Networks 2003 Family nutrition and physical activity study. *Journal of the American Dietetic Association, 103*(11), 1541–1546.

Moen, P. (2003). *It's about time: Couples and careers.* Ithaca, NY: ILR Press.

Morris, J. E., & Coley, R. L. (2004). Maternal, family, and work correlates of role strain in low-income mothers. *Journal of Family Psychology, 18*(3), 424–432.

Nelson, M. (2010, July). When both parents serve, war takes a toll. *Pensacola News Journal (Pensacola, FL).* n.p. *SIRS Researcher.* Retrieved Feb. 28, 2011.

Orthner, D. K., & Rose, R. (2005). *SAF V survey report: Reunion adjustment among army civilian spouses with returned soldiers.* Chapel Hill, NC: University of North Carolina.

Parish, S. L. (2006). Juggling and struggling: A preliminary work-life study of mothers with adolescents who have developmental disabilities. *Mental Retardation, 44*, 393–404.

Parker-Pope, T. (2010). Now, Dad feels as stressed as mom. *New York Times,* June 19. Retrieved March 1, 2011.

Patlak, M. (2005). Your guide to healthy sleep. Washington, DC: U.S. Department of Health and Human Service. Retrieved March 12, 2011 from www.nhlbi.nih.gov/health/public/sleep/healthy_sleep.pdf.

Pituc, S. T., & Lee, S. J. (2007). Asian women and work-family issues. In Sweet, S., & Casey, J (Eds.), *Work and family encyclopedia.* Chestnut Hill, MA: Sloan Work and Family Research Network. Retrieved March 3, 2011, from http://wfnetwork.bc.edu/.

Poelmans, S., Stepanova, O., & Masuda, A. (2008). Positive spillover between personal and professional life: Definitions, antecedents, consequences, and strategies. In K. Korabik, D. S. Lero, & D. L. Whitehead (Eds.), *Handbook of work–Family integration* (pp. 141–156). Amsterdam: Elsevier.

Rapoport, B., & Le Bourdais, C. (2008). Parental time and working schedules. *Journal of Population Economics, 21*, 903–932.

Raskin, P. M. (2006). Women, work, and family: Three studies of roles and identity among working mothers. *American Behavioral Scientist, 49*, 1354–1381.

Raskin, P. M., Kummel, P., & Bannister, T. (1998). The relationship between coping styles, attachment, and career salience in partnered working women with children. *Journal of Career Assessment, 6*(4), 403–416.

Roberts, E. R., Jr. (2010). African American fathers and Afrocentric parenting—factors associated with parenting of their children. *ProQuest Dissertations and Theses, 0452* (2502).

Rosen, R. (2007). The care crisis. *Nation, 284*(10), 11–15.

Shafer, E. F. (2011). Wives' relative wages, husbands' paid work hours, and wives' labor-force exit. *Journal of Marriage and the Family, 73*, 250–263.

Sliver, E., Westbrook, L., & Stein, R. (1998). Relationship of parental psychological distress to consequences of chronic health conditions in children. *Journal of Pediatric Psychology, 23*(1), 5–15.

Taylor, N. E., Wall, S. M., Liebow, H., Sabatino, C. A., Timberlake, E. M., & Farber, M. Z. (2005). Mother and soldier: Raising a child with a disability in a low-income military family. *Exceptional Children, 72*(1), 83–89.

Thein, H. H., Austen, S., Currie, J., & Lewin, E. (2010). The impact of cultural context on the perception of work/family balance by professional women in Singapore and Hong Kong. *International Journal of Cross Cultural Management, 10*(3), 303–320.

Tliyen, U., Terres, N., Yazdgerdi, S., & Perrin, J. (1998). Impact of long-term care of children assisted by technology on maternal health. *Journal of Developmental and Behavioral Pediatrics, 9*(4), 273–282.

Van Dyck, P., Kohan, M., McPherson, M., Weissman, G., & Newacheck, P. (2004). Prevalence and characteristics of children with special health care needs. *Archives of Pediatrics & Adolescent Medicine, 158*(9), 884–890.

Voydanoff, P. (2005). Toward a conceptualization of perceived work—Family fit and balance: A demands and resources approach. *Journal of Marriage and Family, 67*, 822–836.

White House Forum on Workplace Flexibility (2010, April 1). Retrieved March 1, 2011 from http://Whitehouse.Gov.

Williams, J. (1999). *Unbending gender: Why family and work conflict and what to do about it.* New York: Oxford University Press.

Williams, J. C., & Boushey, H. (2010). *The three faces of work-family conflict: The poor the professionals, and the missing middle.* San Francisco: Center for American Progress/Work Life Law, Hastings College of the Law.

Yohalem, A. (1978). *The careers of professional women.* New York: Columbia University Press.

Zhang, J. (2011). Antecedents of work-family conflict: Review and prospect. *International Journal of Business and Management, 6*(1), 89–103.

Adjusting Intervention Acuity in School Mental Health: Perceiving Trauma Through the Lens of Cultural Competence

18

Leslie K. Taylor, Heather L. Lasky, and Mark D. Weist

Over the past decade, the linkage among traumatized youth's school performance, and specifically the impact of posttraumatic stress disorder (PTSD) symptoms on learning, has garnered increasing attention. Traumatized youth with PTSD report significant deficits in verbal abilities (Saigh, Yasik, Oberfield, Halamdaris, & Bremner, 2006), learning, and memory in comparison to their peers (Yasik, Saigh, Oberfield, & Halamandaris, 2007). This may be due to the impact of traumatic experiences on brain development; some of which include slowing brain cell growth (Cook et al., 2005; Davies, 2002), reduced neurogenesis (e.g., Teicher, Polcari, Andersen, Anderson, & Navalta, 2003), suppression of the immune system (Cook et al., 2005; Davies, 2002), and interference among parts of the brain responsible for the development of affect regulation (van der Kolk, 2005). Thus, it is not surprising that traumatized youth struggle to adapt to the demands of school. Within the classroom, traumatized youth may present with fear, hyperactivity, aggression, somatic problems, and depression (Gabowitz, Zucker, & Cook, 2008), all of which can interfere with learning. Moreover, given the presentation of these problems, teachers and school counselors may falsely classify traumatized youth as oppositional, defiant, or having attention deficit hyperactivity disorder (ADHD), leading to the erroneous suspension, expulsion, or referral of these youth to special education services for emotional disabilities. Notably, none of these classifications or disciplinary actions will likely result in an intervention plan that addresses past trauma exposure.

This is particularly concerning when taken together with data indicating that many youth are unlikely to receive mental health interventions unless they are provided in schools (Burns et al., 1995; Leaf et al., 1996; Weist, 1997). Consequently, research regarding the implementation of school mental health (SMH) programs has grown rapidly over the past two decades. Schools are uniquely positioned to provide mental health services to youth and their families (Stephan, Weist, Kataoka, Adelsheim, & Mills, 2007; Weist, Evans, & Lever, 2003), have been implicated in improving youth accessibility to services (Soleimanpour, Geierstanger, Kaller, McCarter, & Brindis, 2010) while decreasing stigma (Atkins, Adil, Jackson, McKay, & Bell, 2001), and have been shown to facilitate the generalization of intervention effects across settings (Evans, Langberg, & Williams, 2003). In as much, school-based interventions for traumatized youth have become a pressing agenda item among key stakeholders (i.e., educators, researchers, policymakers, mental health professionals; see Dean et al., 2008; Kataoka et al., 2009). This is encouraging given many traumatized youth remain

---

L.K. Taylor (✉) • H.L. Lasky • M.D. Weist
University of South Carolina, Columbia, SC, USA
e-mail: taylorlk@mailbox.sc.edu; laskyh@mailbox.sc.edu; weist@mailbox.sc.edu

unidentified unless formally assessed and treated (Stein, Jaycox, Kataoka, Wong, et al., 2003; Taylor & Weems, 2011).

In spite of this progress, there is a continued strong need to expand the knowledge base on helping youth experiencing trauma and its related challenges succeed in school through effective and culturally competent programs and services (Clauss-Ehlers, Weist, Gregory, & Hull, 2010; New Freedom Commission, 2003). Minority youth not only represent a population with higher levels of trauma exposure than other groups (Pole, Gone, & Kulkarni, 2008), but an underserved population (Pumariega, Rogers, & Rothe, 2005). Mental health services provided in community settings, such as schools, facilitate comfortability in accessing services for minority and culturally diverse populations (Pumariega et al.). Indeed, school-based interventions are a key mechanism for engaging these youth in treatment (see Ngo et al., 2008; Stein, Jaycox, Kataoka, Wong, et al., 2003). This, taken together with data suggesting that culture influences individual reactions to trauma, and can potentially exacerbate the development of posttraumatic stress symptoms (Zayfert, 2008), emphasizes the need for cultural competence in the delivery of school-based trauma-focused interventions.

Cultural competence is a key ingredient in the delivery of effective mental health care broadly (New Freedom Commission, 2003; U.S. Department of Health and Human Services, 2001) and for developing and conducting child and adolescent trauma interventions specifically (see Silverman et al., 2008). Cultural influences pervade youth ecology (Yasui & Dishion, 2007). For example, cultural values influence child rearing practices and developmental norms (e.g., toileting, when to leave a child unsupervised, readiness for sexuality/intimacy, and readiness to leave the parental home; Pumariega et al., 2005). Moreover, culture may also impact frequency of health maintenance behaviors (e.g., preventative practices and risk behaviors), the role of family in facilitating help-seeking behavior, and expectations regarding the roles of healers in their recovery (e. g., some may expect a more authoritarian healer, others a more egalitarian healer; Pumariega et al., 2005). Taken together, culture not only influences potential exposure to traumatic events, but accessibility and effectiveness of intervention. Yet, cultural influences on treatment outcomes, and as informants to intervention development, are scarcely acknowledged and investigated within intervention research. This presents a notable limitation within the trauma-focused intervention research. Minority representation is relatively higher in trauma populations than in other child and adolescent treatment research, and there is scant information regarding the adaptation of these interventions to cultural context (Silverman et al., 2008) thus compromising the impact and generalizability of interventions.

An identified barrier to realizing these adaptations is methodological; the gap between philosophical definitions of cultural competence and their application in practice and research settings has been linked to slowed progress in this area (see Sue, 2006). For example, conceptual frameworks, such as those developed by the American Psychological Association (2003), provide guidance on three critical domains of cultural competence (i.e., cultural awareness and beliefs, knowledge, and skills) but leave ambiguity in terms of the operationalization of these domains, which may explain poor agreement on these topics across key stakeholders (Cunningham, Foster, & Henggeler, 2002). Beyond issues with operationalization, the applicability of these domains to child development and the context in which it occurs are unclear. This affects intervention science, research, and practice. Empirically supported interventions are habitually designed to serve the majority of children and families (typically people of European American descent and culture) and then altered post hoc to serve the needs of specific groups (Yasui & Dishion, 2007). New frameworks, which take into consideration the cultural influences on normative and adaptive developmental pathways relative to intervention science, help facilitate the development of theories, methods, and research paradigms for addressing the influences of ethnicity or culture (see Yasui & Dishion). Often though, there is substantial time lag from theory testing to cross over in mental health practice. While correcting this issue is beyond the scope of this chapter, review of cultural influences on the experience of trauma and the effectiveness of existing culturally sensitive trauma-focused interventions have the potential to forward intervention science. Such a review could facilitate identification of culture-specific factors contributing to treatment effectiveness and potential culture-specific treatment alterations in need of further empirical investigation.

An additional contribution of this chapter includes recommendations for building capacities necessary for supporting and sustaining culturally competent trauma-focused intervention within schools. Inadequate intervention staffing and training, lack of administrative support, and budget needs are common barriers to sustainability of SMH programs (Horner, Sugai, Lewis-Palmer, & Todd, 2001). Building capacities through the development of school policies and partnerships can circumvent these barriers. For example, by facilitating administrative support, helping to increase resources and funding, and assuring well trained and supported staff (Anderson-Butcher et al., 2010; Flaspohler, Anderson-Butcher, & Wandersman, 2008). This chapter offers guidance in the consideration of cultural factors impacting cognitive and perceptual responses to trauma (as thought patterns as behavioral reactions are focused intervention targets; see Silverman et al., 2008) and review of school- and community-based culturally competent trauma interventions. This information can be used to identify cultural competence needs, the development of school policies, and potential school–community partnerships for the sustainability of these interventions. Thus, the aims of this chapter are to (1) provide a review of research regarding cultural influences on the experience of traumatic reactions as informants to clinical work, (2) discuss the effectiveness of different types of school-based trauma-focused interventions in diverse populations, (3) and building school capacities to support the interventions. Finally, conclusions drawn from this review set up a discussion of testable alterations to interventions to provide a roadmap for developing and implementing culturally competent treatment programs for traumatized youth in schools.

The Intersection Among Culture, Trauma, and Posttraumatic Responses

Trauma and posttraumatic stress symptoms are not culturally bound, but a cross cultural phenomenon impacting people and communities of all ethnicities and heritages (see Ford, 2008; Pumariega et al., 2005; Ruchkin et al., 2005). Traumatic events typically occur and are embedded within a cultural context and culture may influence an individual's interpretation (Tummala-Narra, 2007) and responses to that event (Zayfert, 2008). Thus, some have argued that culture influences the experience, understanding, behavioral and emotional expression of distress (Pumariega et al., 2005). Perhaps because of this, culture has been posited as a highly relevant factor in the development, maintenance, and treatment of emotional distress symptoms in the wake of trauma (Zayfert, 2008).

However, identifying cultural influences as contributors to the development and maintenance of symptom expression is complicated. Discerning unique cultural influences, in contrast with factors commonly associated with traumatized youth, can be difficult to untangle. For example, increased likelihood of trauma exposure can be influenced by factors unrelated to culture specifically, such as contextual/community level factors (McKay, Lynn, & Bannon, 2005) with a very prominent one being violence exposure (see Attar, Guerra, & Tolan, 1994; Stein, Jaycox, Kataoka, Rhodes, & Vestal, 2003) and its significant impact on emotional/behavioral functioning (Stein, Jaycox, Kataoka, Rhodes, et al., 2003; Stein, Jaycox, Kataoka, Wong, et al., 2003). Similarly, symptom development posttrauma can depend upon risk and protective factors such as social support networks or individual coping responses (e.g., La Greca, Silverman, Vernberg, & Prinstein, 1996), and while these factors may be influenced by culture, the onset and development of PTSD symptoms is not necessarily culturally bound (Zayfert, 2008). Moreover, many traumatized youth are at high risk for substance abuse problems, violent, or suicidal behaviors regardless of ethnocultural background (Schwab-Stone et al., 1999).

Research methods used to investigate potential cultural influences on posttraumatic adjustment are of further concern. Empirical investigations of heterogeneously traumatized ethnic samples can significantly decrease treatment effects for minority youth (see Silverman et al., 2008). Using these types of methods, it is difficult to make statistical comparisons regarding symptomatology across different cultures (i.e., Latino/Hispanic, American Indian, Asian individuals) due to statistical power. Because of these methodological issues, trauma researchers have made a general call for designing studies with sufficient statistical power to fully evaluate the role of ethnicity (see Silverman et al.).

Notable recommendations for future intervention studies also include taking into consideration the level of youth and family level of acculturation. Acculturation level can impact the ability to communicate with others, perceptions of mental health, and help seeking for mental health concerns (Tata & Leong, 1994). A related design concern is that ethnicity groupings are heterogeneous and can cover a large number of nationalities (e.g., Hispanic/Latino refers to 20 different countries of origin; U.S. Census Bureau, 2001), and within group trends may not necessarily speak to all of these nationalities (e.g., Piña & Silverman, 2004). Lastly, children and adolescents have been less widely examined within the trauma research base than adults generally, and within intervention research specifically.

Because of all of these issues, the intersection of culture and trauma relative to youth intervention may not be as well known or understood. Limitations notwithstanding, conducting a review and meaningful synthesis of trauma and traumatic responses is an important foundation to the discussion of school-based trauma-focused interventions. Traumatized youth are at increased risk for many of the same psychological problems (e.g., suicide, substance abuse, guilt). However, it is plausible that pathways to these problems are mediated or moderated by cultural influences (see Ford, 2008; Pole et al., 2008; Zayfert, 2008), and given youth are more likely to receive intervention in schools rather than in community mental health agencies (Burns et al., 1995; Leaf et al., 1996; Weist, 1997), it is important for SMH professionals to develop an understanding of these influences as potential risk and protective factors for poor posttraumatic outcomes (Zyromski, 2007). Further, growing evidence suggests the need to adapt evidence-based treatments (EBTs) to specific ethnocultural groups regarding terms of service use, treatment preferences, and beliefs about health (Cauce et al., 2002). Relative to trauma and posttraumatic symptomatology, knowledge of the types of traumas commonly experienced by minority youth, as well as cultural influences on psychological adjustment posttrauma, allow for movement toward conducting and implementing culturally adapted interventions. In the proceeding paragraphs, a review of the commonly experienced traumas in minority youth, and potential cultural influences on the development and maintenance of these symptoms, are explored.

African American Youth

As previously indicated, minority youth are exposed to potentially traumatic events at a higher frequency than other youth. Simply being a part of an ethnic minority group increases risk for exposure to prejudice and discriminatory practices which can be considered traumatic (Ford, 2008), and possibly contribute to intergenerational transmission of risk for the development of PTSD (Kellermann, 2001). For many African American youth, and among their families, the perceptions of traditional safeguards (e.g., the police department, related government agencies) are contaminated by experiences of discrimination and prejudice (see Graves, Kaslow, & Frabutt, 2010). Given traditional safeguards are not perceived as protective, youth and families may not call upon these sources when criminal or violent acts occur in their communities, and in turn African American youth may be at increased risk of violence exposure (see Fitzpatrick & Boldizar, 1993).

Violence exposure has many impacts on urban youth, including increased emotional and behavioral problems, and impaired school behavior and performance (see Warner & Weist, 1996; Warner, Weist, & Krulak, 1999; Weist & Cooley-Quille, 2001). Across gender, African American youth are at risk for exposure to violence (Attar et al., 1994; Crouch, Hanson, Saunders, Kilpatrick, & Resnick, 2000; Warner & Weist, 1996). However, African American females are at increased risk of sexual victimization (abuse or assault) relative to their male counterparts. A strong consensus regarding the role of ethnicity as a risk factor for sexual victimization remains unclear given these types of events are generally associated with underreporting. Reported rates indicate that sexual victimization is higher (2.3%) among African American adolescent females than Caucasian Americans (1.8%; Ackard & Neumark-Sztainer, 2002). Of further concern are the implications of childhood sexual victimization for African American females. African American women reporting childhood sexual abuse experiences are at increased risk of sexual assault as adults (Goodman & Fallot, 1998; Miner, Flitter, & Robinson, 2006) and are significantly more likely to be assaulted by their partners than non-African American counterparts (Campbell & Soeken, 1999). In particular, findings indicate that African American couples report twice the rate of sexual aggression than Caucasian couples (Ramisetty-Mikler, Caetano, & McGrath, 2007).

Sexual victimization, either through assault or repeated abuse is a particularly significant form of trauma (Low & Organista, 2000; Monroe et al., 2005). In making this conclusion, it seems that African American youth are at increased risk of exposure to both interpersonal (violence that occurs between individuals in ongoing relationships) and situational violence (violence that occurs due to social factors such as the availability of guns or drugs, poverty; Acosta, Albus, Reynolds, Spriggs, & Weist, 2001; Weist & Cooley-Quille, 2001). Moreover, the interplay among exposure and victimization may contribute to the continuation of aggressive behavior patterns from childhood to adulthood (Warner & Weist, 1996). Findings from a sample of ethnically diverse, trauma exposed high school students suggest that African American youth are more likely to experience a pattern of emotional dysregulation resulting from trauma exposure than Caucasian youth, and that this emotional dysregulation is linked to the manifestation of overt, aggressive behavior (Marsee, 2008). This underlying emotional dysregulation may also explain the manifestation of violent behavior in African American adolescent males and suicidal behavior in females (Dulmus & Hilarski, 2006). As noted, contextual factors, such as neighborhood disadvantage and high experiences with racism, can interact with and exacerbate the impact of trauma. These factors, coupled with poor emotion regulation, may lead African American youth to believe they have fewer options for resisting violence, leaving them more inclined to react aggressively, either toward others or themselves (see Albus, Weist, & Perez-Smith, 2004; Weist, Acosta, & Youngstrom, 2001; Youngstrom, Weist, & Albus, 2003).

American Indian Youth

Despite the disproportionate burden of mental health problems experienced by American Indian youth, there has been a lack of epidemiology and surveillance regarding mental health (U.S. Public Health Service Office of the Surgeon General, 2001). To date, the research base regarding American Indian mental health continues to grow, and suggests this group is at increased risk of being exposed to traumatic experiences relative to their contemporaries. Prevalence from American Indian youth samples suggests trauma exposure rates of 55% (Kaufman, Beals, Mitchell, LeMaster, & Fickenscher, 2004) to 61% (Jones, Dauphinais, Sack, & Somervell, 1997). Moreover, American Indians reportedly experience violent victimization at rates greater than other ethnic minority groups (Tjaden & Thoennes, 2000).

A concerning theme within the lives of American Indian youth, and one that has been posited as a risk factor or cause for mental health problems and risk behaviors generally, includes historical and generational traumas experienced by American Indians resulting from boarding school experiences (Boyd-Ball, Manson, Noonan, & Beals, 2006; Kawamoto, 2001; Yasui & Dishion, 2007). The overarching objective of the boarding school system has been to civilize American Indian children by destroying their Indian cultural identity. To achieve this, American Indian youth experienced mandatory separation from their families of origin, which prevented generations of youth from learning their native culture and communication/language practices, spiritual traditions, and heritage (Kawamoto, 2001). At these boarding schools, youth received harsh discipline practices, and in some cases youth were physically and sexually abused (Horejsi, Heavy Runer-Craig, & Pablo, 1992; Ishisaka, 1978; Merriam, 1977). Exposure to this abuse has been implicated not only in the development of unresolved psychological issues for survivors, but the introduction to harsh discipline practices for their own children (Horejsi et al., 1992). Given generations of American Indians experienced boarding schools and that traditional cultural transmission processes were disrupted, many grandparents and parents failed to learn or gain exposure to parenting skills and roles beyond what was observed in school (Horejsi et al.). The boarding school system continues to be implicated as a context for trauma exposure. Youth attending American Indian boarding schools are at increased risk of witnessing and experiencing interpersonal violence than those who do not attend (Boyd-Ball et al., 2006), suggesting that without reformation and intervention, the cycle of trauma exposure will continue unaddressed.

Given the cultural trauma history, it is not surprising that many American Indian youth struggle with substance abuse issues (Beauvais, 1992, 1996; Goodkind, Ross-Toledo, et al., 2010; May, 1996), and alarmingly, have the highest rate of suicide among 15–24-year-olds in the United States (Health US, 2004). Fortunately, culturally specific factors have been associated with decreased likelihood of mental health problems. Youth more strongly aligned with their American Indian culture evidence lower rates of substance use (Gray & Nye, 2001). In as much, ethnic identity has been identified as a resiliency factor.

Ethnic identity (i.e., efforts to learn about one's culture and become involved in traditional cultural activities, establish relationships with those in one's ethnic group, and adopt aspects of a specific identity; Marcia, 1980) has been associated with increased levels of self-esteem and for Navajo (Jones & Galliher, 2007), Lakota/Dakota, and Sioux youth (Pittinger, 1998), and Northern Plains, Southwest, and Pueblo American Indian adolescents across time (Whitesell, Mitchell, Kaufman, & Spicer, 2006; Whitesell, Mitchell, & Spicer, 2009). Moreover, strong ethnic identity is also tied to decreased level of substance use (Jones & Galliher, 2007).

Taken together, these findings suggest the importance of conducting school-based trauma interventions that incorporate cultural practices particularly given American Indian families are likely to look toward traditional health practices to heal youth's problems (see Goodkind, Ross-Toledo, et al., 2010). A limitation of current trauma-focused intervention research is the scarcity of American Indian youth in these studies and the exclusion of traditional healing practices from these programs (Miranda et al., 2005). Intervention researchers are answering this call through the development and implementation of culturally adapted evidence-based practices for traumatized youth and report promising decreases in anxious and depressive symptoms postintervention (Goodkind, LaNoue, & Milford, 2010).

Asian American Youth

While there are several different Asian American subgroups, each with unique linguistic, cultural, and sociodemographic backgrounds (Sue & Morishima, 1982), there are overarching similarities across groups that may present barriers to SMH professional working with traumatized youth (Zhou, Siu, & Xin, 2009; see Mock, 2012, Chap. 8). Asian Americans are among the most rapidly growing ethnic minority group in the United States (U.S. Census Bureau, 2004). Sadly, research indicates that these youth are more reluctant than other groups to disclose psychological difficulties (Abe-Kim et al., 2007; Zhou et al., 2009), and particularly traumatic experiences (Tjaden & Thoennes, 1998; Tracy, 2002), to mental health professionals (Sue & Kirk, 1975). In cases where help is sought, youth and families may first consult with physicians rather than mental health professionals (Leong & Lau, 2001) given subscription to body mind-holism, or belief in indistinct demarcation between psychological and physical illnesses (Zhou et al., 2009).

Cultural values may impact proneness to adopt avoidant coping and wishful thinking (Hung-Bin & Sedlacek, 2004). In contrast to Western views of healthy family functioning, which advocate clear boundaries and individuation from the family, Asian cultures place high value on collectivity and interdependence with the family as the primary source of social support. Asian youth are taught to consider their behavior as a reflection on the family unit and to view individual identity as secondary to family identity. In addition, Asian families are traditionally patriarchal, and youth are taught to uphold harmony within the social hierarchy (Uba, 1994), employ self-control and restraint, and are discouraged to display direct and open expression of emotions (e.g., the ability to suppress emotions is seen as an indication of emotional maturity; Zhou et al., 2009). Moreover, whereas communication styles in Western society focus upon expression of direct, verbal communication, Asian communication styles rely more strongly upon context, nonverbal cues, and other subtleties to convey messages (Zhou et al.). Taken together, Asian youth may not feel comfortable reporting traumatic events, or discussing feelings about what happened, with their caregivers or siblings as it may cause disharmony within the family unit. This is problematic given caregivers may not know if their child has witnessed or experienced unless directly told by the child. Further, Asian youth may use avoidant strategies to cope with traumatic events and posttraumatic psychological problems given the importance of showing restraint and control of their emotional states.

Perhaps due to trends in coping styles, and in desire to suppress emotional events (Park, Brody, & Wilson, 2008), and emotional responses to these events (Arkoff, Thaver, & Elkind, 1996), assessment of youth trauma exposure and posttraumatic stress symptoms among Asian youth may not accurately capture symptoms and impairment. Research suggests that these youth may underreport exposure to potentially traumatic events (i.e., exposure to violence) and internalizing symptoms in their aftermath (Chen, 2010). Levels of biculturation (adherence to values of the dominant culture and their cultural heritage; LaFromboise, Coleman, & Gerton, 1993) may also influence youth report and emotional expression in response to trauma exposure. Violence exposed youth with higher levels of bicultural orientation have reported lower externalizing and traumatic stress symptoms, regardless of number of exposure events, compared to those reporting lower levels of biculturation (Ho, 2008). It is plausible that youth with high levels of biculturation are relying upon more direct methods of communicating, open expression of emotion, and employing less avoidant/wishful thinking coping strategies and that this is contributing to their responses to trauma exposure.

Although more research is needed to better understand the intersection of cultural values and trauma within Asian youth (see Mock, 2012, Chap. 8), there are similarities in posttrauma psychological responses across ethnic minority groups. For example, Asian American females with histories of sexual victimization report high levels of helplessness, shame, and embarrassment (Luo, 2000), substance use (Tracy, 2002), and suicidal ideation (Rao, DiClemente, & Ponton, 1992). Of these problems, cultural influences on pathways to suicidality differ in Asian American trauma survivors. Although spirituality can serve as a barrier to committing suicide, it can also be perceived as a rationale for completing suicide (Leong, Leach, Yeh, & Chou, 2007). Cultural and spiritual emphasis on group suppression of conflict, avoidance of social shame, and indirect communication have been implicated as contributing factors in the belief that suicide will allow for self or family protection (Zane & Mak, 2003).

Hispanic and Latino (a) Youth

Taken together, the terms Hispanic and Latino refer to people from approximately 20 different nations; representing diverse races, ethnicities, sociopolitical histories, and cultures (U.S. Census Bureau, 2001). Though there are categorical distinctions between the two terms, overlap in cultural constructs shaping the response and impact of potentially traumatic events may not be. In particular, consideration of key themes such as dignity and respect, family values/value of family, *personalismo, machismo, marianismo,* and religion and spirituality have been identified when working with Hispanic/Latino clients (Andrés-Hyman, Ortiz, Añez, Paris, & Davidson, 2006). Given the role of family in childhood and adolescence, cultural influences (i.e., family values and value of family) within the family are key to understanding Latino youths responses to traumatic events. For example, Latinos traditionally look toward informal, but established, family-based support networks where immediate and extended family members provide support to those in need (Starrett, Bresler, Decker, Walters, & Rogers, 1990). Because of this, rather than accessing mental health centers, Latinos may be more likely to consult with family or trusted members within their community (McMiller & Weisz, 1996; Woodward, Dwinell, & Arons, 1992). Thus, it is plausible that for traumatized Latino youth, schools present an ideal context for providing effective interventions in the wake of trauma (see Acosta, Weist, Lopez, Shafer, & Pizarro, 2004).

Without intervention, emotional and behavioral problems among traumatized youth can worsen. In particular, the experience of emotions such as shame, blame, and guilt (see Diagneault, Tournigy, & Hebert, 2006; Greenberg & Keane, 2001; La Greca et al., 1996) contribute to the maintenance of posttraumatic symptoms and impairment. These emotions are particularly salient in the wake of sexual victimization, and to Latinas specifically. National data suggest that Latinas (14.6%) are less likely to be assaulted than non-Latina women (18.4%; Tjaden & Thoennes, 1998); however, sexual victimization is generally underreported (Rennison, 2000), and potentially more so in Latinas given cultural subscription to sex and sexuality as private matters rather than topics for open discussion (Low & Organista, 2000). In addition, research indicates Latinas are more likely to endorse rape scripts holding women as contributors to sexual assault (i.e., through their clothing, behavior, and or lack of control over men's sexuality) and have more punitive attitudes toward women coming forward as rape victims in comparison to Caucasian and African American females (Lefley, Scott, Llabre, & Hicks, 1993).

Marianismo may serve as a foundation for this linkage among trends in Latina responses to sexuality and sexual victimization. *Marianismo* encompasses values of worshiping and emulating the Virgin Mary (the connotation of this implying that women are morally superior to men and can more easily endure the suffering inflicted on them by men; Comas-Diaz & Duncan, 1985), and sexual purity, sexual suppression, and responsibility for keeping oneself pure before marriage (Morales & Reyes, 1998). Given *marianismo* implicates Latinas in controlling the sexual responses and behaviors of men, it is plausible that this belief potentially contributes to the development of shame and blame in the wake of sexual assault, and other emotional responses such as feeling guilt over the loss of purity or the inability to control what occurred during the assault. Factors of shame, blame, and guilt may also render Latinas less likely to seek help from professionals generally and may lead them to feel uncomfortable talking about what happened to them specifically (see Low & Organista, 2000). Sadly, and perhaps because of beliefs held, Latinas who do speak out, and seek support from those in their social network may not be met with sympathy (Jimenez & Abreu, 2003).

Although further research is needed to explore direct links among the development of posttraumatic adjustment and associated feelings of shame blame and guilt in minority groups (Bryant-Davis, Chung, & Tillman, 2009), findings suggest cultural trends in Latina responses to trauma. For example, greater adherence to Latina/o cultural norms has been associated with greater peritraumatic dissociation posttrauma

(Marshall & Orlando, 2002). Dissociation is a robust risk factor for the development of PTSD (Weller, Baer, da Alba Garcia, & Rocha, 2008). In particular, high levels of peritraumatic dissociation (an immediate reaction traumatic events, consisting of disturbances in memory, depersonalization and derealization, alterations in time perception, and an overall sense of detachment from people and surroundings; Marmar et al., 1994) among Latinos have been implicated as one of the most important variables accounting for PTSD differences between Latino and non-Latino European Americans (Pole et al., 2005). Latinas may describe dissociative symptomatology as *ataque de nervious*, or complain of depersonalization, identity alteration, and trance-like states (Lewis-Fernandez et al., 2002), and believe that these dissociative spells have spiritual or religious influences (Wirtz, 2005).

Consistent with research regarding other minority groups, Hispanic/Latino youth are also at increased risk for exposure to violence (Crouch et al., 2000), with unique issues complicating the impact of this exposure. For example, Latino youth and their families may face other stressors such as lack of support (e.g., positive role models), family instability in the form of unemployment and marital conflict compounded by language barriers, acculturations issues, and discrimination issues (Acosta et al., 2004).

The Effectiveness of School-Based Trauma-Focused Interventions in Diverse Populations

In a recent meta-analysis, Silverman et al. (2008) evaluated treatment studies conducted in samples of traumatized youth for methodological rigor and evidence level. Results of this meta-analysis identified school-based group cognitive behavioral treatments and trauma-focused cognitive behavioral therapies (TFCBTs) as the most rigorously tested and effective interventions for posttraumatic stress, depression, and anxiety symptom reduction in traumatized youth (see Silverman et al.). Notably, trials of these two types of interventions have occurred in predominately ethnic minority samples (i.e., school-based group cognitive behavioral treatments, Kataoka et al., 2003; Stein, Jaycox, Kataoka, Wong, et al., 2003; TFCBTs Jaycox et al., 2010) and have shown similar, effective patterns of symptom reduction in comparison to nonminority samples (see Silverman et al., 2008).

In particular, the school-based group treatment, Cognitive Behavioral Intervention for Trauma in Schools (CBITS; Jaycox, 2003) remains one of the most widely examined trauma interventions for ethnic minority youth. CBITS is a ten-session group intervention (with individual pull out sessions for trauma narrative development) specifically designed for traumatized multicultural youth and implementation in school settings (Stein, Jaycox, Kataoka, Wong, et al., 2003). CBITS has been recognized by the Substance Abuse and Mental Health Services Administration's National Registry of Evidence Based Programs and Practices (SAMHSA's NREPP), the Office of Juvenile Justice and Delinquency Program's Model Programs Guide, and has been identified as a Promising Practices Network Proven Program. The intervention incorporates skills such as psychoeducation, relaxation, enhancing safety, affective modulation, cognitive coping skills, in vivo mastery of trauma reminders, and the development of the trauma narrative (see Stein, Jaycox, Kataoka, Wong, et al.). CBITS effectiveness has been tested and supported in diverse samples of urban youth who have experienced various trauma exposure including community violence (Stein, Jaycox, Kataoka, Wong, et al.) and natural disasters (Jaycox et al., 2010).

As this emerging knowledge base regarding intervention effectiveness continues to grow, SMH professionals may be concerned about which interventions to conduct with ethnic minority youth. The consensus regarding enhanced treatment effects for youth receiving culturally modified treatments (in comparison to unmodified approaches) remains unclear, and mental health professionals are cautioned against use of untested culturally adapted treatments (Lau, 2006). CBITS and TFCBTs have been identified as EBTs for traumatized youth and EBTs are suggested as first-line interventions for ethnic minority youth (Huey & Polo, 2008). Specific application of EBTs to particular cultural/ethnic groups is an important research and practice agenda. For example, the CBITS program has been culturally adapted for American Indian youth through replacing European focused CBITS examples (e.g., Chicken Little) with characters better understood by this population (Goodkind, LaNoue, et al., 2010). Results from these culturally adapted interventions show effective symptom reduction traumatized youth (Goodkind, LaNoue, et al., 2010; Kataoka et al., 2003).

Building School Capacities to Support the Intervention

Review from the previous section indicates the importance of cultural influences in presentation of psychological distress symptoms and when conducting interventions with traumatized youth. However, despite a movement towards integration of evidence-based interventions into real-world practice (Hennessy & Levin, 2010), there are many issues associated with implementing these interventions in the school setting (Domitrovich et al., 2008; Forman, Olin, Hoagwood, Crowe, & Saka, 2009; Langley, Nadeem, Kataoka, Stein, & Jaycox, 2010). Notable examples of these include funding, time, school personnel beliefs about the intervention, competing priorities within the school, and the No Child Left Behind Act (i.e., school personnel focused more on results of testing).

Similar barriers are evident when looking specifically at the implementation of CBITS (Langley et al., 2010). The four most common implementation barriers were lack of parent engagement, competing responsibilities, logistical barriers, and lack of support from school personnel. To overcome these barriers, Langley et al. (2010) emphasized the importance of professional networks. Successful CBITS implementers report having a supportive professional network with fellow implementers; network participation was not reported by nonsuccessful implementers. In addition, financing is obviously a critical need for culturally responsive and effective SMH interventions (see Evans, Glass-Siegel, et al., 2003) and thus successful implementation of CBITS is linked to fund allocation (Langley et al., 2010).

In contrast, facilitators such as teacher support, principal support, support from other administrators, and good training have been implicated in the successful implementation of evidence-based practice in schools (Forman et al., 2009). These facilitators point toward the importance of preintervention activities aimed at building relationships among key stakeholders. In order for schools to implement and sustain interventions generally, and trauma interventions for ethnic minority youth specifically, school–family–community partnerships are critical (Andis et al., 2002). In particular, developing this type of partnership has been implicated as a centralizing force for the dissemination, program development, preintervention planning, and delivery of trauma-focused intervention programs in ethnically diverse youth (Ngo et al., 2008). Moreover, ongoing communication among stakeholders during these processes allows for culturally sensitive tailoring of trauma intervention programs based on community needs and developing adaptations for empirical investigation and intervention sustainability (Ngo et al.).

Conclusions

Schools play a pivotal role in identifying and providing mental health services to youth (Burns et al., 1997; Weist & Warner, 1997) and are particularly instrumental for intervening in underserved populations, such as ethnic minority youth (see Goodkind, LaNoue, et al., 2010; Kataoka et al., 2003). As school performance become more strongly linked to mental health generally (see Atkins, Hoagwood, Kutash, & Seidman, 2010; Rones & Hoagwood, 2000) and trauma specifically (dropout rates, McGloin & Widom, 2001; achievement scores, Weems et al., 2010), so does the salience of mental health screenings that include inquiry of trauma exposure. Relatedly, sustaining effective school-based interventions for identified youth involves developing strong community partnerships (Ngo et al., 2008) and maintaining ongoing training and implementation support (Forman et al., 2009; Langley et al., 2010). Beyond screening and intervention, the importance for building competency in SMH professionals regarding the impact of culture on the interpretation of traumatic events also emerges. Movement of trauma-focused intervention research from research settings to real-world settings, such as schools, allows for systematic identification of cultural factors that differentially contribute to posttraumatic adjustment and response to intervention. Continued development and testing of culturally adaptive trauma-focused interventions based on these identified factors could potentially expedite trauma recovery in youth while allowing for promising long-term outcomes (see McGloin & Widom, 2001).

References

Abe-Kim, J., Takeuchi, D. T., Hong, S., Zane, N., Sue, S., Spencer, M. S., et al. (2007). Use of mental health-related services among immigrant and US-born Asian Americans: Results from the National Latino and Asian American study. *American Journal of Public Health, 97*(1), 91–98.

Ackard, D. M., & Neumark-Sztainer, D. (2002). Date violence and date rape among adolescents: Associations with disordered eating behaviors and psychological health. *Child Abuse & Neglect, 26*, 455–473.

Acosta, O. M., Albus, K. E., Reynolds, M. W., Spriggs, D., & Weist, M. D. (2001). Assessing the status of research on violence related problems among youth. *Journal of Clinical Child and Adolescent Psychology, 30*, 152–160.

Acosta, O. M., Weist, M. D., Lopez, F. A., Shafer, M. E., & Pizarro, L. J. (2004). Assessing the psychosocial and academic needs of Latino youth to inform the development of school-based programs. *Behavior Modification, 28*, 579–595.

Albus, K. E., Weist, M. D., & Perez-Smith, A. M. (2004). Association between youth risk behavior and exposure to violence: Implications for the provision of mental health services in urban schools. *Behavior Modification, 28*, 548–564.

American Psychological Association. (2003). Guidelines on multicultural education, training, research, practice, and organizational change for psychologists. *American Psychologist, 58*, 377–402.

Anderson-Butcher, D., Lawson, H. A., Iachini, A., Flaspohler, P., Bean, J., & Wade-Mdivanian, R. (2010). Emergent evidence in support of a community collaboration model for school improvement. *Children and Schools, 32*(3), 160–171.

Andis, P., Cashman, J., Praschil, R., Oglesby, D., Adelman, H., Taylor, L., et al. (2002). A strategic and shared agenda to advance mental health in schools through family and system partnerships. *International Journal of Mental Health Promotion, 4*, 28–35.

Andrés-Hyman, R. C., Ortiz, J., Añez, L. M., Paris, M., & Davidson, L. (2006). Culture and clinical practice: Recommendations for working with Puerto Ricans and other Latinas(os) in the United States. *Professional Psychology: Research and Practice, 37*, 694–701.

Arkoff, A., Thaver, F., & Elkind, L. (1996). Mental health and counseling ideas of Asian and American students. *Journal of Counseling Psychology, 13*, 219–223.

Atkins, M., Adil, J., Jackson, M., McKay, M., & Bell, C. (2001). *An ecological model for school based mental health services*. In 13th annual conference proceedings: A system of care for children's mental health: Expanding the research base. Tampa: University of South Florida.

Atkins, M. S., Hoagwood, K. E., Kutash, K., & Seidman, E. (2010). Toward the integration of education and mental health in schools. *Administration & Policy in Mental Health & Mental Health Services Research, 37*(1/2), 40–47.

Attar, B., Guerra, N., & Tolan, P. (1994). Neighborhood disadvantage, stressful life events, and adjustment in urban elementary school children. *Journal of Clinical Child Psychology, 23*, 391–400.

Beauvais, F. (1992). Characteristics of Indian youth and drug use. *American Indian and Alaska Native Mental Health Research, 5*, 50–67.

Beauvais, F. (1996). Trends in drug use among American Indian students and dropouts. *American Journal of Public Health, 86*, 1594–1599.

Boyd-Ball, A. J., Manson, S. M., Noonan, C., & Beals, J. (2006). Traumatic events and alcohol use disorder among American Indian adolescents and young adults. *Journal of Traumatic Stress, 19*, 937–947.

Bryant-Davis, T., Chung, H., & Tillman, S. (2009). From the margin to center: Ethnic minority women and the mental health effects of sexual assault. *Trauma, Violence & Abuse, 10*, 330–357.

Burns, B. J., Costello, E. J., Angold, A., Tweed, D., Stangle, D., Farmer, E. M. Z., et al. (1995). Data watch: Children's mental health service use across service sectors. *Health Affairs, 14*(3), 147–159.

Burns, B. J., Costello, E., Erkanli, A., Tweed, D. L., Farmer, E. Z., & Angold, A. (1997). Insurance coverage and mental health service use by adolescents with serious emotional disturbance. *Journal Of Child & Family Studies, 6*(1), 89–111.

Campbell, J. C., & Soeken, K. (1999). Forced sex and intimate partner violence: Effects on women's risk and women's health. *Violence Against Women, 5*(2), 1017–1035.

Cauce, A., Paradise, M., Domenech-Rodriguez, M., Cochran, B. N., Shea, J., Srebnik, D., et al. (2002).

Cultural and contextual influences in mental health help seeking: A focus on ethic minority youth. *Journal of Consulting and Clinical Psychology, 70*(1), 44.

Census Bureau, U. S. (2004). *We the people: Asians in the United States.* Washington, DC: U.S. Government Printing Office.

Chen, W. (2010). Exposure to community violence and adolescents' internalizing behaviors among African American and Asian American adolescents. *Journal of Youth and Adolescence, 39*(4), 403–413.

Clauss-Ehlers, C., Weist, M. D., Gregory, W. H., & Hull, R. (2010). Enhancing cultural competence in schools and school mental health programs. In C. Clauss-Ehlers (Ed.), *Encyclopedia of cross-cultural school psychology* (pp. 39–44). New York: Springer.

Comas-Diaz, L., & Duncan, J. W. (1985). The cultural context: A factor in assertiveness training with mainland Puerto Rican women. *Psychology of Women Quarterly, 9*, 463–475.

Cook, A., Spinazzola, J., Ford, J., Lanktree, C., Blaustein, M., Cloitre, M., et al. (2005). Complex trauma in children and adolescents. *Psychiatric Annals, 35*(5), 390–398.

Crouch, J. L., Hanson, R. F., Saunders, B. F., Kilpatrick, D. G., & Resnick, H. S. (2000). Income, race/ethnicity, and exposure to violence in youth: Results from the national survey of adolescents. *Journal of Community Psychology, 28*(6), 625–641.

Cunningham, P. B., Foster, S. L., & Henggeler, S. W. (2002). The elusive concept of cultural competence. *Children's Services: Social Policy, Research, and Practice, 5*, 231–243.

Davies, M. (2002). A few thoughts about the mind, the brain, and a child with early deprivation. *The Journal of Analytical Psychology, 47*(3), 421–435.

Dean, K. L., Langley, A. K., Kataoka, S. H., Jaycox, L. H., Wong, M., & Stein, B. D. (2008). School-based disaster mental health services: Clinical, policy, and community challenges. *Professional Psychology: Research & Practice, 39*(1), 52–57.

Diagneault, I., Tournigy, M., & Hebert, M. (2006). Self-attributions of blame in sexually abused adolescents: A mediational model. *Journal of Traumatic Stress, 19*(1), 153–157.

Domitrovich, C. E., Bradshaw, C. P., Poduska, J. M., Hoagwood, K., Buckley, J. A., Olin, S., et al. (2008). Maximizing the implementation quality of evidence-based preventive interventions in schools: A conceptual framework. *Advances in School Mental Health Promotion, 1*(3), 6–28.

Dulmus, C., & Hilarski, C. (2006). Significance of gender and age in African American children's response to parental victimization. *Health and Social Work, 31*, 181–188.

Evans, S. W., Glass-Siegel, M., Frank, A., Van Treuren, R., Lever, N. A., & Weist, M. D. (2003). Overcoming the challenges of funding school mental health programs. In M. D. Weist, S. W. Evans, & N. A. Lever (Eds.), *Handbook of school mental health: Advancing practice and research* (pp. 73–86). New York, NY: Springer.

Evans, S. W., Langberg, J., & Willimas, J. (2003). Achieving generalization in school-based mental health. In M. D. Weist, S. W. Evans, & N. A. Lever (Eds.), *Handbook of school mental health: Advancing practice and research* (pp. 335–348). New York: Kluwer Academic.

Fitzpatrick, K. M., & Boldizar, J. P. (1993). The prevalence and consequence of exposure to violence among African American youth. *Journal of the American Academy of Child and Adolescent Psychiatry, 32*(2), 424–430.

Flaspohler, P., Anderson-Butcher, D., & Wandersman, A. (2008). Supporting implementation of expanded school mental health services: Application of the Interactive Systems Framework in Ohio. *Advances in School Mental Health Promotion, 1*(3), 38–48.

Ford, J. D. (2008). Trauma, posttraumatic stress disorder, and ethnoracial minorities: Toward diversity and cultural competence in principles and practices. *Clinical Psychology: Science and Practice, 15*(1), 62–67.

Forman, S. G., Olin, S. S., Hoagwood, K. E., Crowe, M., & Saka, N. (2009). Evidence-based interventions in schools: Developers' views of implementation barriers and facilitators. *School Mental Health, 1*(1), 26–36.

Gabowitz, D., Zucker, M., & Cook, A. (2008). Neuropsychological assessment in clinical evaluation of children and adolescents with complex trauma. *Journal of Child and Adolescent Trauma, 1*, 163–178.

Goodkind, J. R., LaNoue, M. D., & Milford, J. (2010). Adaptation and implementation of cognitive behavioral intervention for trauma in schools with American Indian youth. *Journal of Clinical Child and Adolescent Psychology, 39*(6), 858–872.

Goodkind, J. R., Ross-Toledo, K., John, S., Hall, J., Ross, L., Freeland, L., et al. (2010). Promoting healing and restoring trust: Policy recommendations for improving behavioral health care for American Indian/Alaska native adolescents. *American Journal of Community Psychology, 46*(3/4), 386–394.

Goodman, L., & Fallot, R. (1998). HIV risk-behavior in poor urban women with serious mental disorders: Association with childhood physical and sexual abuse. *The American Journal of Orthopsychiatry, 68*, 73–83.

Graves, K. N., Kaslow, N. J., & Frabutt, J. M. (2010). A culturally-informed approach to trauma, suicidal behavior, and overt aggression in African American adolescents. *Aggression and Violent Behavior: A Review Journal, 15*, 36–41.

Gray, N., & Nye, P. S. (2001). American Indian and Alaska native substance abuse: Co-morbidity and cultural issues. *American Indian and Alaska Native Mental Health Research, 10*(2), 67–84.

Greenberg, H. S., & Keane, A. (2001). Risk factors for chronic posttraumatic stress symptoms and behavior problems in children and adolescents following a home fire. *Child and Adolescent Social Work Journal, 18*(3), 205–221.

Health United States. (2004). *Health, United States, 2004.* Hyattsville, MD: National Center for Health Statistics.

Hennessy, K., & Levin, B. (2010). *Mental health services: A public health perspective* (3rd ed.). London: Oxford University Press.

Ho, J. (2008). Community violence exposure of Southeast Asian American adolescents. *Journal of Interpersonal Violence, 23*(1), 136–146.

Horejsi, C., Heavy Runner Craig, B., & Pablo, J. (1992). Reactions by Native American parents to child protection agencies: Cultural and community factors. *Child Welfare, 62*, 329–342.

Horner, R. H., Sugai, G., Lewis-Palmer, T., & Todd, A. W. (2001). Teaching school-wide behavioral expectations. *Emotional & Behavioral Disorders in Youth, 1*(4), 73–96.

Huey, S. J., & Polo, A. J. (2008). Evidence-based psychosocial treatments for ethnic minority youth. *Journal of Clinical Child and Adolescent Psychology, 37*(1), 262–301.

Hung-Bin, S., & Sedlacek, W. E. (2004). An exploratory study of help-seeking attitudes and coping strategies among college students by race and gender. *Measurement & Evaluation in Counseling & Development (American Counseling Association), 37*(3), 130–143.

Ishisaka, H. (1978). American Indians and foster care: Cultural factors in separation. *Child Welfare, 57*, 299–308.

Jaycox, L. (2003). *Cognitive-behavioral intervention for trauma in schools.* Longmont, CO: Sopris West Educational Services.

Jaycox, L. H., Cohen, J. A., Mannarino, A. P., Walker, D. W., Langley, A. K., Gegenheimer, K. L., et al. (2010). Children's mental health care following Hurricane Katrina: A field trial of trauma-focused psychotherapies. *Journal of Traumatic Stress, 23*(2), 223–231.

Jimenez, J. A., & Abreu, J. M. (2003). Race and sex effects on attitudinal perceptions of acquaintance rape. *Journal of Counseling Psychology, 50*(2), 252–256.

Jones, M. C., Dauphinais, P., Sack, W. H., & Somervell, P. D. (1997). Trauma-related symptomatology among American Indian adolescents. *Journal of Traumatic Stress, 10*, 163–173.

Jones, M. D., & Galliher, R. V. (2007). Ethnic identity and psychosocial functioning in Navajo adolescents. *Journal of Research on Adolescence, 17*, 683–696.

Kataoka, S. H., Nadeem, E., Wong, M., Langley, A. K., Jaycox, L. H., Stein, B. D., et al. (2009). Improving disaster mental health care in schools: A community-partnered approach. *American Journal of Preventive Medicine, 37*(6), S225–S229.

Kataoka, S. H., Stein, B. D., Jaycox, L. H., Wong, M., Escudero, P., Wenli, T., et al. (2003). A school-based mental health program for traumatized Latino immigrant children. *Journal of the American Academy of Child and Adolescent Psychiatry, 42*(3), 311.

Kaufman, C. E., Beals, J., Mitchell, C. M., LeMaster, P., & Fickenscher, A. (2004). Stress, trauma, and risky sexual behaviour among American Indians in young adulthood. *Culture, Health & Sexuality, 6*(4), 301–318.

Kawamoto, W. T. (2001). Community mental health and family issues in sociohistorical context: The Confederated tribes of Coos, Lower Umpqua, and Siuslaw Indians. *American Behavioral Scientist, 44*(9), 1482–1491.

Kellermann, N. P. (2001). Psychopathology in children of Holocaust survivors. *Israel Journal of Psychiatry and Related Sciences, 38*, 36–46.

La Greca, A. M., Silverman, W. K., Vernberg, E. M., & Prinstein, M. (1996). Symptoms of posttraumatic stress after Hurricane Andrew: A prospective study. *Journal of Consulting and Clinical Psychology, 64*, 712–723.

LaFromboise, T., Coleman, H. L. K., & Gerton, J. (1993). Psychological impact of biculturalism: Evidence and theory. *Psychological Bulletin, 114*, 395–412.

Langley, A. K., Nadeem, E., Kataoka, S. H., Stein, B. D., & Jaycox, L. H. (2010). Evidence-based mental health programs in schools: Barriers and facilitators of successful implementation. *School Mental Health, 2*(3), 105–113.

Lau, A. S. (2006). Making the case for selective and directed cultural adaptations of evidence-based treatments: Examples from parent training. *Clinical Psychology: Science and Practice, 13*(4), 295–310.

Leaf, P. J., Algeria, M., Cohen, P., Goodman, S. H., Horwitz, S. M., Hoven, C. W., et al. (1996). Mental health service use in the community and schools: Results from the four community MECA study. *Journal of the American Academy of Child and Adolescent Psychiatry, 35*, 889–897.

Lefley, C. S., Scott, M., Llabre, M., & Hicks, D. (1993). Cultural beliefs about rape and victims' response in three ethnic groups. *The American Journal of Orthopsychiatry, 63*(4), 623–632.

Leong, F. T. L., & Lau, A. S. L. (2001). Barriers to providing effective mental health services to Asian Americans. *Mental Health Services Research, 3*(4), 201–214.

Leong, F. T. L., Leach, M. M., Yeh, C., & Chou, E. (2007). Suicide among Asian Americans: What do we know? What do we need to know? *Death Studies, 31*, 417–434.

Lewis-Fernandez, R., Guarnaccia, P. J., Martinez, I. E., Salman, E., Schmidt, A., & Liebowitz, M. (2002). Comparative phenomenology of ataques de nervios, panic attacks, and panic disorder. *Culture, Medicine and Psychiatry, 26*, 199–223.

Low, G., & Organista, K. C. (2000). Latinas and sexual assault: Towards culturally sensitive assessment and intervention. *Journal of Multicultural Social Work, 8*(1/2), 131–157.

Luo, T. (2000). Marrying my rapist? The cultural trauma among Chinese rape survivors. *Gender and Society, 14*, 581–597.

Marcia, J. E. (1980). Identity in adolescents. In J. Adelson (Ed.), *Handbook of adolescent psychology* (pp. 159–187). New York, NY: Wiley.

Marmar, C. R., Weiss, D. S., Schlenger, W. E., Fairbank, J. A., Jordan, B. K., Kulka, R. A., et al. (1994). Peritraumatic dissociation and posttraumatic stress in male Vietnam theater veterans. *The American Journal of Psychiatry, 151*, 902–907.

Marsee, M. A. (2008). Reactive aggression and posttraumatic stress in adolescents affected by hurricane Katrina. *Journal of Clinical Child and Adolescent Psychology, 37*, 519–529.

Marshall, G., & Orlando, M. (2002). Acculturation and peritraumatic dissociation in young adult Latino survivors of community violence. *Journal of Abnormal Psychology, 111*, 166–174.

May, P. A. (1996). Overview of alcohol abuse epidemiology for American Indian populations. In G. D. Sandefur, R. R. Rindfuss, & B. Cohen (Eds.), *Changing numbers, changing needs: American Indian demography and public health* (pp. 235–261). Washington, DC: National Academy Press.

McGloin, J. S., & Widom, C. S. (2001). Resilience among abused and neglected children all grown up. *Development and Psychopathology, 13*, 1021–1038.

McKay, M. M., Lynn, C. J., & Bannon, W. M. (2005). Understanding inner city child mental health need and trauma exposure: Implications for preparing urban service providers. *The American Journal of Orthopsychiatry, 75*(2), 201–210.

McMiller, W. P., & Weisz, J. R. (1996). Help-seeking preceding mental health clinic intake among African-American, Latino and Caucasian youths. *Journal of the American Academy of Child and Adolescent Psychiatry, 35*(3), 1086–1094.

Merriam, L. (1977). The effects of boarding schools on Indian family life. In S. Unger (Ed.), *The destruction of American Indian families* (pp. 14–17). New York: Association on American Indian Affairs.

Miner, M. H., Flitter, J. M., & Robinson, B. B. (2006). Association of sexual revictimization with sexuality and psychological function. *Journal of Interpersonal Violence, 21*, 503–524.

Miranda, J., Bernal, G., Lau, A., Kohn, L., Hwang, W., & LaFromboise, T. (2005). State of the science on psychosocial interventions for ethnic minorities. *Annual Review of Clinical Psychology, 1*, 113–142.

Mock, M. (2012). Advancing school-based mental health for Asian American Pacific Islander youth. In C. S. Clauss-Ehlers, Z. Serpell, & M. D. Weist (Eds.), *Handbook of culturally responsive school mental health: Advancing research, training, practice, and policy*. New York, NY: Springer.

Monroe, L., Kinney, L. M., Weist, M. D., Spriggs, D., Dantzler, J., & Reynolds, M. (2005). The experience of sexual assault: Findings from a statewide victim needs assessment. *Journal of Interpersonal Violence, 20*, 767–776.

Morales, J., & Reyes, M. (1998). Cultural and political realities for community social work practice with Puerto Ricans in the United States. In F. G. Rivera & J. L. Erlich (Eds.), *Community organizing in a diverse society* (3rd ed., pp. 75–96). Boston: Allyn and Bacon.

Ngo, V., Langley, A., Kataoka, S. H., Nadeem, E., Escudero, P., & Stein, B. D. (2008). Providing evidence based practice to ethnically diverse youths: examples from the Cognitive Behavioral Intervention for Trauma in Schools (CBITS) program. *Journal of the American Academy of Child and Adolescent Psychiatry, 47*(8), 858–862.

Park, S., Brody, L. R., & Wilson, V. (2008). Social sharing of emotional experiences in Asian- and European-American women. *Cognition and Emotion, 22*, 802–814.

Piña, A. A., & Silverman, W. K. (2004). Clinical phenomenology, somatic symptoms, and distress in Hispanic/Latino and European American youths with anxiety disorders. *Journal of Clinical Child and Adolescent Psychology, 33*, 227–236.

Pittinger, S. M. (1998). The relationship between ethnic identity, self esteem, emotional well-being and depression among Lakota/Dakota Sioux adolescents. *Dissertation Abstracts International, 60*, 1311B.

Pole, N., Best, S. R., Metzler, T., & Marmar, C. R. (2005). Why are Hispanics at greater risk for PTSD? *Cultural Diversity and Ethnic Minority Psychology, 11*, 144–161.

Pole, N., Gone, J. P., & Kulkarni, M. (2008). Posttraumatic stress disorder among ethnoracial minorities in the United States. *Clinical Psychology: Science and Practice, 15*(1), 35–61.

President's New Freedom Commission on Mental Health. (2003). *Achieving the promise: Transforming mental health care in America, executive summary* (DHHS Pub. No. SMA-03-3831). Rockville, MD: U.S. Department of Health and Human Services.

Pumariega, A. J., Rogers, K., & Rothe, E. (2005). Culturally competent systems of care for children's mental health: Advances and challenges. *Community Mental Health Journal, 41*, 539–555.

Ramisetty-Mikler, S., Caetano, R., & McGrath, C. (2007). Sexual aggression among White, Black, and Hispanic couples in the U. S.: Alcohol use and other forms of aggression as its correlates. *The American Journal of Drug and Alcohol Abuse, 33*, 31–43.

Rao, K., DiClemente, R. J., & Ponton, L. E. (1992). Child sexual abuse of Asians compared to other populations. *Journal of the American Academy of Child and Adolescent Psychiatry, 31*, 880–886.

Rennison, C. M. (2000). *Criminal victimization 1999: Changes 1998–99 with trends 1993–99*. Washington, DC: Bureau of Justice Statistics, National Crime Victimization Survey, US Department of Justice.

Rones, M., & Hoagwood, K. (2000). School based mental health services: A research review. *Clinical Child and Family Psychology Review, 3*(4), 223–241.

Ruchkin, V., Schwab-Stone, M., Jones, S., Cicchetti, D. V., Koposov, R., & Vermeiren, R. (2005). Is posttraumatic stress in youth a culture-bound phenomenon? A comparison of symptom trends in selected U.S. and Russian communities. *The American Journal of Psychiatry, 16*(2), 538–544.

Saigh, P. A., Yasik, A. E., Oberfield, R. O., Halamandaris, P., & Bremner, D. J. (2006). The intellectual performance of traumatized children and adolescents with or without posttraumatic stress disorder. *Journal of Abnormal Psychology, 115*, 332–340.

Schwab-Stone, M., Chen, C., Greenberger, E., Silver, D., Lichtman, J., & Voyce, C. (1999). No safe haven II: The effects of violence exposure on urban youth. *Journal of the American Academy of Child and Adolescent Psychiatry, 38*(4), 359–367.

Silverman, W. K., Oritz, C. D., Viswesvaran, C., Burns, B. J., Kolko, D. J., Putnam, F. W., et al. (2008). Evidence based treatments for children and adolescents exposed to traumatic events. *Journal of Clinical Child and Adolescent Psychology, 37*(1), 156–183.

Soleimanpour, S., Geierstanger, S. P., Kaller, S., McCarter, V., & Brindis, C. D. (2010). The role of school health centers in health care access and client outcomes. *American Journal of Public Health, 100*(9), 1597–1603.

Starrett, R. A., Bresler, C., Decker, J. T., Walters, G. T., & Rogers, D. (1990). The role of environment awareness and support networks in Hispanic elderly persons' use of formal social services. *Journal of Community Psychology, 18*, 218–226.

Stein, B. D., Jaycox, L. H., Kataoka, S., Rhodes, H. J., & Vestal, K. D. (2003). Prevalence of child and adolescent exposure to community violence. *Clinical Child and Family Psychology Review, 6*(4), 247–264.

Stein, B. D., Jaycox, L. H., Kataoka, S. H., Wong, M., Tu, W., Elliot, M. N., et al. (2003). A mental health intervention for schoolchildren exposed to violence: A randomized controlled trial. *Journal of the American Medical Association, 290*(5), 603–611.

Stephan, S. H., Weist, M., Kataoka, S., Adelsheim, S., & Mills, C. (2007). Transformation of children's mental health services: The role of school mental health. *Psychiatric Services, 58*(10), 1330–1338.

Sue, D. W., & Kirk, B. A. (1975). Asian Americans: Uses of counseling and psychiatric services on a college campus. *Journal of Counseling Psychology, 22*, 84–86.

Sue, S. (2006). Cultural competency: From philosophy to research and practice. *Journal of Community Psychology, 34*(2), 237–245.

Sue, S., & Morishima, J. K. (1982). *The mental health of Asian Americans*. San Francisco: Jossey-Bass.

Tata, S. P., & Leong, F. T. L. (1994). Individualism-collectivism, social-network orientation, and acculturation as predictors of attitudes toward seeking professional psychological help among Chinese Americans. *Journal of Counseling Psychology, 41*, 280–287.

Taylor, L. K., & Weems, C. F. (2011). Cognitive-behavior therapy for disaster exposed youth with post traumatic stress: Results from a multiple-baseline examination. *Behavior Therapy, 42*, 349–363.

Teicher, M. H., Polcari, A., Andersen, S. L., Anderson, C. M., & Navalta, C. (2003). Neurobiological effects of childhood stress and trauma. In S. W. Coates, J. L. Rosenthal, & D. S. Schechter (Eds.), *September 11, trauma and human bonds*. New York: Analytic Press.

Tjaden, P., & Thoennes, N. (1998). *Prevalence, incidence, and consequences of violence against women: Findings from the National Violence Against Women Survey*. Washington, DC: U.S. Department of Justice.

Tjaden, P., & Thoennes, N. (2000). *Full report of the prevalence, incidence, and consequences of violence against women: Findings From the national violence against women survey*. Research report. Washington, DC: U.S. Department of Justice, National Institute of Justice, November 2000, NCJ 183781.

Tracy, L. (2002). Post-traumatic stress disorder, depression and heavy alcohol use among Chinese Americans: The salience of trauma. *Dissertation Abstracts International Section A: Humanities and Social Sciences, 62*, 2574.

Tummala-Narra, P. (2007). Trauma and resilience: A case of individual psychotherapy in a multicultural context. *Journal of Aggression, Maltreatment, and Trauma, 14*, 33–53.

U.S. Census Bureau. (2001). *Profiles of general demographic characteristics 2000. 2000 census of populations and housing*. Washington, DC: U.S. Government Printing Office.

U.S. Department of Health and Human Services. (2001). *Mental health: Culture, race, and ethnicity. A supplement to mental health: A report of the surgeon general*. Rockville, MD: U.S. Department of Health and Human Services, Substance Abuse and Mental Health Services Administration, Center for Mental Health Services.

U.S. Public Health Service Office of the Surgeon General. (2001). *Mental health: Culture, race, and ethnicity: A supplement to mental health: A report of the surgeon general*. Rockville, MD: Department of Health and Human Services.

Uba, L. (1994). *Asian Americans: Personality patterns, identity, and mental health*. New York: The Guilford Press.

van der Kolk, B. (2005). Developmental trauma disorder: Toward a rational diagnosis for children with complex trauma histories. *Psychiatric Annals, 35*(5), 401–409.

Warner, B. S., & Weist, M. D. (1996). Urban youth as witnesses to violence: Beginning assessment and treatment efforts. *Journal of Youth and Adolescence, 25*, 361–377.

Warner, B. S., Weist, M. D., & Krulak, A. (1999). Risk factors for school violence. *Urban Education, 34*, 52–68.

Weems, C. F., Scott, B. G., Taylor, L. K., Cannon, M. F., Romano, D. M., Perry, A. M., et al. (2010). Test anxiety intervention and prevention programs in schools: Program development and rationale. *School Mental Health, 2*, 62–71.

Weist, M. D. (1997). Expanded school mental health services: A national movement in progress. In T. H. Ollendick & R. J. Prinz (Eds.), *Advances in clinical child psychology* (Vol. 19, pp. 319–352). New York: Plenum Press.

Weist, M. D., Acosta, O. M., & Youngstrom, E. (2001). Predictors of violence exposure among inner-city youth. *Journal of Clinical Child Psychology, 30*, 187–198.

Weist, M. D., & Cooley-Quille, M. (2001). Advancing efforts to address violence and youth. *Journal of Clinical Child Psychology, 30*, 147–151.

Weist, M. D., Evans, S. W., & Lever, N. (2003). *Handbook of school mental health: Advancing practice and research*. New York, NY: Kluwer Academic.

Weist, M. D., & Warner, B. S. (1997). Intervening against violence in the schools. *Annals of Adolescent Psychiatry, 21*, 235–251.

Weller, S. C., Baer, R. D., Garcia de Alba Garcia, J., & Salcedo Rocha, A. L. (2008). Susto and nervios: Expressions for stress and depression. *Culture, Medicine & Psychiatry, 32*(3), 406–420.

Whitesell, N. R., Mitchell, C. M., Kaufman, C. E., & Spicer, P. (2006). Developmental trajectories of personal and collective self-concept among American Indian adolescents. *Child Development, 77*, 1487–1503.

Whitesell, N. R., Mitchell, C. M., & Spicer, P. (2009). A longitudinal study of self-esteem, cultural identity, and academic success among American Indian adolescents. *Cultural Diversity and Ethnic Minority Psychology, 15*, 38–50.

Wirtz, K. (2005). 'Where obscurity is a virtue': The mystique of unintelligibility in Santería ritual. *Language & Communication, 25*, 351–375.

Woodward, A. M., Dwinell, A. D., & Arons, B. S. (1992). Barriers to mental health care for Hispanic Americans: A literature review and discussion. *Journal of Mental Health Administration, 19*, 224–236.

Yasik, A. E., Saigh, P. A., Oberfield, R. O., & Halamandaris, P. V. (2007). Posttraumatic stress disorder: Memory and learning performance in children and adolescents. *Biological Psychiatry, 61*, 382–388.

Yasui, M., & Dishion, T. J. (2007). The ethnic context of child and adolescent problem behavior: Implications for child and family interventions. *Clinical Child and Family Psychology Review, 10*(2), 137–179.

Youngstrom, E. A., Weist, M. D., & Albus, K. E. (2003). Exploring violence exposure, stress, protective factors, and behavioral problems among inner-city youth. *American Journal of Community Psychology, 32*, 115–129.

Zane, N., & Mak, W. (2003). Major approaches to the measurement of acculturation among ethnic minority populations: A content analysis and an alternative empirical strategy. In K. M. Chun, P. B. Organista, & G. Maria (Eds.), *Acculturation: Advances in theory, measurement, and applied research* (pp. 39–60). Washington, DC: American Psychological Association.

Zayfert, C. (2008). Culturally competent treatment of posttraumatic stress disorder in clinical practice: An ideographic, transcultural approach. *Clinical Psychology: Science and Practice, 15*(1), 68–73.

Zhou, Z., Siu, C. R., & Xin, T. (2009). Promoting cultural competence in counseling Asian American children and adolescents. *Psychology in the Schools, 46*(3), 290–298.

Zyromski, B. (2007). African American and Latino youth and post-traumatic stress syndrome: Effects on school violence and interventions for school counselors. *Journal of School Violence, 6*(1), 121–137.

Next Steps: Advancing Culturally Competent School Mental Health

19

Zewelanji N. Serpell, Caroline S. Clauss-Ehlers, and Mark D. Weist

Current Status of Culturally Competent School Mental Health

Chapter 19 of this *Handbook* offers some concluding thoughts. The first part of this chapter presents an overview of critical themes and advancements evident in each of the *Handbook*'s major sections (i.e., research, innovation, and specific problems). This part is followed by a discussion of key outstanding issues relevant to culturally competent school mental health (SMH). The chapter concludes with recommendations for next steps and guidelines about how to formulate a call to action for the provision of culturally responsive SMH.

Three critical themes emerged across sections of the handbook: (1) *relevance*—culture is in multiple ways a relevant consideration in SMH; (2) *responsiveness*—efforts to promote SMH must be responsive to the concerns, strengths, and needs of diverse communities of children, adolescents, and their families; and (3) *perspective*—effective SMH policy, research, training, and practice all require a culturally-integrated perspective.

Z.N. Serpell (✉)
Virginia State University, Petersburg, VA, USA
e-mail: zserpell@vsu.edu

C.S. Clauss-Ehlers
Rutgers, The State University of New Jersey, New Brunswick, NJ, USA

M.D. Weist
University of South Carolina, Columbia, SC, USA

Relevance. Writings in Part I exemplify the first theme by illustrating that cultural considerations cut across diverse school settings. We know that children learn in a host of different educational environments, and chapters in this section discuss the relevance of culture in contexts that range from overseas military base schools to rural communities within the U.S. Chapters throughout Part I also demonstrate that cultural consideration is relevant to the roles held by school personnel and their resulting diversity of experience. For instance, in Chap. 3 discussion of school-based mental health services in a rural context illustrates the challenges faced by a graduate student attempting to provide evidence-based therapy to a client while developing his own skills as a clinician such as the challenges the SMH provider faces in efforts to address multiple issues; and consultation with educators about the extent and nature of problems identified in the school setting. Similarly, Chap. 4, *From Guidance to School Counseling: New Models in School Mental Health,* discusses challenges associated with collaborating across educational and counseling cultures. This chapter addresses cultural shifts in the school counselor role as the approach increasingly considers the child's social/emotional development.

Responsiveness. The second theme evident in the *Handbook* comes across most clearly in *Part II: Innovative Approaches in Work with Diverse Children and Adolescents in Schools.* Being responsive to diverse communities of youth requires innovation. In this chapter, Clauss-Ehlers refers to culturally innovative responders as systems that develop creative programmatic strategies that respond to and are implemented within a specific cultural context. Two types of responsiveness are conceptualized in the chapters that comprise Part II: responsiveness through program development and/or adaptation, and being responsive to diverse communities of youth.

The first type of responsiveness occurs through program development/adaptation and is the more specific of the two. The central principle is to create/adapt programs in ways that attend specifically to the cultural values embedded in the community the program was designed to serve. This is complex work, as illustrated in Chap. 6, where researchers tackle the difference between issues of fidelity versus cultural specificity in the Black Parents Strengths and Strategies (BPSS) program-a cultural adaptation of an existing evidence-based intervention.

The second type of responsiveness entails being responsive to particular communities of youth by attending to the fact that their experiences in school contexts may be unique. For example, Chaps. 7 and 9 underscore the need to acknowledge that schools may be uniquely hostile and compromise the mental health of particular groups of youth. Hence, for schools to ensure all their students can learn and thrive, contextual and school climate issues must be systematically addressed. For example, Chap. 7 demonstrates how many lesbian, gay, bisexual, and transgender (LGBT) youth feel unsafe, harassed, and unsupported in school. As such, it is imperative that schools address climate issues for LGBT youth and through systemic changes in policy related to dealing with bullying, supporting teachers, training school personnel, community organizing, and involving parents. Similarly, readers will recall that Chap. 9 discusses the importance of positive school climate for the mental health of African American boys. The chapter illustrates how school context issues such as racial discrimination, overrepresentation in remedial education classes, and being more likely than their non-Black counterparts to be accused by teachers of misbehaving; predisposes African American males to negative mental health and academic outcomes. The take home message from this chapter is that effective policies, programs, and practices require researchers and practitioners to consider what it is like to be an African American male in the school context.

Culturally Integrated Perspective. The third major theme is evident throughout *Part III* and captures the overarching purpose of the *Handbook,* which is to advocate for a comprehensive perspective to addressing culture in SMH. This approach requires that cultural considerations be infused throughout all facets of SMH work. This process starts at the outset, with the training of school personnel, but extends to meet the larger societal goal by advocating for change through public policy initiatives.

Highlights from chapters that comprise Part III are provided below to illustrate how an integrated cultural perspective can be manifested in research, training, practice, and policy.

Research. Chapter 15, *Culturally Integrated Substance Abuse and Sex Education: Prevention Programming for Middle School Students*, provides an excellent example of cultural integration in program development. Authors discuss the research design implemented at each intervention site to create programs that are infused with cultural content, but also consider cultural variables among youth and their families. Chapter 15 also highlights efforts to create direct linkages to practice.

Training. Chapter 14, *Training Transformed School Counselors*, provides an important example of how training can incorporate a cultural perspective. Chapter authors present a program model based on the philosophy that "there is a direct correlation between academic success and optimal mental health. This philosophy posits that if barriers to optimal mental health are effectively challenged and removed, then the likelihood of academic success increases" (Ostvik-deWilde, Park, & Lee, Chap. 19, this volume). Critical to the program is training school counselors to work towards closing the United States (U.S.) educational achievement gap. Readers will recall that the chapter continues with a discussion about how the University of Maryland at College Park's Urban School Counseling Program mentors and trains graduate students committed to social justice, multiculturalism, and work within an urban school context.

Practice. Chapter 16, *Promoting Culturally Competent Assessment in Schools*, addresses how to incorporate a cultural perspective in assessment. Chapter authors discuss the reality of cultural bias in school assessment that leads to disproportionate placement in special education classes among youth of color, bias in social/emotional behavior ratings, bias in referral and disciplinary action, and test bias overall. Readers will recall that the authors present best practices that integrate a cultural perspective in assessment. A case illustration is provided and the use of strengths-based assessments, such as the Behavioral Assessment for Children of African Heritage (BACAH) and the Behavior and Emotional Rating Scale-2 (BERS), are described.

Policy. Chapter 17, *Work–Family Balance: Challenges and Advances for Families,* illustrates the cultural integration theme within the policy arena. The author discusses current issues associated with work/family balance and resulting policy implications within the cultural context of American society. Author Patricia M. Raskin writes: "The absence of societal support, the fact that Americans work more hours, and have fewer days off than any other developed countries, means that our attempts to balance work and family result in individual solutions rather than broad policy changes" (Chap. 19, this volume).

In sum, the three advancements: *relevance*, *responsiveness*, and *integrated cultural perspective* permeate all sections of the *Handbook*. While some sections may place more emphasis on a theme than others, each has the three themes at its core. These advancements do not operate in isolation. Rather, they are linked and connected throughout the *Handbook*.

Key Outstanding Issues

As is evidenced by the richness of the content of the chapters that comprise this handbook, a lot of progress has been made. Culturally competent SMH is increasingly embraced as a mechanism through which to eliminate mental health and educational disparities (New Freedom Commission, 2003), and schools are in many ways the ideal context to reach a good number of diverse and underserved groups (Weist, Myers, Hastings, Ghuman, & Han, 1999). Yet, significant challenges abide (Adelman & Taylor, 2002). Highlighted in the next section of this chapter are some outstanding issues relevant to achieving culturally competent SMH that warrant attention if the field is to move forward, and if the goal of effectively serving culturally diverse youth is to be met.

Operationalizing Cultural Competence in Ways that Are Measurable and Useful

Advancing culturally competent SMH requires a concrete articulation of how best to meet the needs of culturally diverse youth, which is contingent on understanding what constitutes their uniqueness. At the center of this challenge, is defining "culture" and "competence" in ways that are measurable and useful. The field is unfortunately replete with definitional ambiguities, particularly about culture. Culture is frequently defined too broadly, and in school contexts, mostly relegated to the constructs of race, ethnicity, or language (Carpenter-Song, Schwallie, & Longhofer, 2007). Furthermore, culture is often conceptualized as static, homogenous, and not subject to contextual influence (Kleinman & Benson, 2006).

An additional critique levied by anthropologists against traditional cultural competence models is their failure to attend to the dynamic ways in which sociopolitical constructs like race and socioeconomic status play in the conceptualization, provision, and access of mental health care (Carpenter-Song et al., 2007). This failure is particularly evident in schools—where long standing and unresolved racial disparities in referral, special education placement, disciplinary practices, and service provision are rife (Losen & Orfield, 2002; Skiba et al., 2008).

Defining competence. A key issue in defining competence is whether it is a unidimensional or multidimensional construct. If examined as a multidimensional construct, competence likely includes knowledge, awareness, and emotive components (Sue & Torino, 2005). However, how these components relate to one another and which is more or less important in the developing of "competence" is still largely unknown. Historically, knowledge and awareness have been the dimensions most heavily emphasized in multicultural training. Yet, experts in the field are quick to highlight the importance of caring in actuating changes in practitioner beliefs and attitudes (Sue, 2006). Knowing, caring, and acting likely follow a hierarchical order, such that knowledge and caring may be necessary prerequisites to action.

Increasingly embraced is the notion that competence is a dynamic and ongoing process that cannot be pursued as an outcome nor achieved as a result of a single training event (Cunningham, Ozdemir, Summers, & Ghunney, 2006). Moreover, newer frameworks that identify the critical elements of cultural competence note the importance of recognizing that sometimes culture may not be central to understanding students' mental health problems (Yamada & Brekke, 2008). In fact, cultural competence could more appropriately be defined as the ability to recognize when cultural factors *are* at play or relevant, and working in a manner that attends to these factors (Ortiz & Flanagan, 2002). Others have emphasized that culture and cultural factors can actually promote resilience and positive mental health outcomes for youth (Clauss-Ehlers, 2008b; Clauss-Ehlers & Wibrowski, 2007; Clauss-Ehlers, Yang, & Chen, 2006). While these perspectives are gaining traction in the field, actualizing their use in school contexts requires attention to institutional factors and policies that dictate the behavior of people operating within schools.

Eliminating Barriers Embedded in the "Culture" of School

Several models of culturally competent practice arise from the health sector, and while many issues are cross cutting; addressing mental health in school contexts entails its own set of challenges. Culture is embedded in the structure of schools. Part of the culture of schools is a long-standing debate about whether mental health is an integral and inseparable part of education (Adelman & Taylor, 2011; Clauss-Ehlers, 2008a). That is, an implicit necessity in efforts to promote SMH is engaging teachers to take on as part of their identities as educators, helping schools meet students' mental health needs (Burke & Paternite, 2007; Rones & Hoagwood, 2000). Achieving culturally competent SMH will require a transformation in the school environment and to the policies that reinforce existing structures that contribute to inequities experienced by culturally diverse students and their families. Part of this transformation involves building stronger collaborations between the educational and the counseling factions within schools (see Chap. 4; Clauss-Ehlers, 2008a).

Improving Cultural Competence Training Models

The skills necessary to successfully navigate diverse social contexts and to be more receptive and sensitive to the unique needs of culturally diverse students and their families are complex. Multicultural counseling training is the basis for much of what today is encompassed in cultural competence training. Multicultural counseling competencies were developed more than three decades ago and provide a set of guidelines for enhancing service delivery with racial and ethnic populations, including an articulation of a tripartite model defined in terms of counselors ability to: (1) recognize their personal attitudes and values around race and ethnicity; (2) develop their knowledge of diverse cultural worldviews and experiences; and (3) identify effective skills in working with diverse populations (Sue, Arredondo, & McDavis, 1992). This framework was expanded to include three key characteristics that culturally competent counselors should have: an awareness of personal assumptions, values, and biases; an understanding of the worldviews of culturally diverse clients; and developing abilities to use and create culturally appropriate intervention strategies (Sue et al. 1992). The key part of the expansion was the inclusion of action—using and creating appropriate strategies.

Cultural competence training is increasingly a standard part of preprofessional training of teachers and other school personnel. However, it frequently functions as a separate add-on, rather than as an underlying theme across preservice courses (see Ostvik-deWilde, Park & Lee, Chap. 19, this volume, for a rare example of a program that uses cultural competency as the foundation for an entire program curriculum).

Once preservice teachers, counselors, psychologists, and others are integrated into the profession, opportunities for developing cultural competence most often take the form of professional development workshops. These workshops are frequently built into schools as a one-time professional development experience. While an important mechanism to provide training to school personnel, this practice can foster a belief that participating in a single training event is sufficient. The fact that there is rarely an effort within schools to provide continuous professional development in this domain is problematic. It is a significant problem because cultures evolve quickly, and the cultural diversity in schools is becoming far more nuanced than has been the case in the past. In fact, many teachers report that they rarely utilize much of what is covered in such workshops and that they rely mostly on experience to inform their multicultural practice (Gallavan, 2007).

Also worthy of note is that the focus of cultural competence workshops is typically knowledge and awareness, which may prompt some changes in the caring dimension of competence, but will rarely actuate change in the acting dimension. This is because the latter is quite resistant to change, as there are many things that get in the way of acting on multicultural issues. For example, one might choose not to act because one does not recognize the relative benefit of action or alternatively the risk associated with nonaction. Furthermore, practitioners may be uncomfortable or not confident about the appropriate course of action.

Hence, training for action appears to be a neglected but critical component of cultural competence training in schools. Actuating real change requires an explicit confrontation—one that entails understanding and acknowledging ones own biases (Arredondo, Tovar-Blank, & Parham, 2008). As such, almost by definition cultural competence training entails some level of discomfort, which is not usually present in professional development workshops. It is a fine balance because training must be structured to, while uncomfortable, not be threatening.

Social scientists have noted that as a result of *stereotype threat*, multicultural training can sometimes yield the opposite effect—that is, rather than promoting competence in interactions with culturally diverse others, it yields behaviors that are antithetical to positive and productive interactions (Steele, 2003). Steele defines stereotype threat simply as "the threat of being viewed through the lens of a negative stereotype or the fear of doing something that would inadvertently confirm that stereotype" (Perry, Steele, & Hilliard, 2003, p. 111). Practitioners need to develop "full competence, rather than just sensitivity, in the skills and knowledge bases related to these areas and be able to integrate them in a manner that guides cross-cultural interactions" (Ortiz, Flanagan, & Dynda, 2008, p. 1722).

Lastly, while there is much guidance about specific methods to improve cultural competence among practitioners, there is little empirically supported work that justifies or "proves" the utility of attending to culture in mental health care (Bhui, Warfa, Edonya, McKenzie, & Bhugra, 2007). Given the relatively early stage of research and development on multicultural competence training for teachers, much more work is needed to fully integrate cultural competence training into SMH efforts. Much of the wider literature on training is descriptive and focused on justifying why multicultural competence is an important goal for practitioners.

A consideration that will become increasingly important as work in this domain progresses is examining whether training translates not only to shifts in knowledge and attitude, but also shifts in comfort, ease, and specific changes in practice. More research is also needed to assess whether multicultural training has a long-term impact on practice as well as on student outcomes.

Improving Measures of Cultural Competence

Cultural competence, cultural responsiveness, and cultural proficiency are all used interchangeably but are arguably quite different in their operational form, and measuring each of these indices within school contexts is difficult. A critical area of need in the field is research that helps define or guide efforts to measure cultural competence among SMH providers and teachers. There is a plethora of measurement scales examining personal attitudes, behaviors, and skills of individual care providers (see Cunningham et al., 2006 for a summarized list), including the Cross-Cultural Counseling Inventory (CCCI), Multicultural Awareness/Knowledge/Skills Survey (MAKSS), Multicultural Counseling Awareness Scale—Form B (MCAS-B), Multicultural Counseling Inventory (MCI), and the Self-Inventory for Educators Promoting Multicultural Efforts in Schools.

However, the assessment of cultural competence frequently occurs at the individual level, is short term, and relies on self-reports of attitude and knowledge. We know that assessments of knowledge alone are insufficient and there are substantial measurement problems with some widely used scales. For example, Davis and Phiney (2006) found that the Cross-Cultural Adaptability Inventory (CCAI) demonstrates poor reliability and factor structures that are uninterpretable when used with preservice college students. Additionally, although institutional structures are critical to establishing policy and ensuring the necessary support for culturally competent practice, few instruments assess competence at the institutional level.

Addressing Critical Gaps in the Knowledge Base

Research and practice in child, adolescent, and SMH are increasingly emphasizing evidence-based practice (EBP) or implementing prevention and intervention programs based on the science of what has been proven to be associated with valued outcomes. As this emphasis plays out, it is becoming clear that research-based EBPs, associated with infrastructure and implementation support (such as significant training, incentives, ongoing coaching, and fidelity monitoring) are quite different from implementing EBPs in real-world settings such as schools, where there is little if any infrastructure and implementation support (see Weist et al., 2009). This is promoting research and practice strategies on *achievable* EBP, or strategies that can actually be implemented in real-world settings such as schools, with clinicians contending with real-world issues such as fluidity in the environment, poor infrastructure support, and significant deficits in service capacity to meet the needs of the many children and youth presenting mental health challenges (see Evans & Weist, 2004).

Adding to this problematic context is the recognition that many EBPs have not been developed and tested with a range of groups varying along dimensions such as race/ethnicity, socioeconomic status, age, local geography, and culture (see Alegria, Atkins, Farmer, Slaton, & Stelk, 2010). This can lead to the erroneous conclusion that because a particular EBP has not been tested with a particular group, then it is not appropriate or relevant to that group. If many were to adopt this view, movement toward culturally competent and EBP would come to a standstill. Jensen and Foster (2010) emphasize a significant and multidimensional research-to-practice gap in child and adolescent mental health. To help bridge this gap they call for purposeful attention to and measurement of aspects of the gap, for example, looking at research translation problems across parameters of (a) disorder, (b) intervention type, and (c) setting type. They suggest gathering information on aspects of the gap through "consensus conferences" during which diverse stakeholder groups would identify areas where gaps are prominent, identifying areas of "low hanging fruit" where the most progress could be made. We would recommend that culture/ethnicity is a fourth dimension of this framework, and we agree with Jensen and Foster's call for such consensus conferences to identifying key strategies to advance research and practice, ideally in ways that are linked together. The University of Maryland Center for School Mental Health (CSMH) held such a consensus conference on Cultural Competence in SMH (see Cunningham et al., 2006), with a number of fruitful recommendations generated (see discussion that follows for examples). Similar and regular consensus conferences are needed, with active methods for generating ongoing dialogue and collaboration among relevant stakeholders and professional groups.

An alternative direction is for research to consider the added value of training and emphases on cultural competence to the effectiveness of EBPs delivered in schools. For example, providing training and support for culturally competent strategies simultaneous to the training and delivery of established EBPs for particular groups, and exploring the added value of such complementary training and support (see Alegria et al., 2010). A similar strategy can be taken in practice, where practitioners use established EBPs while at the same time receiving guidance on their implementation from local cultural experts. For example, implementing evidence-based anger management training for youth in the Baltimore schools, while receiving guidance from local stakeholders with experience in working effectively with African American youth.

It is also important to distinguish between focused EBPs, often associated with manualized intervention, and *empirically supported* strategies, which are based on science, but not as prescriptive as EBPs (see Evans & Weist, 2004). Here, building interventions based on knowledge of risk and protective factors is a particularly important approach. For example, continuing the theme of working with youth in Baltimore, guided by local stakeholders, interventions could be implemented focused on reducing hanging out in dangerous neighborhoods (especially at potentially dangerous times such as late at night on the weekend), avoiding involvement with peers involved with drug using or dealing, and increasing involvement in activities clearly shown to have a protective influence, such as athletic, extracurricular, and spiritual involvements; enhancing connections with positive adults; and enhancing connections with positive resources in the neighborhood, such as after-school programs and recreation centers (see Warner & Weist, 1996). Research is also needed that compares these empirically supported strategies with implementation of more focused EBPs.

Another critical avenue for research and practice is clarifying the provider characteristics that contribute to culturally competent and effective prevention and intervention. Unfortunately, there is little research to provide answers to this question. As mentioned, the University of Maryland CSMH convened a panel in 2006 on cultural competence in SMH. A key conclusion was a major factor contributing to provider cultural competence is *empathy* manifested in many different ways. For example, openly acknowledging differences in race/ethnicity and background with youth and families served by the school and expressing and demonstrating genuine eagerness in learning about local culture; seeking understanding of strengths and needs of the community and its families; and adjusting prevention and intervention approaches to match what is learned (Cunningham et al., 2006). Such an empathic approach to SMH would also mean identifying various cultural groups, reaching out to their members and leaders, and explicitly seeking recommendations on the delivery of programs and services, and ongoing feedback to continuously improve them.

Integrating Research, Practice, and Policy

The aforementioned strategies for effective research and practice should ideally occur within an environment characterized by diverse stakeholders and disciplines coming together to advance effective SMH within a true system of care (see Chap. 1). This usually means developing a *coherent* and progressively evolving agenda for SMH that involves systems leaders and staff from education, mental health, child welfare, juvenile services, health services, developmental disabilities, and others working together to better connect programs and services, with SMH often serving as a uniting influence since it is already positioned in the nexus of these systems (Weist & Paternite, 2006). However, the reality is that SMH initiatives are usually not coherent, instead reflecting an ad hoc arrangement of different partnerships and approaches in different schools.

Here, the Community of Practice framework (see Chap. 1) can be very helpful. A key factor is for one group that has legitimacy to step forward and provide the convening and supportive functions for diverse stakeholders to come together to move from discussion to dialogue to collaboration on key dimensions of growing and increasing the cultural competence and effectiveness of SMH. Universities are uniquely positioned to be in this convening and supportive role. Ideally, these coherent initiatives occur in areas with logical boundaries, such as school districts or counties, as supported by state leaders, and again, all of the work should reflect a *shared agenda* or partnership among education, families, mental health, and other community systems (Andis et al., 2002). Often a Steering Team of 4–8 leaders reflecting this shared agenda comes together for initial planning; holds successive discussion and planning meetings, with a larger Advisory Board for the initiative emerging from these meetings. The group will then work on developing an identity, with a name, common goals, development of Memoranda of Agreement (MOAs) between schools and provider organizations in communities, standardized approaches for training and evaluation, and a plan for growing funding and expanding programs and services.

These coherent SMH initiatives are emerging at the local level (e.g., the Baltimore Expanded SMH initiative) and at the state level (e.g., the Ohio Mental Health Network for School Success, Montana's Integrated SMH Initiative). Importantly, they provide a vehicle for advancing training, practice, research, and policy in SMH while at the same time promoting interconnections among these realms. As mentioned, examples of this work can be found at http:\\www.sharedwork.org, a website organized by a National Community of Practice on SMH (see Chap. 1).

Seven Steps to Devising an Action Plan for Culturally Responsive School Mental Health Services

We have come full circle. From a discussion of critical advancements to consideration of challenges—we now face the question, "What's next?" What are the next steps for those of us involved with research, training, practice, and policy in our respective school communities? How does what we have learned apply to the environments in which we live and work? The rationale for culturally competent SMH is often present in an unresolved issue or challenge encompassed in our individual and collective experiences in schools. The question is how to move forward. What are the essential steps in designing and implementing culturally competent SMH in one's community?

The National Community of Practice on Collaborative School Behavioral Health provides a practical lens from which to organize one's action plan. As discussed in Chap. 1, a key goal of the Collaborative is to support multiscale learning, and in so doing, organize community stakeholders in efforts to move from discussion to action to advocate for positive change. The Collaborative currently includes over 3,000 members that represent professional organizations, states, and practice groups. The Collaborative has identified 12 key themes for the SMH field (see Chap. 1). There are several lessons to be learned from the success of the Collaborative and the *Handbook* overall. Lessons learned have implications for developing action plans that promote culturally responsive school-based mental health. They are:

1. *Involve key stakeholders in the development of your action plan from the outset.* The program development and adaptation chapters in the *Handbook* illustrate the importance of working with key stakeholders to promote change. Stakeholders bring knowledge, resources, and buy-in for the change.
2. *Do not work in isolation—collaborate with others to address your goals.* Not unlike the first step in the action plan, collaborating with others goes a step further. This step encourages active collaboration and participation across stakeholder groups. Creating a community of participants, similar to the Collaborative, can provide support and brain power in accomplishing action plan items.
3. *In a climate of scarce resources work with stakeholders and other organizations to identify overlap in services and where resources can be*

shared. The question here concerns where to best put one's resources to address action plan items. One starting point is to examine where overlap in services exist. How can duplication be decreased and those additional resources be channeled to address action items?

4. *Identify barriers to change and strategies to address them.* What are the attitudes, views, and policies that create barriers to change? How can the community of action plan participants address these barriers?
5. *Make your plan comprehensive, not an add-on.* A culturally responsive SMH services action plan gains credibility and is effective when it is infused throughout the school. School climate issues are best addressed through a comprehensive approach that involves all aspects of the system to promote positive change.
6. *Examine and expand upon the interconnections between the action plan and research, training, practice, and policy.* In building a comprehensive culturally responsive SMH action plan, what are the interconnections between research, training, practice, and policy? For instance, how does training future professionals in evidence-based practice further the action plan? How do positive outcomes from this work influence policy?
7. *Integrate the three advancements, relevance, responsiveness, and integration of a cultural perspective throughout the plan.* The community of participants can step back and ask themselves about the extent to which they are moving towards their action items. Is the approach relevant to students and the community? Does it respond to the specific needs of the diverse students the action plan is designed to support? Is a cultural perspective integrated throughout the plan?

Translating theory into action is not an easy task. Readers are encouraged to draw from these seven steps and reflect back to the chapters for models of change. These models can provide a foundation for the particular issue a school needs to address. In so doing, it is likely that the school will tailor the model to better reflect the needs of its own community. This is culturally responsive SMH in action.

References

Adelman, H. S., & Taylor, L. (2011). Expanding school improvement policy to better address barriers to learning and integrate public health concerns. *Policy Futures in Education, 9*(3), 431–436.

Adelman, H. S., & Taylor, L. (2002). *Impediments to enhancing availability of mental health services in schools: Fragmentation, overspecialization, counterproductive competition, and marginalization.* ERIC/CASS Clearinghouse. Accessible at http://www.smhp.psych.ucla.edu/pdfdocs/impediments.pdf

Alegria, M., Atkins, M., Farmer, E., Slaton, E., & Salk, W. (2010). One size does not fit all: Taking diversity, culture and context seriously. *Administration and Policy in Mental Health and Mental Health Services Research, 37*(1, 2), 48–61.

Andis, P., Cashman, J., Praschil, R., Oglesby, D., Adelman, H., Taylor, L., et al. (2002). A strategic and shared agenda to advance mental health in schools through family and system partnerships. *International Journal of Mental Health Promotion, 4,* 28–35.

Arredondo, P., Tovar-Blank, Z. G., & Parham, T. A. (2008). Challenges and promises of becoming a culturally competent counselor in a sociopolitical era of change and empowerment. *Journal of Counseling and Development, 86*(3), 261–273.

Bhui, K., Warfa, N., Edonya, P., McKenzie, K., & Bhugra, D. (2007). Cultural competence in mental health care: a review of model evaluations. *BMC Health Services Research, 7,* 15.

Burke, B., & Paternite, C. E. (2007). Teacher engagement in expanded school mental health. In S. Evans, Z. Serpell, & M.D. Weist (Eds.), *Advances in school-based mental health, Volume 2.* Kingston, NJ: Civic, Research Institute, Inc. Also appeared in *Report on Emotional and Behavioral Disorders in Youth,* Winter 2006–2007, *7(1),* 3–4, 22–27.

Carpenter-Song, E. A., Schwallie, M. N., & Longhofer, J. (2007). Cultural competence reexamined: Critique and directions for the future. *Psychiatric Services, 58,* 1362–1365.

Clauss-Ehlers, C. S. (2008a). Creative arts counseling in schools: Toward a more comprehensive approach. In H. L. K. Coleman & C. Yeh (Eds.), *Handbook on school counseling* (pp. 517–530). Newbury Park, CA: Sage Publications.

Clauss-Ehlers, C. S. (2008b). Sociocultural factors, resilience, and coping: Support for a culturally sensitive measure of resilience. *Journal of Applied Developmental Psychology, 29,* 197–212.

Clauss-Ehlers, C. S., & Wibrowski, C. (2007). Building resilience and social support: The effects of an educational opportunity fund academic program among first- and second-generation college students. *Journal of College Student Development, 24*(5), 574–584.

Clauss-Ehlers, C. S., Yang, Y. T., & Chen, W. J. (2006). Resilience from childhood stressors: The role of cultural resilience, ethnic identity, and gender identity.

Journal of Infant, Child, and Adolescent Psychotherapy, 5, 124–138.

Cunningham, D. L., Ozdemir, M., Summers, J., & Ghunney, A. (2006). *Cultural competence*. Baltimore, MD: Center for School Mental Health Analysis and Action, Department of Psychiatry, University of Maryland School of Medicine.

Davis, S. L., & Finney, S. J. (2006). Examining the psychometric properties of the Cross Cultural Adaptability Inventory. *Educational and Psychological Measurement, 66*, 318–330.

Evans, S. W., & Weist, M. D. (2004). Implementing empirically supported treatments in schools: What are we asking? *Child & Family Psychology Review, 7*, 263–267.

Gallavan, N.P. (2007). Seven perceptions influencing novice teachers' efficacy and cultural competence. *Journal of Praxis in Multicultural Education, 2*, 1, Article 1. Available at: http://digitalcommons.library.unlv.edu/jpme/vol2/iss1/1

Jensen, P. S., & Foster, M. (2010). Closing the research to practice gap in children's mental health: Structures, solutions and strategies. *Administration and Policy in Mental Health AND Mental Health Services Research, 37*(1, 2), 111–119.

Kleinman, A., & Benson, P. (2006). Anthropology in the clinic: The problem of cultural competency and how to fix it. *PLoS Med, 3*(10), e294. doi:10.1371/journal.pmed.0030294.

Losen, D., & Orfield, G. (Eds.). (2002). *Racial inequity in special education*. Cambridge, MA: Harvard Education Publishing Group.

New Freedom Commission on Mental Health. (2003). *Achieving the promise: Transforming mental health care in America*. Final Report. Rockville, MD: DHHS Pub. No. SMA-03-3832.

Ortiz, S. O., & Flanagan, D. P. (2002). Best practices in working with culturally diverse children and families. In A. Thomas & J. Grimes (Eds.), *Best practices in school psychology IV* (pp. 337–351). National Association of School Psychologists: Bethesda, MD.

Ortiz, S. O., Flanagan, D. P., & Dynda, A. M. (2008). Best practices in working with culturally and linguistically diverse children and families. In A. Thomas & J. Grimes (Eds.), *Best practices in school psychology V* (pp. 1721–1738). Washington, DC: National Association of School Psychologists.

Perry, T., Steele, C., & Hilliard, A., III. (2003). *Young, gifted and black: Promoting high achievement among African-American students*. New York: Beacon.

Rones, M., & Hoagwood, K. (2000). School-based mental health services: A research review. *Clinical Child and Family Psychology Review, 3*(4), 223–241.

Skiba, R. J., Horner, R. H., Chung, C., Rausch, M. K., Seth, M., & Tobin, T. (2008). Race is not neutral: A national investigation of African American and Latino disproportionality in school discipline. *School Psychology Review, 40*(10), 85–107.

Steele, C. (2003). *How group stereotypes affect our lives and what we can do about it when those effects aren't good*. Accessible at: http://www.vodium.com/MediapodLibrary/library/stanford_psychology/index.asp

Sue, S. (2006). Cultural competency: From philosophy to research and practice. *Journal of Community Psychology, 34*(2), 237–245.

Sue, D. W., & Torino, G. C. (2005). Racial-cultural competence: Awareness, knowledge and skills. In R. T. Carter (Ed.), *Handbook of racial-cultural psychology and counseling* (pp. 3–9). Hoboken, NJ: Wiley.

Sue, D. W., Arredondo, P., & McDavis, R. J. (1992). Multicultural counseling competencies and standards: A call to the profession. *Journal of Counseling & Development, 70*, 477–486.

Warner, B. S., & Weist, M. D. (1996). Urban youth as witnesses to violence: Beginning assessment and treatment efforts. *Journal of Youth and Adolescence, 25*, 361–377.

Weist, M. D., & Paternite, C. E. (2006). Building an interconnected policy-training-practice-research agenda to advance school mental health. *Education and Treatment of Children, 29*, 173–196.

Weist, M. D., Lever, N., Stephan, S., Youngstrom, E., Moore, E., Harrison, B., et al. (2009). Formative evaluation of a framework for high quality, evidence-based services in school mental health. *School Mental Health, 1*(3), 196–211.

Weist, M. D., Myers, C. P., Hastings, E., Ghuman, H., & Han, Y. (1999). Psychosocial functioning of youth receiving mental health services in the schools vs. community mental health centers. *Community Mental Health Journal, 35*, 69–81.

Yamada, A., & Brekke, J. S. (2008). Addressing mental health disparities through clinical competence not just cultural competence: The need for assessment of sociocultural issues in the delivery of evidence-based psychosocial rehabilitation services. *Clinical Psychology Review, 28*(8), 1386–1399.

About the Editors

Caroline S. Clauss-Ehlers (aka CC) received her Ph.D. from Teachers College, Columbia University and is Associate Professor in the counseling psychology and school counseling programs at Rutgers, The State University of New Jersey. She is a bilingual, practicing, licensed psychologist. Dr. Clauss-Ehlers is Editor of the *Journal of Multicultural Counseling and Development*. Previous books she has authored/edited include: *Encyclopedia of Cross-Cultural School Psychology* (Ed., Springer, 2010), *Diversity Training for Classroom Teaching: A Manual for Students and Educators* (Springer, 2006), and *Community Planning to Foster Resilience in Children* (coedited with M. D. Weist, Kluwer Academic Publishers, 2004). Dr. Clauss-Ehlers is a 2004–2005 Rosalynn Carter Fellow for Mental Health Journalism and currently serves as an advisory board member for this program. She is the Director of the Mental Health Advisory Board for the Jack Kent Cooke Foundation and serves on the boards of the International Alliance for Child and Adolescent Mental Health in Schools (INTERCAMHS) and The Resource for Advancing Children's Health (REACH) Institute. Dr. Clauss-Ehlers presented for the President's New Freedom Commission on Mental Health about the need for population-based community intervention research with diverse youth. She has been a contributor to Spanish language media outlets such as *Univision*, *Ser Padres* (the Spanish language version of *Parents* magazine), and was a columnist for the Chicago Tribune's Spanish language newspaper *HOY* for 6 years.

Zewelanji N. Serpell received her Ph.D. in Developmental Psychology from Howard University in Washington, DC, and is currently an Associate Professor in the Psychology Department at Virginia State University. She is the author of several publications and currently serves on the editorial board for the *Journal of School Mental Health*. She has also coedited two books on school mental health — *Advances in School-Based Mental Health Interventions* (coedited with S. Evans & M. D. Weist, Civic Research Institute, 2007) and this work, the *Handbook of Culturally Responsive School Mental Health: Advancing Research, Training, Practice, and Policy* (coedited with C. S. Clauss-Ehlers & M. D. Weist). Dr. Serpell has an active research program focusing on educational innovations designed to enhance cognitive and social functioning among African American youth, supported over the years by grant funding from the National Science Foundation, Institute for Educational Sciences, American Psychological Association, and the Virginia Tobacco Settlement Foundation.

Mark D. Weist received a Ph.D. in clinical psychology from Virginia Tech in 1991 and is currently a Professor in the Department of Psychology at the University of South Carolina. He was on the faculty of the University of Maryland School of Medicine (UMSM) for 19 years where he helped to found and direct the Center for School Mental Health (http://csmh.umaryland.edu), one of the two national centers providing leadership to the advancement of school mental health (SMH) policies and programs in the United States. He has led a number of federally funded research grants, has advised national research and policy-oriented committees, has testified before Congress, and presented to the President's New Freedom Commission on Mental Health. He helped to found the International Alliance for Child and Adolescent Mental Health in Schools (INTERCAMHS). Dr. Weist has edited four books and has published and presented widely in the SMH field and in the areas of trauma, violence and youth, evidence-based practice, and cognitive behavioral therapy. With colleagues from the Clifford Beers Foundation and the UMSM, he edits the journal *Advances in School Mental Health Promotion* (published now by Routledge of the Taylor & Francis Group).

Index

A
Academic achievement, 83–84
Adolescents
  American Indian adolescents
    acculturation, 158
    mental health professionals, 159
  Arab American adolescents, 159–160
  Asian American adolescents, 160–162
  Asian American Pacific Islander, 110–112
  Black American adolescents (*see* Black American adolescents)
  Latino/Latina adolescents, 165–166
  multiracial/biracial American adolescents, 166–168
  school-based behavioral health, 18–19, 22–23
  White American adolescents, 168–169
Adopting Culturally Competent Practices (ACCP) Project, 116
Advocates For Youth, 104
African American boys, 12, 252
  culturally-relevant measurement and assessment, 128
  culturally-responsive approaches, 126–127
  healthy coping strategies, 121–122
  lack of knowledge and training, 123
  promote coping strategies, 128–129
  PVEST, 125
  racial and gender discrimination, 123
  racial/ethnic literacy
    conflict management and resolution, 128
    CWT project, 128
    self-awareness, 127
    stress appraisal, 127
    stress reappraisal, 127–128
  racial stress and socialization, 124
  RECAST, 125–126
  school contexts, 122
  school policies and practices, 122–123
African American families and youth, 12
  assessment implications, 69
  culturally diverse practice framework
    assessment and diagnoses, 66–67
    contact stage, 65
  intervention, 67
  problem identification, 65–66
  service closure, 67–68
  culture and posttraumatic stress symptoms, 238–239
  diagnosis and treatment, 61–62
  historical and contemporary overview, 60–61
  jargon/language, 61
  policy implications, 70–71
  practice, training, and education implications, 69–70
  premature dropout, 59
  racial identity, 61
  racial socialization, 62–64
  religiosity and spirituality, 62
  research implications, 68–69
  school climate, 64
  sociocontextual issues, 61
Aggression Replacement Therapy (ART), 183
Alcohol and other drug (AOD), 117
Alienation, 12, 214
American Indian adolescents, 157–159
American Indian Life Skills, 116
American Indian youth, 239–240
American Psychological Association (APA), 212
American School Counselor Association (ASCA), 45, 48
Anger, 126, 127, 183
Arab American adolescents, 159–160
ASCA. *See* American School Counselor Association (ASCA)
Asian American Pacific Islander (AAPI), 12
  ACCP Matrix, 116
  BEATZ program, 116–117
  CHAA program, 117
  child and adolescent, 110–112
  cognitive-behavioral approach, 116
  cultural communities, 117
  cultural humility, 115
  diverse population, 108–109
  education, 109–110
  evidence-based practices, 116
  familial belief systems, 114
  holistic perspective, 114

Asian American Pacific Islander (AAPI) (cont.)
   language differences, 114
   physical health, 114
   psychoeducation, 117
   religious institutions, 115
   school
      immigrant families, 112
      learning English, 112
      mental health issues and concerns, 113–114
   stereotype challenges, 108
   teenage antiviolence programs, 116
Asian American Recovery Services (AARS), 116
Assessment, 13
   culturally competent practitioners
      policy, 212
      theoretical and conceptual frameworks, 212–213
   disproportional rates, 209–210
   families, 214–215
   language issues, 214
   racial/ethnic minorities, 213–214
   referral and disciplinary action, 210–211
   social–emotional and behavior ratings, 210
   strength-based assessment, 215
   SWPBIS, 215
   test bias, 211
Asylum seekers, 137

B
Bavaria School-Based Behavioral Health Program (B-SBBH)
   adolescent culture, 22–23
   clinical outcomes, 25
   clinical services, 20
   evidenced-based practice, 26
   feedback informed treatment, 26–28
   German cultural considerations
      bi-cultural families, 23
      billing procedures, 24
      civilians, 23
      legal responsibilities, 23
      parental permission, 24
      self-hatred, 24–25
      SOFA regulations, 23
   getting to outcomes, 25
   multiple role management, 21–22
   rating scale, 25–26
   subjective distress, 26
   therapeutic alliance, 26–27
   U.S. Army MEDCOM model, 20
Behavioral Assessment for Children of African Heritage (BACAH), 215
Behavior and Emotional Rating Scale-2 (BERS), 215
Black American adolescents
   class-conscious, 163
   ethnic socialization, 163
   immersion-emersion stage, 164
   internalization, 164
   pre-encounter stage, 164
   race-conscious family frame, 163
   race-neutral family, 163
   school settings, 164
   self-esteem, 163
Black parents strengths and strategies (BPSS) program, 11, 252
   development process
      academic achievement, 83–84
      adaptation assessment, 80–81
      community engagement, 81–82
      content adaptation, 83
      core components, 80
      delivery adaptations, 85–86
      discrimination, 84–85
      goals, 78
      implementation, 82–83
      program developers consultation, 79–80
      racism and prejudice, 84–85
      social exclusion, 83
      standard intervention, 78–79
      theory and logic, 79
   program fidelity *vs.* cultural specificity, 77–78
Black Racial Dissonance Inventory (BRDI), 128
B-SBBH. *See* Bavaria School-Based Behavioral Health Program (B-SBBH)
Building-level advisory (BLA), 19
Bureau of Vocational Guidance, 44

C
California Institute for Mental Health (CiMH), 116
Can WE Talk? (CWT), 127, 128
CARES. *See* Cultural and Racial Experiences of Socialization (CARES)
CBT. *See* Cognitive-behavioral therapy (CBT)
Child and Family Behavioral Health Office (CAF-BHO), 19
Childcare, 224
Child Outcome Rating Scale (CORS), 26
Cognitive Behavioral Intervention for Trauma in Schools (CBITS), 243
Cognitive-behavioral therapy (CBT), 67
Collaborative culture (CC), 5
Colorism, 163
Community Health for Asian Americans (CHAA), 117
Community-level advisory (CLA), 19
Comprehensive Behavioral Health System of Care-Campaign Plan (CBHSOC-CP), 17–18
Content adaptation, 83
Cultural and Racial Experiences of Socialization (CARES), 128
Cultural competency
   LGBT school intervention, 97
   school mental health
      collaboration, 259
      culture of schools, 254
      definition, 253–254
      evidence-based practice, 256–257
      research, practice and policy, 257–258

stakeholders, 258–259
training models, 254–255
substance abuse and sex education prevention
cultural competence, 200–201
trauma, 236
Culturally competent assessment. *See* Assessment
Culturally diverse youth, 7
Cultural responsiveness, 27, 256

D
Delivery adaptations, 85–86
Depression, 24, 34, 37, 91
Diagnostic Statistical Manual of Mental Health Disorders (DSM-IV TR), 67
Diversity, 97, 140, 255

E
Educational Policies and Accreditation Standards (EPAS), 70
English-as-a-Second-Language (ESL), 115
Essential component of systems of care (EESOC), 5–6
Ethnicity. *See* Race and ethnicity
Evidence-based practice (EBP), 7
Evidence-based treatments (EBTs), 243–244

F
Federation of Parents and Friends of Lesbians and Gays (PFLAG), 104
Feedback informed treatment (FIT), 26
Five-step model, 51–53
Forced migrant children and family, 13
asylum seekers, 137
developmental considerations, 139–140
legal considerations, 140
linguistic considerations, 140–141
mental health considerations, 137–139
refugees, 136
school responsiveness, 141–143
unaccompanied minors, 136
undocumented children, 137

G
Gang Resistance Education and Training (G.R.E.A.T.) Program, 183
Gay Lesbian and Straight Education Network (GLSEN), 89, 104
Gay-Straight Alliance (GSA), 101
GLSEN. *See* Gay Lesbian and Straight Education Network (GLSEN)

H
Hip Hop 2 prevent substance abuse and HIV (H2P), 201
Hispanic and Latino youth, 241–242
Human Rights Campaign, 104

I
Immigration detention, 137
Individualized Education Program (IEP), 54
Institute of Medicine (IOM), 147

J
Juvenile justice and dropout (JJD), 5

L
Learning language (LL), 6–7
Lesbian, gay, bisexual and transgender (LGBT), 252
Advocates For Youth, 104
cultural considerations, 96–97
developmental and contextual considerations, 94–95
evidence-based programs, 100–101
Gay Lesbian and Straight Education Network, 104
Human Rights Campaign, 104
risk factors
athletics, 92
criminal justice system, 92
DSM-IV, 91
faith-based organizations, 92
high-risk sexual behavior, 91
homelessness, 92
homophobia, 93
religion, 92
school personnel and parents, 93
student victimization, 93
role models, 96
school climate
anti-bullying/harassment policy, 101
communities, 102
components, 102
gay-straight alliance, 101
parent support groups, 103
schoolwide support, 103
social media, 103
teacher support, 102
Welcoming Schools, 102
school environments, 95
school intervention
anti-bullying intervention program, 99–100
CDC recommendation, 97–98
cultural competency, 97
engagement and socialization, 97
environmental and behavioral monitoring, 97
Health Care Bill of Rights, 98–99
individual support, 98
mental and physical needs, 97
resources, 104
school counselors, 99
school leadership, 97
LGBT. *See* Lesbian, gay, bisexual and transgender (LGBT)

M

Making proud choices program, 202
Military
    families, 7
    school-based behavioral health (*see* School-based behavioral health (SBBH))
    work–family balance, 229–230
Multifaceted school counselor, 53–55

N

National Association of School Psychology (NASP), 212
National Defense Education Act (NDEA), 45
National Standards for School Counseling Programs, 45

O

Office of Juvenile Justice and Delinquency Prevention (OJJDP), 180
Olweus Bullying Prevention Program, 100
Outcome Rating Scale (ORS), 26

P

Parenting the Strong-Willed Child (PSWC)
    academic achievement, 83
    core components, 80
    program developers consultation, 80
    racism, prejudice, and discrimination, 84
    standard intervention, 78–79
    strategy, 79
Phenomenological Variant of Ecological Systems Theory (PVEST), 125
PLAAY. *See* Preventing Long-term Anger and Aggression in Youth (PLAAY)
Positive behavior supports (PBS), 5
Posttraumatic stress disorder (PTSD), 235, 238, 242
    See also Trauma
Preventing Long-term Anger and Aggression in Youth (PLAAY), 126–127
Psychiatry and schools (PS), 6–7

R

Race and ethnicity
    American Indian adolescents
        acculturation, 158
        mental health professionals, 159
    Arab American adolescents, 159–160
    Asian American adolescents, 160–162
    assessment, 213–214
    Black American adolescents
        class-conscious, 163
        ethnic socialization, 163
        immersion-emersion stage, 164
        internalization, 164
        pre-encounter stage, 164
        race-conscious family frame, 163
        race-neutral family, 163
        school settings, 164
        self-esteem, 163
    conflict management and resolution, 128
    CWT project, 128
    Latino/Latina adolescents, 165–166
    multiracial/biracial American adolescents, 166–168
    self-awareness, 127
    stress appraisal, 127
    stress reappraisal, 127–128
    substance abuse and sex education prevention, 200
    White American adolescents, 168–169
    work–family balance, 221–222
Racial identity, 61
Racial Investment Questionnaire (RIQ), 128
Racial socialization
    child outcomes, 63
    contextual and meaningful guidance, 62
    cultural practice, 63
    definition, 62
    goal, 63
    pro-Black attitudes and therapeutic setting, 64
    reliable and valid scales, 64
    worldviews and ideologies, 64
Reach for health community youth service (RFH CYS), 202–203
Refugees, 136
RIQ. *See* Racial Investment Questionnaire (RIQ)
Rural community, 12, 251
    definition, 31
    ethical challenges
        family relationship, 37
        geographic isolation, 38
        implications and strategies, 38–39
        professional work, 37
    interpersonal connections, 35–36
    mental health correlation and outcomes, 32–33
    quality services, 33–35
Rural schools
    case studies, 152–153
    challenges, 148–149
    integrated care model, 151
    limitations, 151–152
    mental health disorders, 148
    mental health problems, 151
    pediatric primary care, 149
    primary care, 149–150
    professionals communication, 150
    stigma reduction, 150

S

SBBH. *See* School-based behavioral health (SBBH)
School-based behavioral health (SBBH), 12
    adolescents and families, 18–19
    Bavaria program
        adolescent culture, 22–23
        clinical outcomes, 25
        clinical services, 20
        evidenced-based practice, 26

feedback informed treatment, 26–28
German cultural considerations, 23–25
getting to outcomes, 25
multiple role management, 21–22
rating scale, 25–26
subjective distress, 26
therapeutic alliance, 26–27
U.S. Army MEDCOM model, 20
U.S. Army, 19–20
School climate
　African American families and youth, 64
　lesbian, gay, bisexual and transgender
　　anti-bullying/harassment policy, 101
　　communities, 102
　　components, 102
　　gay-straight alliance, 101
　　parent support groups, 103
　　schoolwide support, 103
　　social media, 103
　　teacher support, 102
　　Welcoming Schools, 102
School counselor, 13, 251, 252
　in 21st century
　　five-step model, 51–53
　　multifaceted school counselor, 53–55
　in 20th century guidance counseling *vs.* 21century school guidance
　　advocacy, 46
　　classroom space, 49
　　counseling culture, 47–48
　　cross-cultural awareness and skill, 46
　　educational culture, 47–48
　　national model and standards, 45
　　NDEA, 45
　　ongoing professional development, 46–47
　　schedules, 49
　　social and emotional learning, 49–50
　　social justice and civil rights movement, 45
　　summer vacation, 50–51
　　training requirements, 44
　　vocational guidance, 44
School counselor training, 13, 252
　academic success, 190
　University of Maryland
　　admissions process, 191–192
　　advocacy project, 193–194
　　culminating experience, 194
　　field experiences, 193
　　program curriculum, 192–193
　　training program outcomes, 194–195
School mental health (SMH)
　African American families and youth (*see* African American families and youth)
　collaborative culture, 5
　cross-cultural competence, 8, 9
　cultural competence
　　collaboration, 259
　　culture of schools, 254
　　definition, 253–254
　　evidence-based practice, 256–257
　　research, practice and policy, 257–258
　　stakeholders, 258–259
　　training models, 254–255
　culturally competent assessment (*see* Assessment)
　culturally diverse youth, 7
　culturally responsive strategies (*see* Youth gangs)
　essential component of systems of care, 5–6
　family–school–community partnerships, 6
　historical perspective, 3–4
　juvenile justice and dropout prevention, 5
　learning language, 6
　military families, 7
　positive behavior supports, 5
　psychiatry and schools, 6–7
　quality and evidence-based practice, 7
　rural community (*see* Rural community)
　rural schools (*see* Rural schools)
　school counselor (*see* School counselor)
　school counselor training (*see* School counselor training)
　trauma (*see* Trauma)
　work–family balance (*see* Work–family balance)
　youth involvement and leadership, 7
　youth with disabilities, 6
School responsiveness
　developmental considerations, 142
　legal considerations, 142
　linguistic consideration, 142–143
　mental health considerations, 141–142
School-Wide Positive Behavioral Interventions and Supports (SWPBIS), 215
SEL. *See* Social and emotional learning (SEL)
Session Rating Scale (SRS), 27
Sisters of Nia program, 204
Social and emotional learning (SEL), 49–50
Social class, 163, 213
Sports, 92, 96
Status of Forces Agreement (SOFA), 23, 24
Steps to Respect program, 100
Strength-based assessment, 215
Substance abuse and sex education prevention, 13, 252
　cultural considerations
　　African American youth, 203
　　"Cuidate," 203
　　cultural competence, 200–201
　　ethnic identity, 200
　　gender issues, 200
　　Hip Hop 2 prevent substance abuse and HIV, 201
　　Making Proud Choices program, 202
　　project venture, 201
　　reach for health community youth service, 202–203
　　storytelling, 201–202
　culture, 198–199
　implications, 204–205
　risk and protective factors, 197–198
　in schools, 199–200
　Sisters of Nia program, 204

Suicide, 32, 91, 114, 241
Systems of Care (SOC), 4

T
Trauma, 13
    cultural competence, 236
    culture and posttraumatic stress symptoms
        African American youth, 238–239
        American Indian youth, 239–240
        Asian American youth, 240–241
        Hispanic and Latino youth, 241–242
    intervention, 244
    school-based group treatment, 243–244
Trauma-focused cognitive behavioral therapies (TFCBTs), 243

U
Unaccompanied minors, 136
United Nations High Commission on Refugees (UNHCR), 136

W
Welcoming Schools, 102
Work–family balance, 13, 253
    after-school care, 228–229
    childcare, 224
    class
        coping strategies, 223–224
        nonstandard work hours, 222–223
        working-mother methods, 223
    crossover, 224
    family-to-work conflict, 225
    flexibility, 226–228
    "living wage" law, 221
    low-wage workers, 221
    military families, 229–230
    nutrition and exercise, 229
    race and ethnicity, 221–222
    recommendations, professionals, 230–231
    in school, 228
    spillover, 224–225
    women, 219–220
    work-to-family conflict, 225–226

Y
Youth gangs, 13
    associated problems, 179–180
    awareness and knowledge, 181
    gang reduction, 180
    intervention, 184
    joining gangs, risk factors of, 178–179
    media and popular culture, 179
    prevalence and demographics, 178
    primary prevention, 182–183
    safety issues, 184
    in schools, 180–181
    secondary prevention, 183–184
Youth involvement and leadership (YIL), 7

CPSIA information can be obtained
at www.ICGtesting.com
Printed in the USA
LVOW03*0220010216
473061LV00013BB/534/P

Barrett Library
Allen College Campus
Waterloo, Iowa 50703